ANESTHESIA AT STANFORD
(1983-1992)

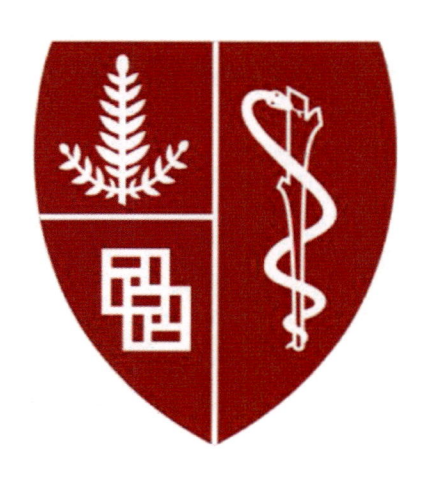

JAY B. BRODSKY

JOHN G. BROCK-UTNE

with

H. BARRIE FAIRLEY

Introduction

ANESTHESIA at STANFORD (1983-1992)

Following Phil Larson's departure as Chair of the Stanford Department of Anesthesiology in 1982, two of the original faculty members, John Bunker (1920-2012) and Ellis Cohen (1919-2010), served as interim department leaders. The search for a new Chair wasn't completed until almost three years later when in 1985 the medical school hired Dr. H. Barrie Fairley to replace Larson. At the time of his Stanford appointment Dr. Fairley was Chief of Anesthesia at San Francisco General Hospital, the same position Larson had held when he was hired by Stanford 10 years earlier in 1972. Fairley's goal was to continue the balance Larson had achieved between teaching, research, and clinical care.

In 1986 the basic anesthesia residency training program in the United States was increased from two to three-years, and many of our residents choose to train for an additional Fellowship year. The size of the anesthesia residency class rose to an average of 16 spots per year, and each of those positions were consistently filled with outstanding applicants. Unfortunately, the period covered by this book also saw a very high incidence of substance abuse among anesthesiology residents.

In 1989 during Fairley's tenure as Chair the Stanford Hospital expansion project was completed at 300 Pasteur Drive. Surgical capacity was markedly increased with the addition of 20 new state-of-the-art operating rooms. The entire anesthesia department had previously been housed in the Grant Building. That space was now converted into laboratories and offices for faculty. The Department's physical footprint was significantly expanded in the new hospital addition with offices, a library, and meeting spaces.

The 1980s was also a time of major changes in medical practice. The role of the anesthesiologist was expanding both inside and outside the operating room. More complex procedures in cardiothoracic surgery, neurosurgery, and transplant surgery were successfully being performed due to the increased sophistication of clinical anesthetic practice. Intraoperative monitoring of patients changed from a simple precordial or esophageal stethoscope, a non-invasive blood pressure cuff and sphygmometer, with a "finger on the pulse", to continuous monitoring with pulse oximetry (introduced into clinical practice by Stanford anesthesiologists William New (1942-2017) and Mark Yelderman) and mass spectrometry and end-tidal carbon dioxide measurements (pioneered by Stanford anesthesiologist Charles Whitcher (1923-2014).

Pre- and post-surgical hospital stays were shortened, and outpatient procedures became much more commonplace. Even patients scheduled for major operations now arrived at the hospital on the day of their surgery. In response, Stanford created the nation's first out-patient pre-anesthesia evaluation clinic under the direction of former resident Stephen Fischer. The clinic began its operation in 1993. Lucile Packard Children's Hospital opened in 1991 with a marked increase in the number of pediatric surgical and perioperative procedures. Stanford anesthesiologist Alvin Hackel is credited with founding the sub-specialty of Pediatric Anesthesia during this period. Stanford residents no longer had to spend their pediatric anesthesia training rotation at Oakland Children's Hospital as they had previously.

In 1992 Dr. Fairley stepped down as Department Chair but remained on the active clinical faculty for several additional years. Dr. Frank Sarnquist served as interim Chair until Dr. Donald Stanski, an in-house candidate working at the Palo Alto Veterans Administration Medical Center took over leadership as the Department's third full-time Chairman later that year.

As with our previous book 'Anesthesia at Stanford – the Larson Years (1972-1982)', this book contains biographical information about the residents, Fellows, and faculty who began their training or started work in the Stanford Department of Anesthesiology in the years 1983-1992. Many of the contributors to this book have submitted their personal memories, anecdotes, and photographs. One-hundred and sixty-two residents and research Fellows started their training or transferred from other anesthesia programs to Stanford during the 1983-1992 period. Several did not complete their residency here. Some resigned and left anesthesia for other specialties, while others were dismissed from the program for a variety of reasons. Sadly, at the time of this writing, 8 former residents have passed away. Of the 130 former residents and Fellows we attempted to contact for this book, we were successful reaching 109 (84%). One-hundred and four of them submitted biographical information and stories about their experience at Stanford and their life and careers after leaving the Farm. The names of those who contributed to this project are highlighted in **blue font** in the text and index. We have accurate biographies from their contribution to the book for these individuals. For those residents who we could not contact or who did not reply to our requests, we were dependent solely on information gathered from the Internet. We apologize for any inaccuracies.

The structure of this book follows that of our previous book. There is one chapter for each of the 10 years covered by this book. We have a chapter devoted to H. Barrie Fairley. The authors thank Dr. Fairley for his help in writing this chapter and for describing the challenges he faced and the successes he achieved as Chair. The authors lost a dear friend, former resident and then colleague Richard Jaffe during the preparation of this book. We wish to honor his memory with a separate chapter. Most of the new attendings joining the faculty during this period were former Stanford anesthesia residents and Fellows, and their information is contained in the chapter for the year they arrived at Stanford as a trainee. Only a few new faculty were recruited from outside Stanford and a single chapter covers new full-time and visiting clinical physicians, research associates, and administrative staff. The transition year from the end of Dr. Fairley's leadership to Dr. Stanski's succession is briefly described in another chapter. Finally, we include with a selection of photographs, many submitted by former residents.

Working on this project enabled us to personally reconnect with dozens of former residents and colleagues, many of whom we hadn't seen or spoken with in years. Learning how much they enjoyed and valued their time at Stanford and what they accomplished after their training was a source of great satisfaction to both of us.

Jay B. Brodsky
John G. Brock-Utne
July, 2024

TABLE OF CONTENTS

Introduction		3-4
Chapter 1	1983	7-18
Chapter 2	1984	19-38
Chapter 3	H. Barrie Fairley	39-55
Chapter 4	1985	57-78
Chapter 5	1986	79-97
Chapter 6	Richard A. Jaffe	99-108
Chapter 7	1987	109-121
Chapter 8	1988	123-135
Chapter 9	1989	137-149
Chapter 10	1990	151-169
Chapter 11	1991	171-191
Chapter 12	1992	193-204
Chapter 13	Clinical and Research Faculty, and Administrative Staff	205-223
Chapter 14	Transition 1992	225-231
Chapter 15	Photographs	233-244
Residents		245-246
Index		247-249

CHAPTER 1
1983

The birth of the "true" Internet began on January 1, 1983, with the official completion of the migration of the Advanced Research Projects Agency Network (ARPANET) to TCP/IP, the framework used for organizing communication protocols to communicate between networks and devices. In March the 3D printer (initially called *'stereolithography'*) was invented. In June the first worldwide mobile telephone, the Motorola DynaTAC was produced. That year the Space Shuttle Challenger was launched on its maiden voyage. Astronauts Peterson and Musgrave performed the first spacewalk of the shuttle program during NASA's STS-6 mission.

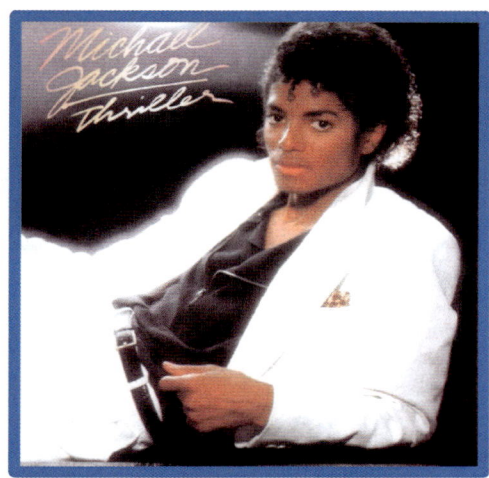

Motorola DynaTAC mobile telephone

On September 26 the Soviet Union's nuclear early-warning system was triggered. Luckily for the world, a technician Stanislav Petrov who was manning the system believed the warning to be a false-alarm and did not report it - thus avoiding a nuclear war. The system was later confirmed to have been malfunctioning. At home Michael Jackson's album *'Thriller'* was released. It remained at #1 on the US *200* Billboard charts for 37 weeks, setting a world record.

In 1983 the most-watched finale of a television show to that date occurred when 105.9 million viewers tuned in to see the final episode of M*A*S*H. It remained the biggest television event in terms of number of viewers until Super Bowl XLIV in 2010. The original 1968 novel by surgeon Richard Hooker, titled "*MASH: A Novel About Three Army Doctors*" was based on the reminiscence of Hooker's army friend, anesthesiologist Dr. Dale Drake. English actor John Orchid played the television series M*A*S*H hospital's sole anesthesiologist 'Ugly John' for only the first season.

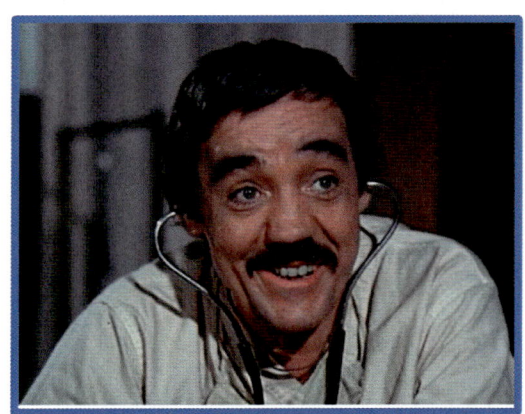

Anesthesiologist "Ugly John" on M*A*S*H

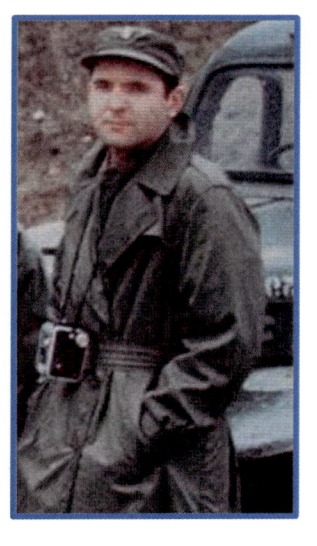

Anesthesiologist Dale Drake, the actual inspiration for M*A*S*H

7

On the medical front, the immunosuppressant drug cyclosporine was approved by the FDA, leading to a revolution in the field of organ transplantation. Two separate research groups, one led by Robert Gallo and the other by Luc Montagnier, independently reported in the journal Science that a novel retrovirus, human immunodeficiency virus (HIV), was infecting people with AIDS. At Stanford, Professor Henry Taube won the Nobel Prize in Chemistry for his work on the mechanisms of electron transfer reactions in metal complexes.

Stanford faculty anesthesiologists William New and Mark Yelderman had formed a company called Nellcor in 1981. In 1983 they released the first commercial pulse oximeter, the Nellcor N-100.

Phil Larson had stepped down in 1982 and was initially succeeded by Dr. Ellis Cohen as interim Chair. Cohen's tenure was short due to health issues, so Dr. John Bunker then served temporarily as department head.

DEPARTMENT OF ANESTHESIOLOGY (1982-1983)

PROFESSOR
John P. Bunker
William H. Forrest
Philip C. Larson Jr
Richard I. Mazze

PROFESSOR OF CLINICAL ANESTHESIA
D. Robert Buechel
Charles E. Whitcher

ASSOCIATE PROFESSOR
Jeffrey M. Baden
Joan E. Kendig
Allen K. Ream
James Trudell

ASSOCIATE PROFESSOR OF CLINICAL ANESTHESIA
George A. Albright
Sheila E. Cohen
Lorne G Eltherington
Thomas W. Feeley
Richard P. Fogdall

ASSOCIATE PROFESSOR OF CLINICAL ANESTHESIA (continued)
J. Kent Garman
Alvin Hackel
Myer H. Rosenthal
Stanley I. Samuels
Edgar O. Yhap

ASSISTANT PROFESSOR
Jay B. Brodsky
Jan Ehrenwerth
Kevin J. Fish
James C. Loomis
Mervyn Maze
Fred Mihm
Frank H. Sarnquist
Robert N. Sladen
Donald R. Stanski
Paul F. White
Janet Wyner
Mark L. Yelderman
Wayne Bellows
Margaret "Pam" Fish
Susan A. Rice

CA2 RESIDENTS (1983)
David Berger
William Cochran
Clayton Horan
David Kaufman
An Kok Lie
Duncan Macdonald
Nicol Mackenzie
Daniel Mcfarland
David Morton
Gary Nitti
Jan Rosnow
James Rushing
Kathleen Sullivan
Lawrence Walsh
William Wilson
Howard Worthen

In the summer of 1983 sixteen CA1 residents joined the Department of Anesthesiology.

David Stuart Anish attended the Mount Sinai School of Medicine of the City University of New York (now the Icahn School of Medicine) (MD, 1982). He interned at Stanford (1982-1983) and then completed his Stanford Anesthesiology residency (1983-1985). He worked at the Sutter Maternity and Surgery Center in Santa Cruz, CA.

James Brian Bird attended UCD (BS, 1978) and graduated from the University of Louisville School of Medicine (MD, 1982). He interned (Transitional, 1982) at Santa Clara County Medical Center (SCVMC)), and then did an Anesthesiology residency at Stanford (1983-1985).

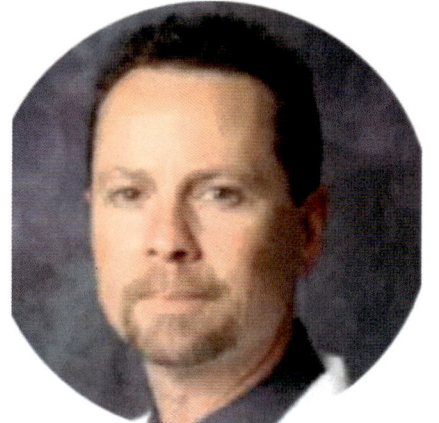

"I was part of a rock band consisting of fellow anesthesia residents. We played at Departmental events."

Following residency, he spent a year at UCSF completing a Fellowship (Neuroanesthesia, 1985-1986).

"I enjoyed working with Dr. Larson. It was Dr. Larson who got me interested in, and eventually doing a Fellowship in Neuroanesthesia at UCSF."

Dr. Bird worked at Kaiser Hospital - Redwood City, CA (1986-1989), then with the Los Gatos Anesthesia Medical Group (1989-1998), before returning to Kaiser - San Jose (1998-2020). He was Director of Perioperative Medicine at San Jose Kaiser (2007-2020). In 2020 he retired from clinical practice. He currently manages Camp Nurse programs for the city of Berkeley's Parks and Recreation Department. He also is a medical consultant for the MAVEN Project. He enjoys hiking, climbing, cooking and music and collects vinyl records.

The MAVEN Project is a nonprofit organization dedicated to correcting social, racial, and economic inequities in the health care system. The all-volunteer specialist physicians support safety net clinics and their patients by connecting clinic providers and specialists via telehealth technology. Physician volunteers guide, teach, encourage, and collaborate with clinical staff to empower them to deliver comprehensive care, relieve burnout, and build healthier communities.

Michael Warren Champeau attended the University of Notre Dame in his native Indiana as an undergraduate (BS, 1971-1975). He received his medical education at Yale (MD, 1980) and then interned (Pediatrics) at UCLA Medical Center (1981). He completed a residency (Pediatrics, 1983) at UCLA and then another at Stanford (Anesthesiology, 1983-1985).

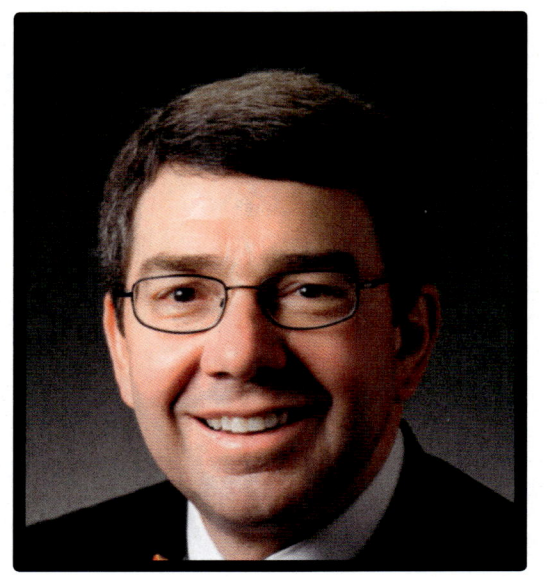

"I am one of several Stanford residents of my era who can trace their inspiration to train in anesthesiology at Stanford directly to the late Bruce Halperin. Bruce and I were close friends at Yale, and following his own residency change from Internal Medicine at Stanford to Anesthesiology, he strongly encouraged me to follow in his footsteps. I think he put in a good word for me with Phil Larson during the application process, and, as a result, Stanford was the only anesthesiology residency to which I applied."

"Overall, changing from Pediatrics to Anesthesiology was the single best professional decision of my life, and, largely due to my long association with Stanford, I've been blessed with a most satisfying and truly rewarding career. My sincere thanks to all who made it possible, particularly Bruce Halperin and Phil Larson."

He served on the faculty at Stanford for two years (1985-1987) and then joined the Associated Anesthesiologist Medical Group (AAMG) of Palo Alto (1987-Present). He has served as the group's President for the past 20 years. His clinical practice is pediatric anesthesia. He is an Adjunct Clinical Professor in Stanford's Department of Anesthesiology.

Dr. Champeau has been extensively involved in anesthesiology organizations for the past 30 years. Beginning in the mid 1990's, he rose through the ranks to be President of the California Society of Anesthesiologists (CSA) (2008-2009). He also served in numerous roles in the ASA, advancing from Director for California (2014-2015), to Assistant Treasurer (2015-2017), to Treasurer (2017-2020), then First Vice-President (2020-2021), and ultimately ASA President (2022-2023).

In addition, Dr. Champeau was President of the Medical Staff at Stanford Children's Health/Lucile Packard Children's Hospital (2014-2016) and is a past President of the Stanford Anesthesia Alumni Association. He served an associate examiner for the American Board of Anesthesiology (ABA) for 27 years (1991-2018)

He is a Fellow of the American Academy of Pediatrics and a recipient of the CSA Distinguished Service Award, and the Lucile Packard Children's Hospital Distinguished Medical Staff Service Award.

"Because of my detour through Pediatrics, both Bruce Halperin and David Gaba, another classmate of mine from Yale, served as Attendings during my anesthesia residency, which was interesting to say the least. Ron Pearl was a fellow resident, and already extremely well-known throughout the hospital due to the fact that he was "stepping down" from his position as an Attending Internal Medicine Intensivist to become an anesthesia resident! In fact, I think half of us in my residency class had already completed other residencies (4 in Internal Medicine and 2 in Pediatrics) and two had even completed Fellowships. Although my class contained many remarkable physicians, I couldn't help but notice that, compared to my Pediatric residency classmates, I never really got to know them as well, simply because we almost always worked in separate ORs, rather than together as a team."

"The Stanford Department had had an extremely strong group of pediatric anesthesiologists that also ran the pediatric intensive care units when I applied, but by the time I arrived all but one had left. Al Hackel took me under his wing during my residency, and Barrie Fairley, who had just recently been appointed Chair, was sufficiently short-staffed in the pediatric area to offer me a position on the faculty when I graduated. I look back on the years I spent on the faculty (as 50% of the Pediatric Anesthesia division!) as two of the most rewarding of my entire career. But, although two residencies can make one an excellent clinician, I quickly realized they didn't provide the research training necessary for a truly successful academic career, so I accepted an offer to join AAMG to remain at Stanford and in Palo Alto."

James Tsung Chang received his undergraduate education at Berkeley (BS, 1975). He is a graduate of the UCSF School of Medicine (MD, 1975-1979). He interned and did a residency (Internal Medicine) at SCVMC (1979-1982) and then his residency in Anesthesiology at Stanford (1983-1985). He began his career as a staff anesthesiologist and Chief of the Department of Anesthesia at Kaiser Permanente Medical Center – San Jose (1985-1990). He was Assistant Physician-in-Chief of The Permanente Medical Group (TPMG) - San Jose (1990-2001) and then Associate Executive Director (TPMG) - Northern California (2001-2020). He retired in April 2020.

Interesting Memories of Stanford – "Point of uniqueness and exclusivity is doing more heart and lung transplants than tonsillectomies at Stanford University Hospital."

Brian Douglas Hershey is a graduate of the Mt. Sinai School of Medicine (MD, 1982). After an internship (Internal Medicine) at Cedars-Sinai Medical Center (CSMC) in Los Angeles (1982-1983), and an Anesthesiology residency at Stanford (1983-1985), he practiced anesthesia in Contra Costa County, CA.

Paul Steven Hummel received his MD from Harvard Medical School (1982) then interned (1982) and trained in Anesthesiology at Stanford (1983-1985). Paul was Chief Resident (1984-1985). He worked in Las Vegas, NV and moved to Seattle after retiring from clinical practice.

Steve Charles Merlone did his undergraduate work at Berkeley (AB, 1977) and graduated medical school from USC (MD, 1981). He interned (Surgery) at UCSF (1981-1982) and completed one year of Orthopedic Surgery residency there (1982-1983). He then did an Anesthesiology residency at Stanford (1983-1986). He was the Chief Resident (1985-1986).

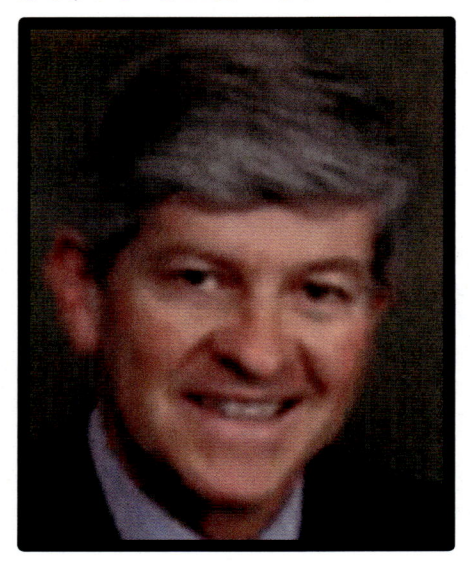

"As a surgery resident at UCSF I became very interested in anesthesia and critical care. I was then able to do an anesthesia rotation at San Francisco General Hospital under H. Barrie Fairley. I had applied to several anesthesia residencies but due to my interest in anesthesia for cardiac surgery I was intrigued with Stanford. I was interviewed by Phil Larson who was the Chair at the time. As I sat on the couch in his office, I noticed a pillow with UC as well as Stanford logos on reverse sides that I thought was unique and showed the common link between these two institutions. At the conclusion of the interview Phil offered me a residency position on the spot. In retrospect the best decision of my entire medical career was the decision to come to Stanford."

After graduation he worked as an Assistant Professor on the faculty (1986-1987) and continued as a volunteer Clinical Assistant Professor and then Associate Professor (1987-2015). He worked as a staff anesthesiologist at PAMF for the remainder of his career (1987-2022).

"My time as an anesthesia resident as well as junior faculty in Cardiac Anesthesia was highlighted by being involved with the Critical Care Transport program with Al Hackel. I had many memorable transport stories including "bucket runs" for organ procurement of heart and heart-lungs for transplantation. Never forget being stranded in Fargo North Dakota on Christmas Eve with Ed Stinson."

Michele Eileen Raney graduated from Keck School of Medicine/USC (MD, 1977) and then did her internship (Surgery) at LAC/USC (1977-1978). In 1979 Dr. Raney became the first woman to stay over winter in Antarctica at the Amundsen-Scott South Pole Station. She served as station's physician (1979). In addition to being responsible for all aspects of medical care, she was a participant and winter-over investigator for a multi-year medical research project supported by the NSF and Veteran's Administration. She studied human immune response in bio-isolation. She also ran the base store and post office.

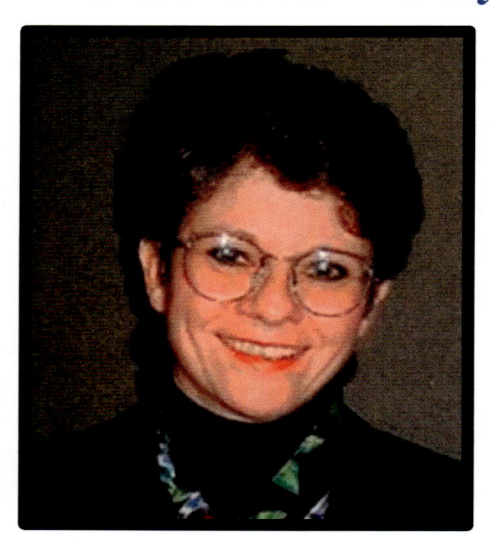

A 2,050-meter-high mountain in Victoria Land, Antarctica, was named 'Raney Peak' by the Advisory Committee on Antarctic Names (US-ACAN) in 2007.

Raney Peak (77°13'02"S 160°31'17"E) is a symmetrical peak rising to 6,730 ft between Rim Glacier and Sprocket Glacier, Victoria Land. It was named after Michele E. Raney, who was a physician with the 1979 winter party at Amundsen–Scott South Pole Station. She was the first female to winter at an Antarctic inland station.

After returning from Antarctica, Dr. Raney practiced Emergency Medicine in Los Angeles. She then completed her Anesthesiology residency at Stanford (1983-1985).

She has served on the faculty at Stanford and UCLA. Raney has also practiced anesthesiology in California, Montana, and New Mexico. Most recently she was associated with the PIH Health Hospital – Downey, Bakersfield, CA (2020).

Michele Raney has been on the board of directors of the California Medical Association (CMA) and on the CSA and has been actively involved in the ASA.

In 1987 she returned to Antarctica to perform site-specific medical facility assessment and training. She continued her association with the American Polar Society as a consultant, trainer, and board member. She has been an invited guest by the Scientific Committee on Antarctica Research (SCAR) Working Group on Human Biology and Medicine on several occasions. She has participated in Oxford University training program for anesthesia in remote and austere environments (including Antarctica).

Like many Stanford anesthesiologists she has served as a volunteer providing education and clinical anesthesia care on numerous medical outreach programs including Interplast (now ReSurge), Rotaplast International, and the International Medical Alliance. Dr. Raney was also a visiting educator for World Federation Societies of Anesthesiologists (WFSA) in Central America.

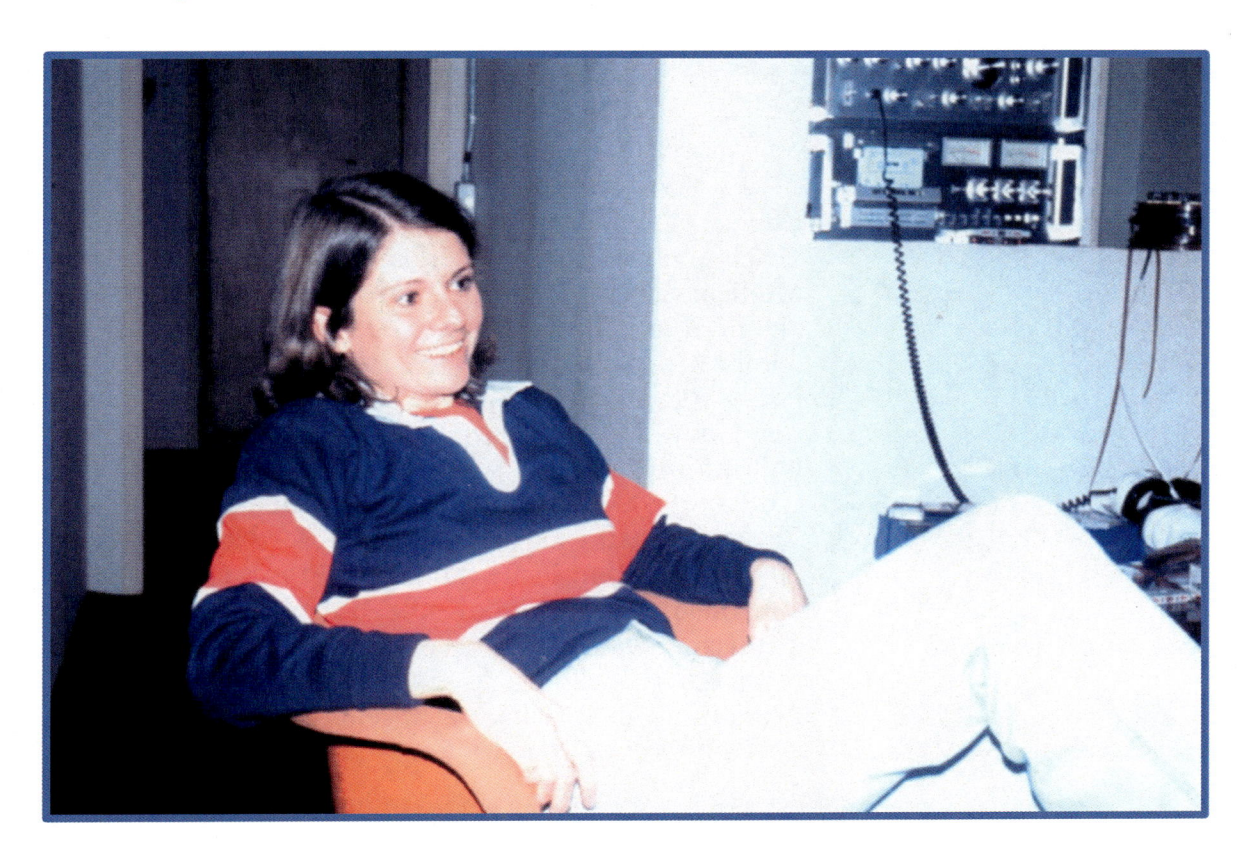

"The picture on the previous page was taken on my 28th birthday. The temperature outside was -100° F. I spoke to my family by ham patch that day, and I was told it was above +100° F where they were. At the time, many people said I "opened the inland stations for women", there having been a lot of interest/concern about a woman wintering at the South Pole (absolutely isolated from February to November, which made South Pole, with its extreme isolation, an analog for long duration space flight). Today it's no longer news."

Thomas Schares was born in New York City. He attended the University of Texas – Austin as an undergraduate (BA, 1976). He is a graduate of the Baylor College of Medicine (MD, 1980). He completed a residency (Pediatrics) at Stanford (1980-1983) and then a residency in Anesthesiology (1983-1985). After that he did a seven-month Fellowship (Pediatric Anesthesiology and Critical Care) at Boston Children's Hospital (1986-1987). Dr. Schares received a Master of Business Administration (MBA, International Business) from the University of Minnesota - Carlson School of Management (2001-2002) and an Executive MBA from Vienna University of Economics and Business.

Following training he joined Bill New at Nellcor as a medical consultant for European operations. Schares has worked at several hospitals during his career. He was clinical Chief of Anesthesiology at the Kaiser Permanente Medical Group - Santa Clara (1985-2001) and then Clinical Chief of Anesthesiology at Kaiser Permanente - Woodland Hills (2001-2006). He is President and Chief Medical Officer (CMO) for Wing Medical Associates, Goleta, CA (2007-2024). During his career Dr. Schares has worked at Kern Medical, Bakersfield, Highland Hospital, Oakland, CA, St. Bernadine Medical Center and Community Medical Center, San Bernadino, CA, and St. John Regional Medical Center, Oxnard, CA.

Barry Nathaniel Swerdlow was born in Los Angeles. He graduated Yale College (BS summa cum laude, Molecular Biophysics and Biochemistry, 1971-1975), and then attended Harvard Medical School in the Harvard-MIT Program in Health Sciences and Technology (MD, 1979). He interned and completed a residency (Internal Medicine) at Stanford (1979-1983). He then did a Stanford Anesthesiology residency (1983-1985) followed by an additional Fellowship (Clinical Pharmacology) at the PA-VAH (1985-1986). He has been a member of the adjunct Clinical Anesthesia Faculty at Stanford since 2011 and is now an Assistant Professor (2018-Present). He was a staff anesthesiologist at Los Robles Regional Medical Center, Thousand Oaks, CA (1987-2018). At Los Robles he received the Chief of Staff Recognition Award for Leadership in Advancing Excellence in Patient Care. In 2018 he joined the Oregon Health & Science University

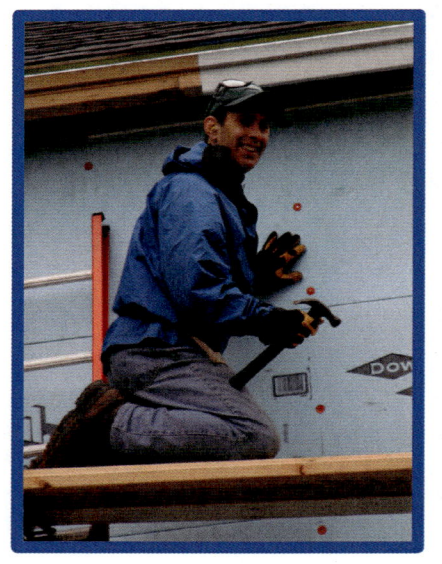

(OHSU) nurse anesthesia program as an Assistant Professor in the School of Nursing. In his free time, he enjoys bird watching.

"My fondest memory of my time at Stanford was talking with Dr. Shumway during surgery."

Paul Ying-Si Wong graduated from the Saint Louis University School of Medicine (MD, 1982), interned at Stanford (1982-1983), and then completed his Stanford residency (Anesthesiology, 1983-1986). He was affiliated with Kaiser Permanente - San Jose and Mercy General Hospital, Los Gatos. Dr. Wong is retired.

Lorna Yoshi Yamaguchi attended UCLA (BA, Psychology, 1970-1973) and then Stanford Medical School (MD, 1973-1977). She did her internship and a residency (Internal Medicine) at SCVMC (1977-1979) followed by a Fellowship (Respiratory Medicine/Critical Care) at Stanford (1979-1982). During that Fellowship she spent several months training in CCM at Stanford. She then worked for Kaiser - San Jose as a staff physician in. medicine (1982-1983).

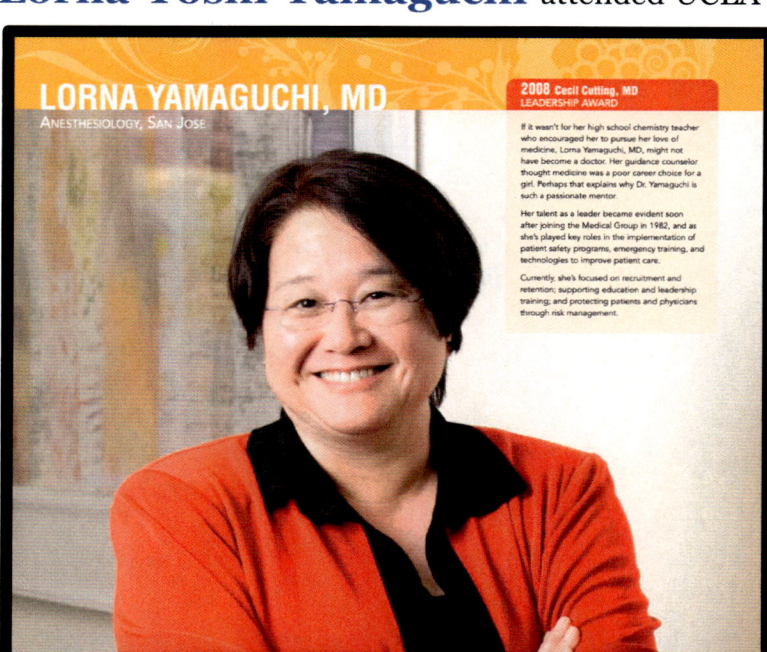

"Prior to entering my anesthesia residency at Stanford I had completed a Pulmonary/Critical Care Fellowship with the Division of Respiratory Medicine at Stanford which included multiple months in the ICU. During one of my clinical rotations as an ICU Fellow I had several residents of varying specialties on my service. One month the anesthesia resident was Kathy Demas (Stanford Anesthesia, 1980-1982) and the internal medicine resident was Ellen Finch (Stanford Anesthesia 1981-1983). They were a great team. Kathy spent the entire month trying to convince Ellen (and me) to pursue anesthesia as a career. She was clearly quite persuasive."

"Rob Sladen was instrumental in shaping my thinking regarding the specialty of anesthesia. He had been one of my attendings in ICU during my Pulmonary Fellowship. We discussed anesthesiology on several occasions . Rob encouraged me to apply to the Anesthesia program after (or despite) the Pulmonary Fellowship. I never forgot his kindness ... or his good advice."

She left her position at Kaiser to do her Anesthesiology residency at Stanford (1983-1985). After finishing her anesthesia training, she returned to Kaiser – San Jose as a staff physician (Pulmonary/Anesthesia/ Palliative Care) (1985-2014). At Kaiser she was ICU Medical Director (1986-1994), PACU Medical Director (1986-1990), and Assistant

Physician-in-Chief with administrative responsibilities for medical legal affairs, risk management and physician HR and professional development (1994-2014). She then served as Regional Director, Operations Design for TPMG - Northern California (2014-2017). One of her most challenging roles was participating in the development of Kaiser's electronic medical record. She was lead for clinical content development for ICUs for the TPMG - Northern California Region – convincing intensivists, ICU managers and nursing staff at 22 Kaiser hospitals to agree to build common ICU documentation, procedures and order sets across the Kaiser Northern California Region (2004-2012).

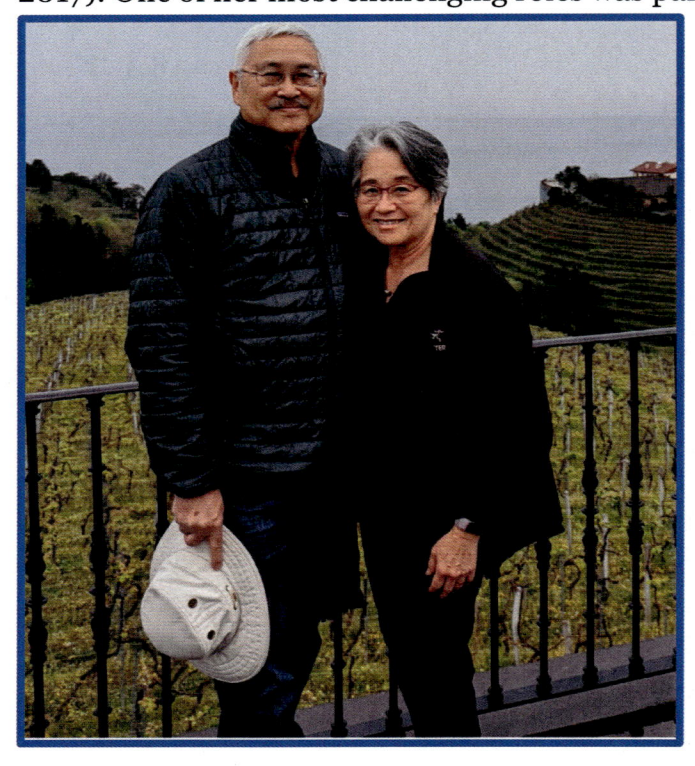

Lorna is board certified by the ABA in both Anesthesiology and Critical Care Medicine (CCM), and the American Board of Internal Medicine (ABIM) in both Internal Medicine and Pulmonary Disease.

After leaving clinical practice she was District Medical Consultant, San Jose for the California Division of Investigation's Health Quality Investigation Unit (on behalf of the Medical Board of California) (2020-2023) until her retirement in August 2023.

She enjoys reading, spinning (Peloton), hiking, and avidly following any team that has one of her children or grandchildren on the roster.

"Becoming a resident in Anesthesia, after being in practice in Pulmonary/ICU was bewildering. The transition from Attending to trainee in a new specialty is particularly unsettling, perhaps more so than having continuity between training programs. My memories of Stanford Anesthesia include many acts of kindness: Mike Lam and Mark Schulman who were rotating interns with me during my medicine internship, were now my Attendings in anesthesia. They were very patient, answering questions and providing reassurance that this was not "a terrible mistake". Mike and Mark were correct, the decision to do an Anesthesia residency at Stanford was one of the best decisions I made."

"Rob Sladen and Fred Mihm who were my Attendings in ICU when I was a Pulmonary Fellow continued to be major support and advisors during my anesthesia training. Stanley Samuels could always be depended on to provide optimism in any situation. I still remember Jay Brodsky patiently teaching double-lumen tube placement. SCVMC was also great learning experience. My first night on call as an anesthesia resident was at SCVMC. I was very relieved to see Carter Cherry, whom I knew from Internal Medicine, was the on-call attending. We and the patients managed to survive that night."

Milford Alan Zasslow
attended UCSD (MD, 1981). He interned and did a residency (Internal Medicine) at Stanford (1981-1983) and then an Anesthesiology

residency (1983-1986). He is listed on the Department's faculty in 1986-1987, most likely as a Clinical Instructor doing an additional CA3 clinical year.

Ronald Gary Pearl was an undergraduate at Yale (BS, Psychology, 1971). He then attended the University of Chicago Division of the Biological Sciences (PhD, Pharmacology and Physiology, 1975). He completed his medical training at the Pritzker School of Medicine (MD, 1977). He interned (1977) and did a residency (Internal Medicine) (1978-1980), followed by a Fellowship (CCM) (1981) all at Stanford. He was an attending physician in Internal Medicine before becoming an Anesthesiology resident (1983-1985). Following residency, he was appointed an Assistant Professor (Anesthesiology) (1985) and has remained on the faculty at Stanford for his entire career (1985-Present).

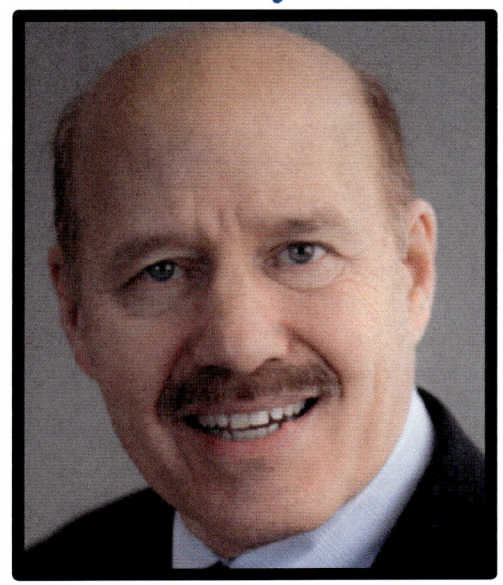

Dr. Pearl served as the Associate Chair for Clinical Affairs and Finance, Associate Medical Director of Medical Transport Program, and Associate Medical Director of the Intensive Care Units at Stanford Hospital. He was elected to the FAER Academy of Anesthesia Mentors. In 1999 he was appointed Chair of the Stanford Anesthesiology Department (1999-2021). He is the Richard K. and Erika N. Richards Professor in the Department of Anesthesiology, Perioperative and Pain Medicine.

Dr Pearl is board certified by the ABA (Anesthesiology and CCM) and by the ABIM (Internal Medicine). He is a Fellow of the ASA, of the American College of Critical Care Medicine (ACCM), and the American College of Physicians (ACP), and is a member of the Cardiovascular Institute.

In his clinical role he has worked as a member of the Cardiothoracic group in the operating rooms and in the ICU as an intensivist. His research has focused on mechanisms (molecular and cellular) of pulmonary hypertension, treatment of pulmonary hypertension, treatment of respiratory failure, treatment of septic shock, and hemodynamic monitoring.

Dr. Pearl is a past President of the CSA (2021). He has been a President of the Society of Academic Associations of Anesthesiology and Perioperative Medicine (SAAAPM), of the Association of Academic Anesthesiology Chairs

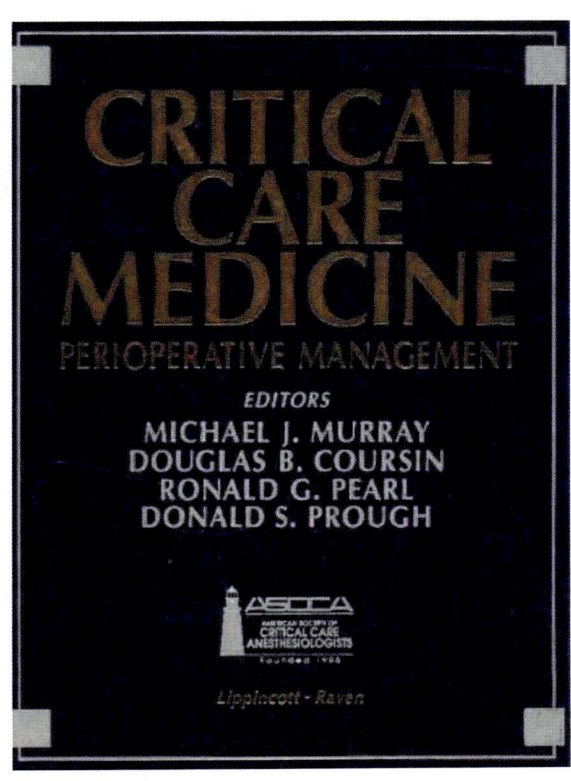

(AAAC), of the Association of University Anesthesiologists (AUA), and the California chapter of the Society of Critical Care Medicine (SCCM). He was Chair of the ASA Committee on Innovation, serves on the ASA's Committee on Academic Anesthesiology, the Committee on Critical Care Medicine, the Educational Track Subcommittee on Critical Care, and the Educational Track Subcommittee on Perioperative Medicine.

He currently remains active in research and clinical care.

"After four decades at Stanford, I remain impressed with three aspects of my residency training. The first is the incredible changes that occurred in anesthesiology at that time. When I began residency, thiopental was the primary induction agent, neuromuscular blockade was limited to pancuronium, metocurine, tubocurarine and succinylcholine, anesthesia maintenance frequently used halothane and enflurane, and pulse oximetry, capnography and transesophageal echocardiography were not available. When I finished residency two years later (residency was only two years back then), anesthesia had transformed into the safer practice we have today. Second, I was impressed with the caliber of my fellow residents, many entering anesthesia training after completing Internal Medicine and Pediatric residencies. The majority of these talented individuals became leaders in Anesthesiology. Finally, although the faculty size was small, they were the quadruple threat (education, clinical care, research, and leadership) that is so rare in anesthesia today. Residency was an incredible experience and the cornerstone of my academic career. My residency experience was nothing short of extraordinary and served as the bedrock upon which I built my academic career."

CHAPTER 2
1984

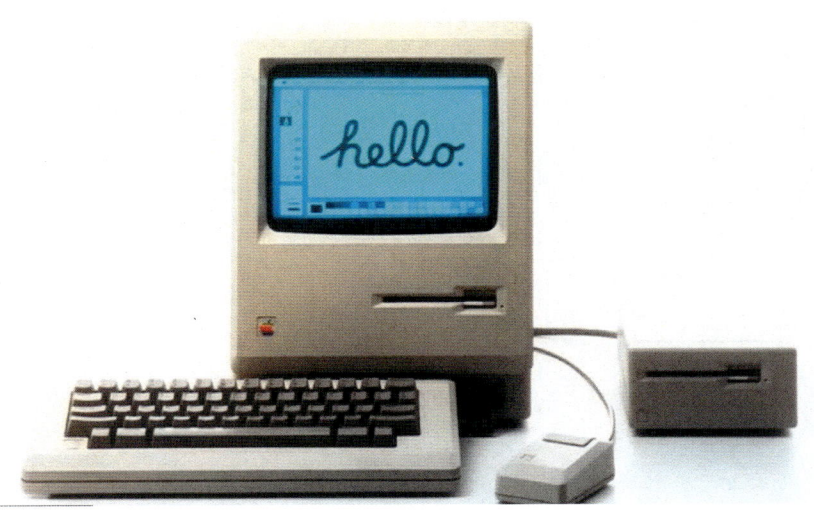

In early 1984 Steve Jobs at Apple launched the Macintosh personal computer, considered the most anticipated personal computer release ever. Ridley Scott directed a one-minute commercial for the Mac based on George Orwell's novel '*1984*'. The commercial aired during Super Bowl XVIII on January 22, 1984. The role of Big Brother was portrayed by a man dictating to the masses from a giant screen (below), only to have a hammer-wielding woman run up and destroy the screen, thus freeing the people. The "Big Brother" motif was a reference to Apple's main competitor IBM. The now famous commercial has been shown only that once. The Macintosh was the first successful mouse-driven computer with a graphical user interface and was based on the Motorola 68000 microprocessor. Its price was $2,500 in 1984, an amount equivalent in purchasing power to about $7,387 in 2023.

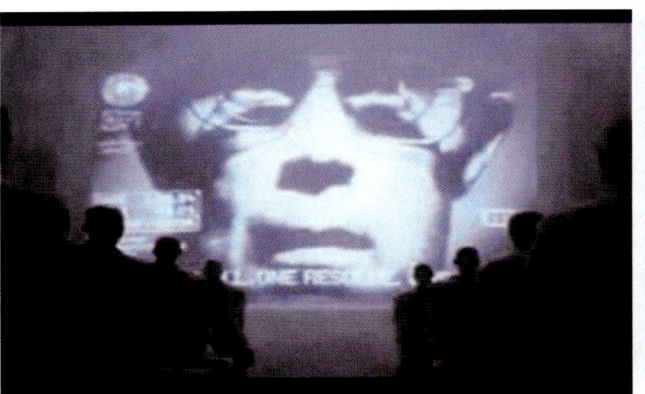

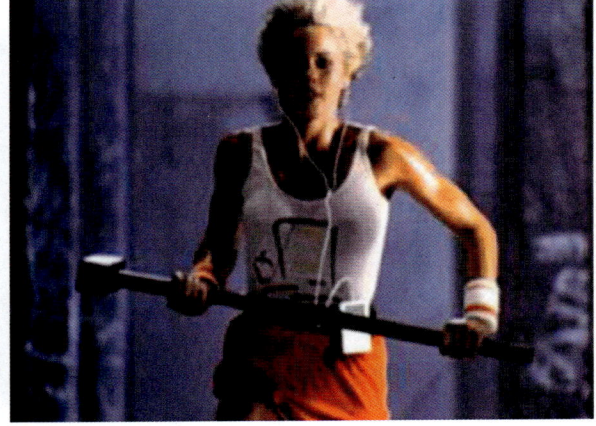

Harbor-UCLA Medical Center in Los Angles announced the first successful embryo transfer from one woman to another. In unrelated obstetrical news, on May 14th 1984, Mark Zuckerberg, the co-founder of Facebook was born.

The Soviet Union boycotted the 1984 Summer Olympics that were also held in Los Angeles, while the United States invaded Grenada. In November, Ronald Reagan overwhelmingly defeated his Democrat opponent former Vice-President Walter Mondale and was re-elected President. At the close of 1984 the Dow Jones was 1,211, the average cost of a new house was $86,700 and average annual income was less than $22,00.

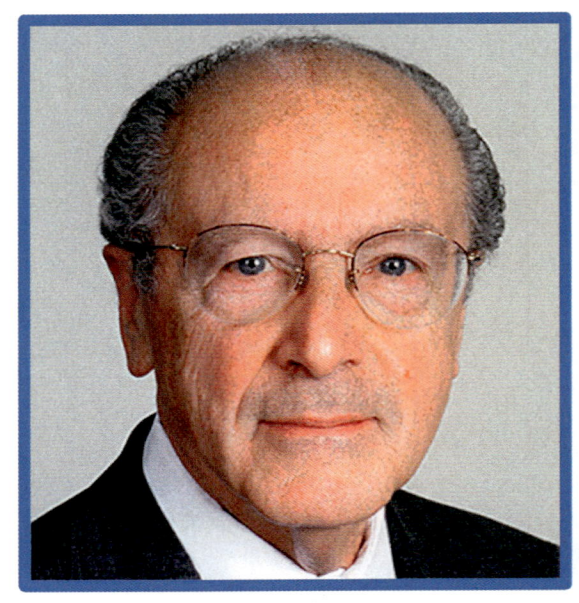

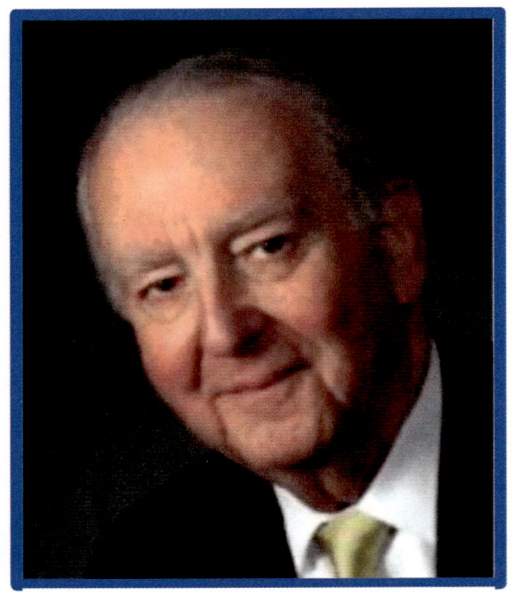

Dominick Purpura (1982-1984)   **David Korn (1984-1995)**

After serving for only 2 years as Dean of the School of Medicine, Dominick P. Purpura left Stanford for the Albert Einstein College of Medicine in 1984. He was replaced that same year by David Korn, a professor of Pathology at Harvard Medical School and Vice Provost for Research at Harvard University. Korn served as Carl and Elizabeth Naumann Professor and Dean of the Stanford University School of Medicine from October 1984 until April 1995 and was Vice President of Stanford University from January 1986 to April 1995.

Several of the CA1 Anesthesiology residents recruited in 1984 had very successful careers in medicine, while others had serious problems with legal difficulties and substance abuse.

Bryan Dirk Bohman attended UCD as an undergraduate (1977) and medical school at the University of Chicago Pritzker School of Medicine (MD, 1981). He interned (Internal Medicine) (1981-1982), followed by a residency (Internal Medicine) (1982-1984) at Stanford Hospital. He then completed his training in Anesthesiology (1984-1986). He has been a member of AAMG in Palo Alto (1990-Present). While in community practice he was a District delegate to the CSA and was Deputy Chief of the Stanford Department of Anesthesiology. (Deputy Chief is a position for a non-academic faculty anesthesiologist working at Stanford Hospital). He is currently both a Clinical Professor of Anesthesiology and a Clinical Professor of Medicine (Primary Care and Population Health) at the Stanford University School of Medicine.

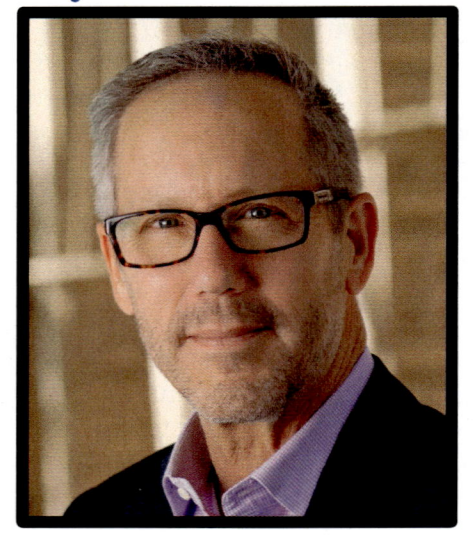

Dr. Bohman was the first elected Chief of the Medical Staff at Stanford Health Care (2008-2011). In that capacity he served as Chair of the Medical Executive Committee and was a member of the Stanford University Hospital Board of Directors.

He was subsequently appointed Associate Chief Medical Officer (CMO) at Stanford Hospital (2011-2021). He established Stanford's Wellness Committee and led the founding of the Stanford WellMD Center (2015). The Center's aim is to advance faculty, trainee and care team wellbeing across Stanford Medicine while also serving as an international leader of scholarship in the field. He served as the Center's interim Director until 2017. Bryan also led the establishment of the Clinical Effectiveness Leadership Program (CELT) which serves as a driver of clinical quality improvement across Stanford Medicine (2014-Present). He continues as co-Director of the CELT program and Senior Advisor to the WellMD Center.

Dr. Bohman was also CMO and Associate Dean for Stanford Medicine Partners (a community health network subsidiary of Stanford Health Care) (2014-2021). He currently serves as Associate CMO for Workforce Health and Wellness for Stanford Health Care and continues his clinical practice in anesthesiology and occupational health.

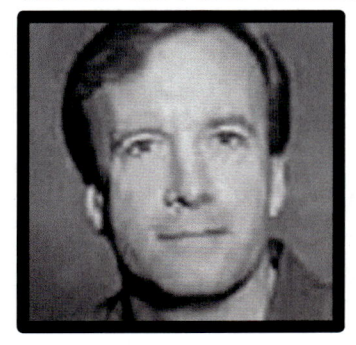

Michael Dale Cully attended medical school at Stanford (MD, 1981), and then completed a residency (Internal Medicine) at the UCLA/David Geffen School of Medicine (1981-1984) and a residency (Anesthesiology) at Stanford (1984-1986). He worked at Hoag Memorial Hospital, Newport Beach, CA, and was President of Newport Harbor Anesthesia Consultants Medical Group. He retired in 2021.

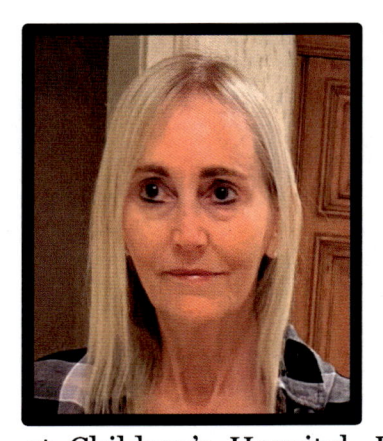

Anne Arbetter Fischell was born in Boston. She graduated from Harvard (BA cum laude with honors, Biology, 1977). During college she was a Teaching Assistant in Neurobiology at Harvard University's Marine Biological Laboratory in Woods Hole, MA (1974). She had grants from Massachusetts Lupus Erythematosus Foundation (1976) and the Georgia Department of Human Resources (1977). She attended UCSF for her medical training (MD, 1981). She interned and completed a residency (Pediatrics) at Children's Hospital, Boston (1981-1984). She was a resident (Anesthesiology) at Stanford (1984-1986). Her first position was as a staff anesthesiologist at Kaiser - Oakland, where she was a partner and Senior Anesthesiologist (1989). At Kaiser she was the Director of Resident Teaching and started the hospital's first labor

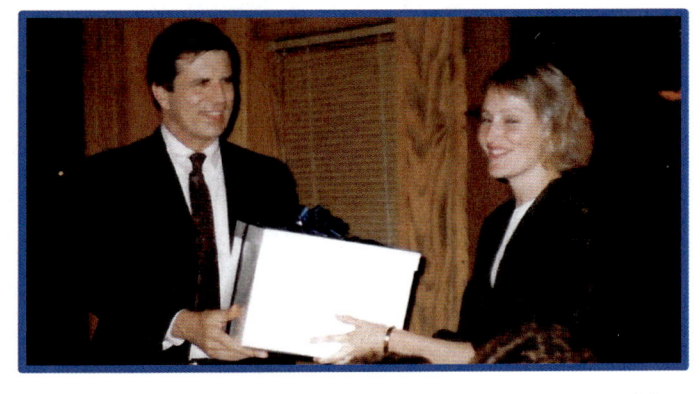

Dr. Donald Sass, Chief of Anesthesia presents Anne with plaque at her farewell dinner leaving Oakland Children's Hospital

epidural service. In 1989 she returned to Stanford as an Assistant Professor (Pediatrics and Anesthesia) (1989-1992).

"Stanford was my last job practicing anesthesia. My husband Tim was extremely busy with private clinical practice, starting and running the cardiology research program at Borgess Hospital, starting and running the Fellowship program, investing biomedical devices, and starting several startup companies. I stayed at home to raise the children and create the family culture. Children are my passion."

Anne has been part of the Greta Berman Arbetter Kazoo School, an independent preschool, elementary, and middle school, for 28 years. She was Vice-Chair of the Kazoo School Board of Trustees (2016-2023) and continues as Honorary Trustee and Vice-Chair, emerita. She was the recipient of the Kazoo School Community Leadership Award (2011). She was on the board of the Congregation of Moses Religious School (2000-2014). For her service and work as a religious schoolteacher, she received the Principal's Award (2004) and the Rabbi's Certificate (2005). Anne served on the Harvard Schools Committee (2005-2021) interviewing applicants for Harvard College. She was the Canvassing Coordinator in Southwest Kalamazoo for the Obama Coalition for Change (2008). Anne now works in refugee resettlement under the auspices of Samaritas. Her focus is with children, working on acquisition of English language skills, development of academic skills, and communication/collaboration between home and school.

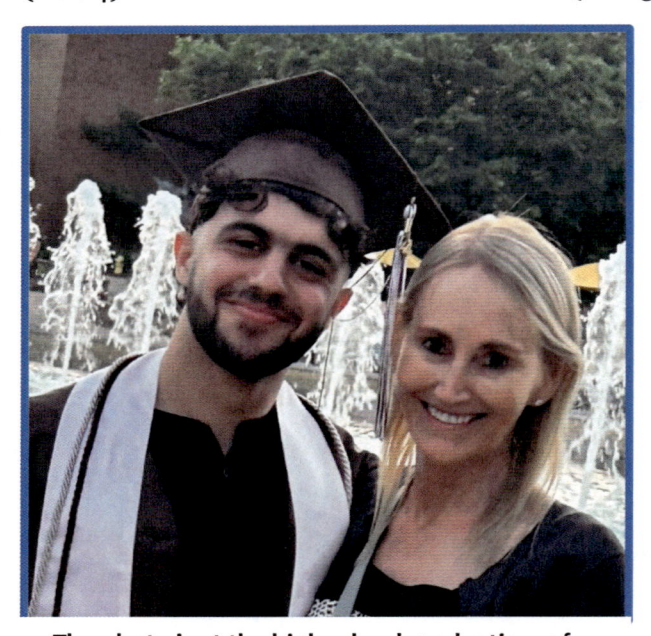

The photo is at the high school graduation of a student who escaped the Syrian Civil War with his family and then spent 5 years in a refugee camp in Jordan. Anne worked with him since he moved to the US in 2016 at the age of 10. He graduated with High Honors and scholar athlete recognition.

"My son Jonathan is Chief Neurology Fellow at the NIH. His clinical interest is in movement disorders, and his research is in gene therapy for Parkinson's Disease. My other son Evan is Senior Director of Analytics for Luminis Hospital Group in Maryland, and my daughter Emma is a recent graduate from Cornell with an Engineering degree."

Interesting Anecdotes/Memories of Time at Stanford:

- *Our favorite attending was Dr Samuels. He was so kind and funny. He used to say, "You make your bed, you sleep in it." Whatever anesthetic technique or procedure you chose, you needed to deal with whatever ensued.*
- *As a resident, cardiac anesthesia was a lot of fun. My husband, Tim Fischell, was a Fellow in Cardiology. We would go to the Cath lab and review the films of my patients for the following day, and we'd discuss the physiology. So, I was always well prepared on that rotation."* ☺
- *Janet Wyner was a great teacher and fun to work with and the cardiac surgeons always played "closing music" at the end of the case. I even kinda got to like country music on those rotations.*

- *For the delivery of my twins, one of our Attendings put in my epidural. This wasn't going to be easy because of my scoliosis. Only my leg became numb. I still felt every labor pain. The Chief of OB Anesthesia, Sheila Cohen was called, and without delay she popped in the most wonderful epidural. I was able to enjoy, pretty much, the rest of my labor and delivery. I had often worked with Sheila, but, during my hour of need, I got to experience firsthand her outstanding technical skill and wonderful way with patients!*

Steven Roy Ford was born in Oklahoma City. He attended the University of Oklahoma (BA, 1978) and the University of Oklahoma College of Medicine (MD with distinction, 1983). He was an intern at SCVMC (1983-1984) and then completed his Stanford Anesthesiology residency (1984-1986) followed by a Fellowship (CCM) (1987). He was Chief Resident (1985-1986). After leaving Stanford he was appointed Assistant Professor (Anesthesia) at the University of Texas Medical Branch (UTMB Health), Galveston, TX (1987-1994) and was promoted to Associate Professor (1994-1995). He was Medical Director of the SICU (1991-1995) at UTMB and won the Walter Bernard Teaching Award (1992).

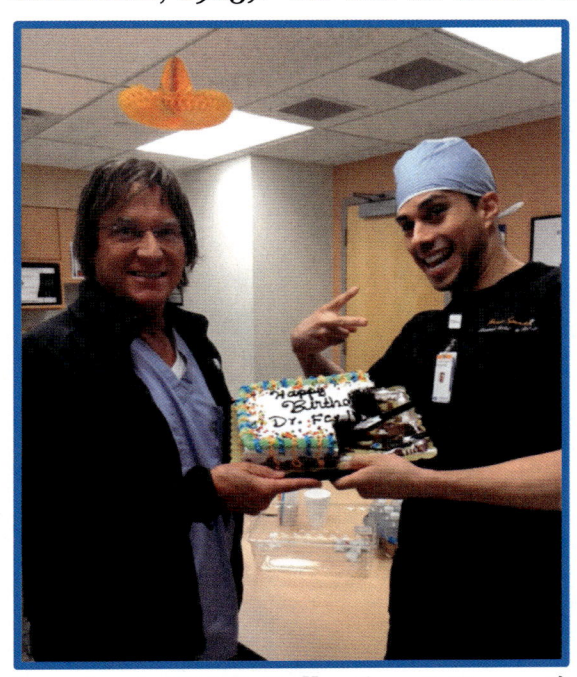

He left for private practice initially with Anesthesia Consultants of Longview, Longview, TX (1995-2001), then joined East Texas Anesthesia Consultants, Tyler, TX (2001-2003). He moved to Dallas with Txan Anesthesia (2003-2014) and then Atlas Anesthesia (2014-2016). Since 2016 he has been Managing Partner and owner of Optima Anesthesia PLLC, Dallas (2016-Present).

Dr. Ford was a member of the Legislative Affairs Committee of the Texas Society of Anesthesiologists (TSA) (1989-1995). He has been a 4-time declarant for the Texas Medical Association (TMA) with amicus briefs for the ASA, TSA, and other medical organizations in the U.S. Federal Court of the Eastern District of Texas, all 4 with favorable summary judgements (2022-2023).

He worked as a part-time sound engineer at Ford Audio-Video (1972-1979). He was a technician in the Endocrinology lab at the University of Oklahoma Health Science Center (1978-1979). He has been a singer, songwriter, and guitarist for the musical groups Hard Rock Candy (1973-1978), The Epidemic (1988-1995), VTac (1995-2003), and currently Punk Ass Mo

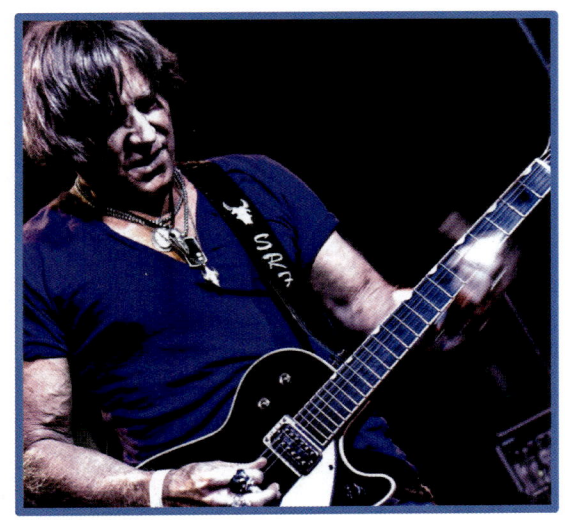

Fo (2012-Present). He is a published singer/songwriter with copyrighted, recorded songs that have enjoyed radio airplay. He has performed with nationally acclaimed artists.

Punk Ass Mo Fo is an American punk blues band from Dallas, TX. Their sound is heavy on fuzzy guitars, driving bass and solid drumbeats, with the vocals slid in just on top. Chuck Berry, the "father of rock'n roll" said "the blues had a baby and they called it rock'n roll " and Punk Ass Mo Fo came from blues, rock and punk. Steven Ford, singer, guitarists, and songwriter for Punk Ass Mo Fo over many years has had the opportunity to perform and do shows with such blues and rock greats as ZZ Top, Chuck Berry and Kenny Wayne Shepherd, and has used those influences in Punk Ass Mo Fo to make a Texas punk blues band. The name Punk Ass Mo Fo was suggested personally to Steven at a show at the House of Blues by guitarists extraordinaire, Earl Slick, as a cool band name and Steven went with it.

Ford is also co-owner of Ford Insurance & Financial Services LLCF in Dallas, TX (2015-Present), and the principal owner and CEO of Formula Autosport Enterprises LLC, Dallas, TX (2016-Present). He is a semi-pro race car driver. He has been a high-performance race car driving instructor and motocross racer for Steve Ford Racing (1970-1975). He has SCCA, NASA, and INDYCAR licenses with multiple wins and podium finishes. He also is a tournament water skier in the slalom event for Steve Ford Waterskiing (1990-2006).

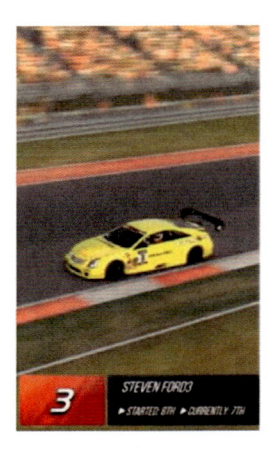

Top 10 Finish for Steven Ford

Another Top 10 finish for Steven Ford in the Hoosier eSports SCCA Super Series driving the yellow #3 Optima Anesthesia TOPSPEED Cadillac CTS-V race car in the GT1 class at Circuit of the Americas in Austin, Tx this evening broadcast live on YouTube on the SCCA channel

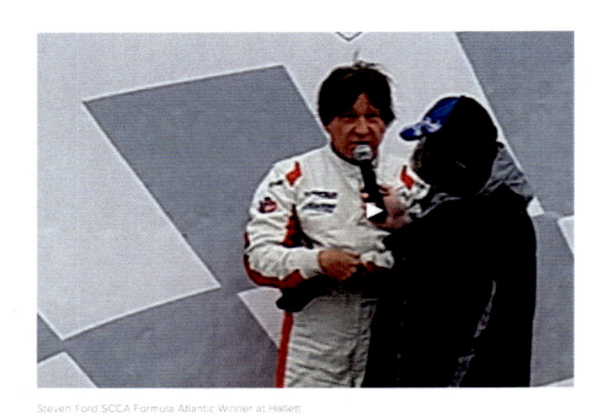

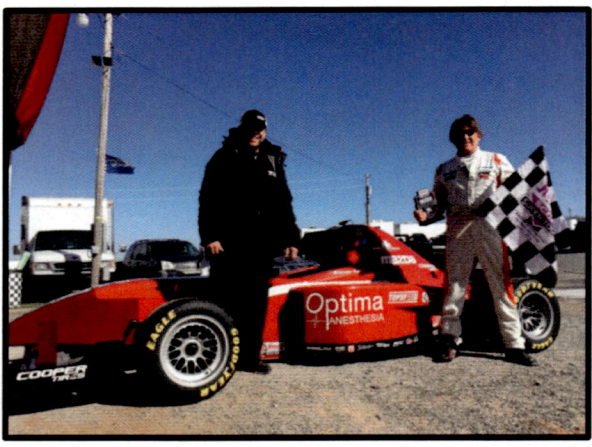

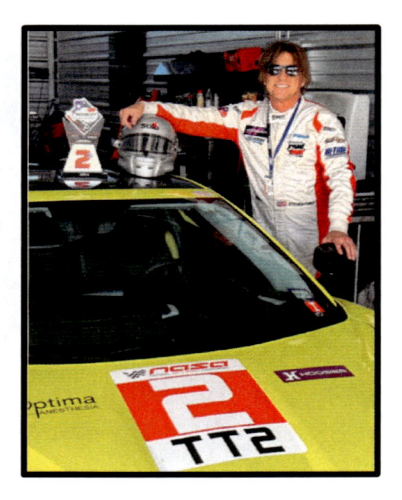

Steven Ford SCCA Formula Atlantic Winner at Hallett

"I am very happily married to a wonderful woman, and we have 3 sons and a daughter, Despite all my outside activities, my best times have always been when I get to spend time with them."

Stanford memories:
- *Critical care rounds and teaching by Myer Rosenthal and Fred Mihm and many other awesome faculty in the department at that time.*
- *Musical performance with David Anish, Jim Byrd and myself for David and Jim's graduation at the end-of-the-year banquet.*
- *Very "spirited" driving one day with Mike Rosenthal riding shotgun around the time of my finishing up at Stanford in a new corvette I had purchased prior to heading to Texas.*

Thomas Lloyd Gaston

was born in Frankfurt Germany. He was an undergraduate at Dartmouth College (BA, 1976). He received his medical education at the University of Minnesota Medical School (MD, 1976-1980), spending time at the University of Nairobi, Kenya during medical school (1980).

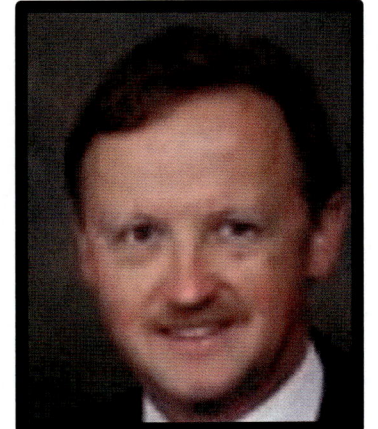

"I spent a year split between doing bench research in hematology and a trip to Africa where I did a pediatric rotation at the University of Nairobi medical school (4 months), and general surgery at University of Witwatersrand, South Africa (1 month)."

He interned and did a residency (Internal Medicine) at Stanford (1981-1984), followed by his Stanford Anesthesiology residency (1984-1986). After training he was briefly on the faculty at the PA-VAH (1986). He worked as a staff anesthesiologist at Washington Hospital, Fremont (1987-1993) and at Sequoia Hospital doing cardiovascular anesthesia (1993-2000). He was a member of PAMF (1993-2020). He was the Medical Director of Menlo Park Surgical Hospital (2001-2008) and then the Vice-Chief of Staff there. He retired in 2020.

Dr. Gaston was active with Interplast and participated on 14 trips to Ecuador, Bolivia, Honduras, Mexico, Nepal, Myanmar, and Vietnam.

In retirement he enjoys traveling with his wife Julie and visiting his 3 children. When home, he spends many hours woodworking and wood turning. He has built a variety of furniture, turned hundreds of bowls, and built outdoor structures. He also teaches woodworking classes at Palo Alto Adult School. His other activities include swimming, biking, hiking, and running.

Richard John Novak was born in Hibbing, MN. He attended Carleton College, Northfield, MN (BA magna cum laude, Chemistry, 1976). While at college he played on the United States Junior Men's Curling championship teams in 1974 and 1975. He graduated from the University of Chicago (MD, 1980). He completed a residency (Internal Medicine) at Stanford (1980-1983) then worked as a medicine Attending in the Emergency Room at Stanford Hospital (1983-1984). He then completed Anesthesiology residency at Stanford (1984-1986).

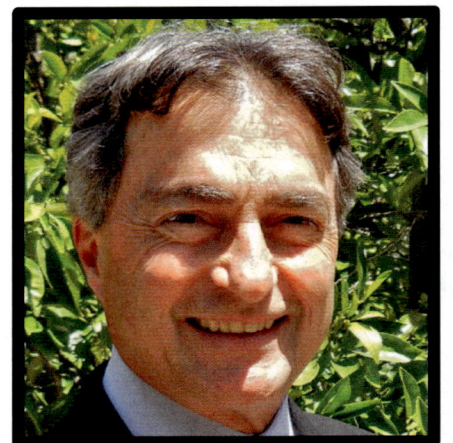

Dr. Novak has been a member of the AAMG since 1989. He is Medical Director of the Waverley Surgery Center, Palo Alto (2002-Present). He is an adjunct Clinical Professor of Anesthesiology, Perioperative and Pain Medicine on our clinical volunteer faculty (2001-Present). He served as Deputy Chief of Anesthesiology at Stanford (2001-2015).

While Deputy Chief he authored a column in the Department's newsletter. The theme of each monthly essay centered on the differences between the private practice of anesthesia and the university-based teaching practice of anesthesia. He began posting these essays on his theanesthesiaconsultant.com website. The Anesthesia Consultant was named the world's number one anesthesiology blog in 2024 by Feedspot. As of March 2024 it had 2.9 *million* views, with readers in over 100 countries around the world.

As 'Rick' Novak he has established himself as a successful novelist publishing three fiction novels with medical themes – *'The Doctor and Mr. Dylan'*, *'Doctor Vita'*, and *'Call From the Jailhouse'*.

He has been a Delegate from District 4 to the CSA. Novak has authored several chapters in anesthesia textbooks and is an Expert Reviewer for the Medical Board of California.

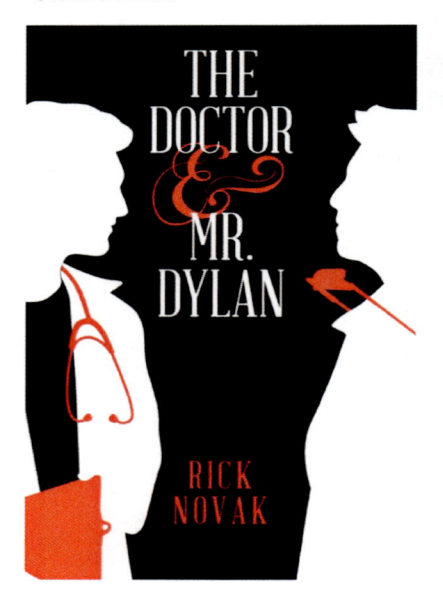

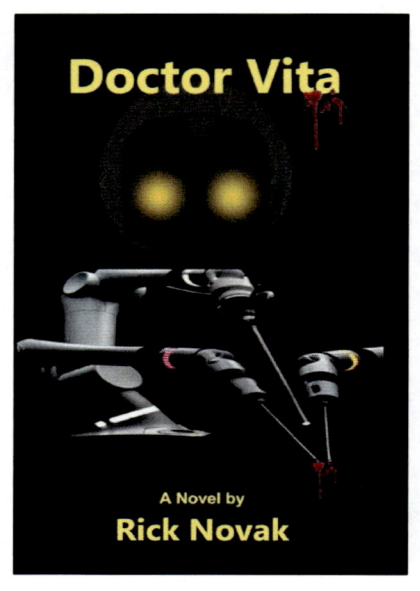

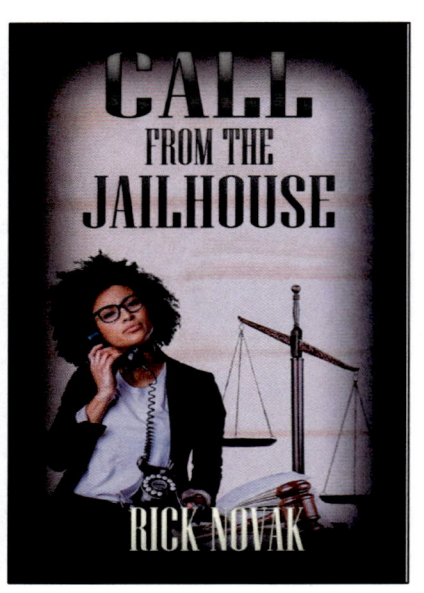

"I remember performing with a moustache and a trumpet as the comedian Father Doctor Guido Sarducci at Department functions as a resident."

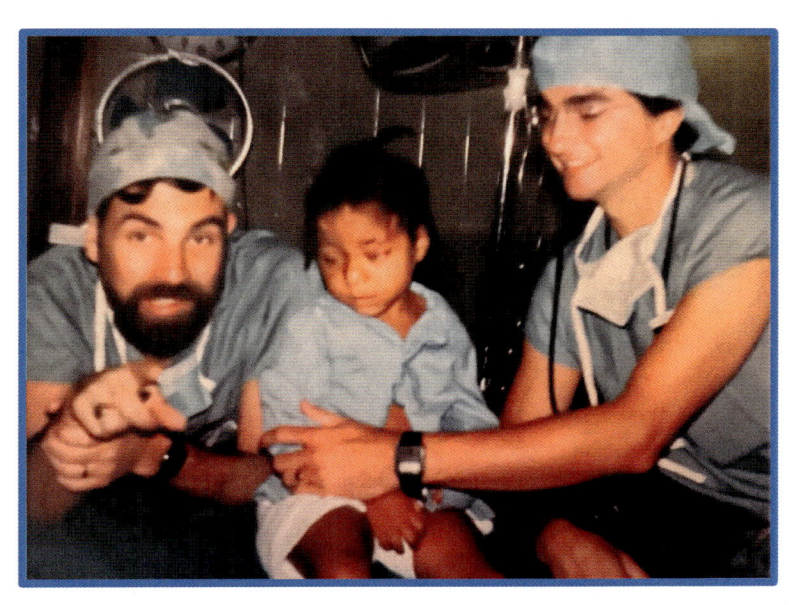

Jay Brodsky and Rick Novak on an Interplast trip to Montego Bay, Jamaica (1986)

Joshua P. Prager was born in New York City and completed his pre-medical studies at Stony Brook University (BS, Chemistry, 1972) before attending graduate school at Harvard University where he studied planning, analysis, and administration and pre-medical courses (1973-1976). He was Special Assistant to Executive Director for Capital Development and Public Services of the Consumer Action Program of Bedford Stuyvesant, Brooklyn, NY (1972-1973). He was a Planning Analyst for the Boston Department of Health and Hospitals (1974-1976) and a Special Assistant to the General Director of Beth Israel Hospital, Harvard (1977). He was President of the Harvard Graduate Student Council.

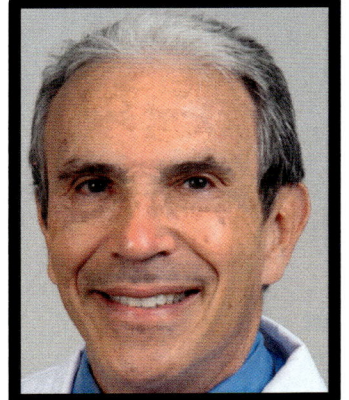

He graduated from the Stanford University School of Medicine (MD, 1977-1981). While there he simultaneously received a master's degree in management/health services research while attending Stanford Graduate School of Business (1979-1981). He has been President of the Board of Governors of the Stanford Medical Alumni Association (2001-2002). He interned and did a residency (Internal Medicine) at the David Geffen School of Medicine/UCLA (1981-1984), followed by starting an Anesthesiology residency at Stanford (1984). He completed his anesthesia residency after returning to Boston for the remainder of his training and a Clinical Fellowship at the MGH (1984-1986).

Dr. Prager has held full-time positions on the faculty of Harvard Medical School/MGH (1986-1987). He was Medical Director and National Consultant for Anesthesiology for CIGNA Health Plans (1991-1993). He was responsible for management of anesthesiology and pain services for half a million lives. He was Medical Director of the operating room and acting Hospital Medical Director of CIGNA's flagship hospital. He has worked at The David Geffen School of Medicine at UCLA (1992-Present). He is a faculty member in the Department of Internal Medicine and Anesthesiology at UCLA and is Director of the Center for the Rehabilitation of Pain Syndromes (CRPS) at UCLA (1997-Present). He is a past president of the North American Neuromodulation Society (NANS).

Dr. Prager's clinical practice focuses on CRPS, neuromodulation, and precision spinal diagnostics and therapeutics. He has run an active ketamine infusion program there for years and has administered over 8000 ketamine infusions. Since 1998 he has managed a comprehensive interdisciplinary functional rehabilitation program designed to return normal function to patients with CRPS and other pain problems that involve central sensitization. He participated in a research study examining brain activity before and after ketamine infusions utilizing functional magnetic resonance imaging (fMRI). In 2016, he was involved in writing guidelines for ketamine treatment under the aegis of the Reflex Sympathetic Dystrophy Syndrome Association (RSDSA).

He has received an award for leadership and contributions by the CSA and is editor of its continuing medical education program on pain and end-of-life care. In 2012 he received the lifetime achievement award and later the distinguished service award from the North American Neuromodulation Society and another award for his dedication and contributions to the field of neuromodulation. Dr. Prager has twice received awards in the Department of Anesthesiology at UCLA for support in teaching in the Fellowship in pain medicine. He has received the Bounty of Hope award from the RSDSA for patient care and contributions to the CRPS community (2007) and two other awards from patient organizations related to CRPS. He chaired a blue ribbon international multispecialty best practices project for the use of intrathecal medications to treat pain. He is analyzing data related to the management of ketamine infusion side effects for the treatment of CRPS as well as depression He served as a pain expert for the California Department of Worker's Compensation in developing treatment guidelines for the injured worker.

In 2005 Prager joined the Medical Evidence Evaluation Advisory Committee (MEEAC), a group appointed by the Governor of California to develop treatment guidelines for medical care of the injured worker. He continued in that role for six years. He served two consecutive 2-year terms as Chair of the CRPS group of the International Association for the Study of Pain (2008-2012). He is also Chair of the End-of-Life CME program of the CSA.

Dr. Prager has provided internal medicine care at the Haight-Ashbury Free Clinic and anesthesia care on medical missions with Interplast. He served as a consultant to Medicare on a local level and currently serves on the national level. He serves as the volunteer Director of pain management and as a volunteer physician for Veterans in Pain (VIP).

Prager plays blues harmonica under the pseudonym Dr. Lester "Les" Payne (a pun) and has played alongside famous musicians and had won an award at the House of Blues in Chicago for best performance by an amateur.

"My most memorable time in the residency at Stanford was having the opportunity to work with Dr. William New, inventor of the pulse oximeter. I was so fascinated with the oximeter and the science behind it that I purchased an oximeter on a resident's salary from Dr. New, which at the time listed for

$5,000. I couldn't imagine providing anesthesia without it at a time when it was barely available. I brought the pulse oximeter with me when I transferred residencies to Massachusetts General Hospital with the encouragement of acting chair John Bunker who had trained there and served on the faculty. The oximeter was extremely controversial. I did have the opportunity to give Grand Rounds about pulse oximetry, a technology that was unknown in Boston at the time. My grand rounds about oximetry as a resident created considerable resentment among the old school faculty who doubted its accuracy and value. Oximetry was a giant step to improve safety in anesthesia and is now standard of care despite the resistance I faced at MGH. Were it not for my opportunity to have met and worked with Dr. New, I would not have had been able to help with the acceptance and adoption of pulse oximetry."

Wendy Rabinov received an MS (Mechanical Engineering) and a medical degree from Stanford (MD, 1982). After an internship (Internal Medicine) at Kaiser Permanente Northern California - Santa Clara (1982-1983) she was an Anesthesiology resident at Stanford (1984-1986). After graduating she worked in TPMG hospitals.

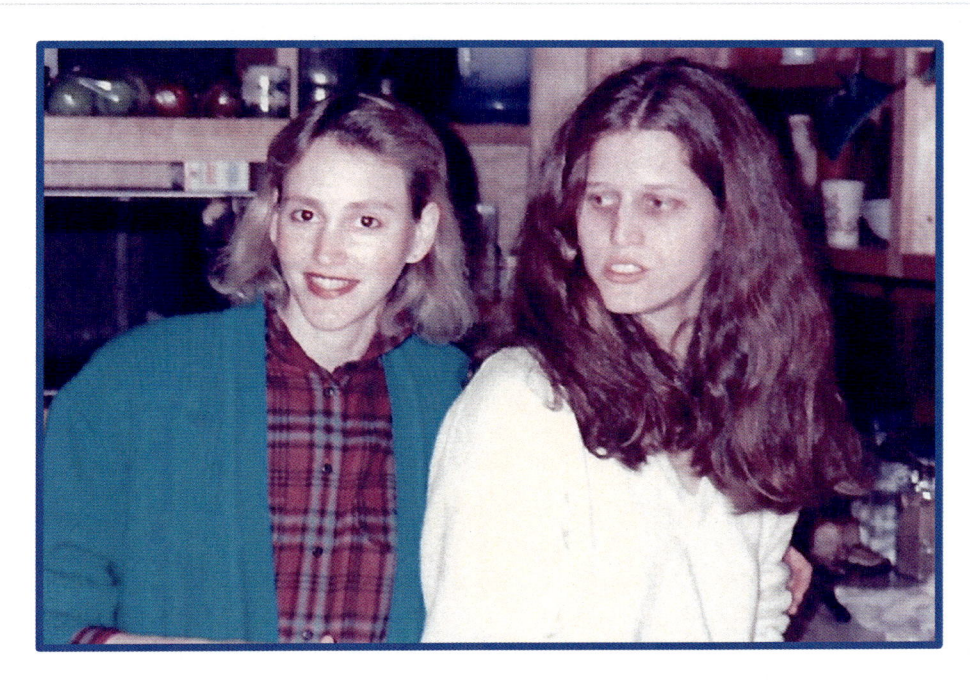

Anne Arbetter Fischell and Wendy Rabinov

Lisa Dianne Saunders was born in Ft. Leavenworth, KS. She attended Dartmouth College (AB summa cum laude, Engineering Sciences, 1979). She graduated from Stanford Medical School (MD, 1983), and did an internship (Rotating) at SCVMC, followed by her Anesthesiology residency at Stanford (1984-1986).

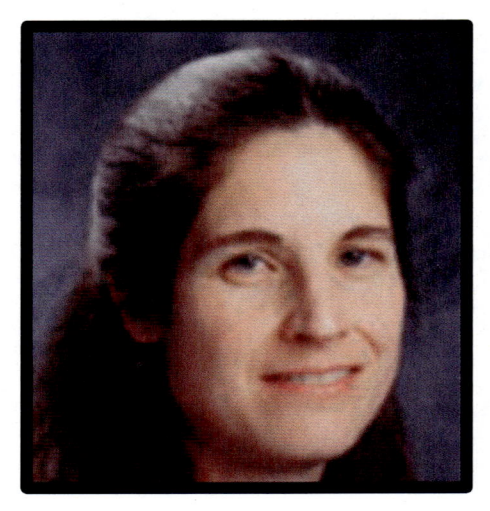

"I used the Army's Health Professions Scholarship Program to pay for medical school. My dad was career Army, so there was a bit of parental coercion. When the time came for me to apply for a residency, I was informed that only those graduates pursuing "high demand" specialties could train in a civilian program. My choices were - anesthesia, general surgery, or oddly enough psychiatry. Not wanting to double my payback obligation, I applied at Stanford in both surgery (thank you Dr Collins!) and anesthesia (thank you Dr Larson!) and was offered spots at both programs. (Given my situation, I did not participate in the match.) Thankfully, I realized early on I would've been a crappy surgeon. That's how I ended up in anesthesia, and what a stroke of luck!"

She was a combined clinical Fellow (Pediatrics and Cardiovascular Anesthesiology) at Stanford (1986-1987).

"Later, I wanted to stay in the SF Bay area, but the Army would only put me at LAMC, a military medicine teaching center if I had three years of anesthesia training (recall back then residency was only two years after internship). That's why I did the weird "fellowship" which was an extra year of advanced cases in cardiac and pediatrics. So, Stanford bailed me out twice!"

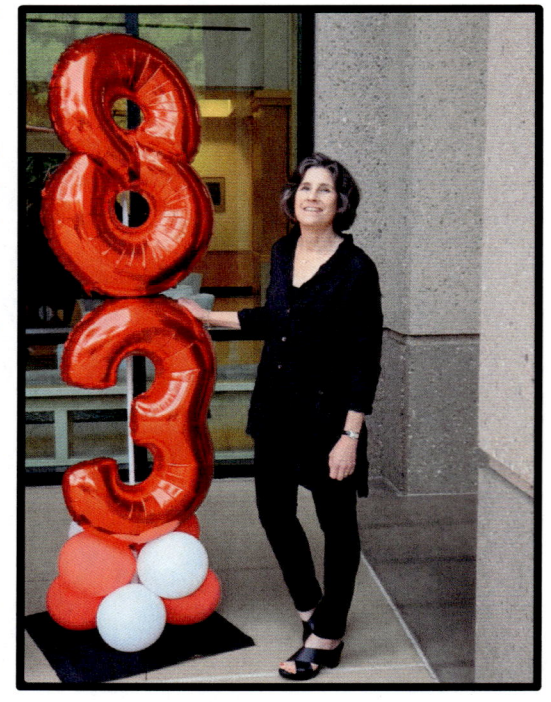

At Stanford Medical Class 40th reunion 2023

She worked as an Attending physician at Letterman Army Medical Center (LAMC) on the Presidio of San Francisco (1987-1992). In 1992 she joined the AAMG (1992-Present). She has also been on the Department's volunteer adjunct faculty since 1989.

"When I started my anesthesia residency in 1984, we were taking intraoperative blood pressures manually and neither O2 Sat monitors nor ETCO2 were available. To my great good fortune, my Attending for my entire first week of training was Dr. Chuck Whitcher. He instructed me to do every single case that week, some of them generals lasting an hour or more, by just mask ventilation. I think he said, "you have a leak!" about a hundred times, but I learned more about airway management in those five days than I did the rest of the year. Soon after, of course, Dr. Whitcher became infamous for

the wacky monitors he rolled around on his "Chuck Wagon" - crazy things like CO2 monitors that eventually became standard, and that we can't practice without today."

"These two pictures are from residency during a neuro case at SCVMC, circa 1985. Note the glass IV bottles!"

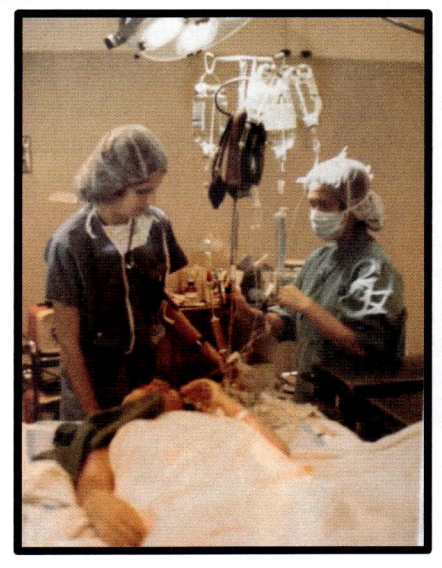

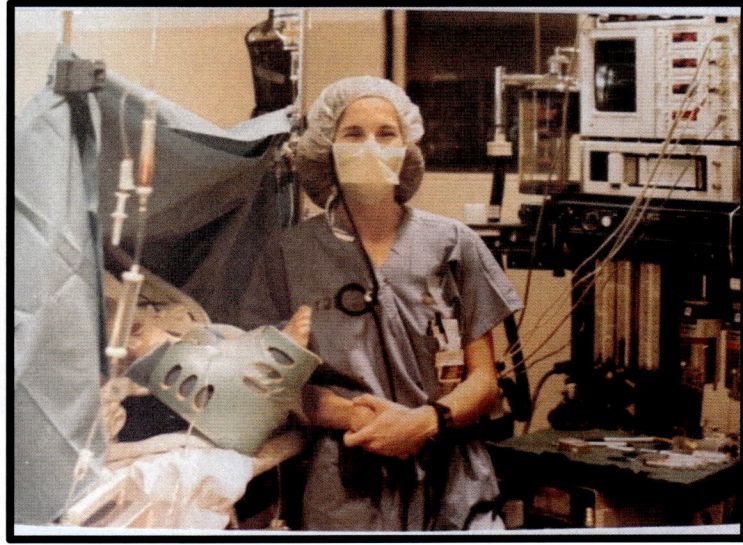

"I was active duty for four years, starting as a Captain and ending as a Major. Being on staff at Letterman was great. My tour was 1987-1991 which spanned the first Gulf War in 1989. For several weeks I had to show up at work every day with my bags packed. I was never deployed but it was stressful. I did an additional year with the Army as an independent contractor, prior to joining AAMG in 1992, and I was on inactive reserve status for four more years after that but never got called. These photos are one just after I got promoted to Major, the other suffering through basic training at Fort Sam Houston while still in medical school."

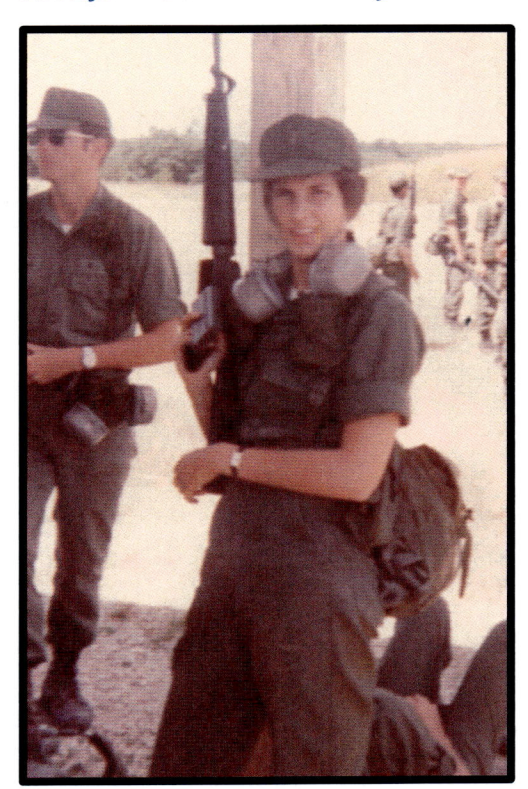

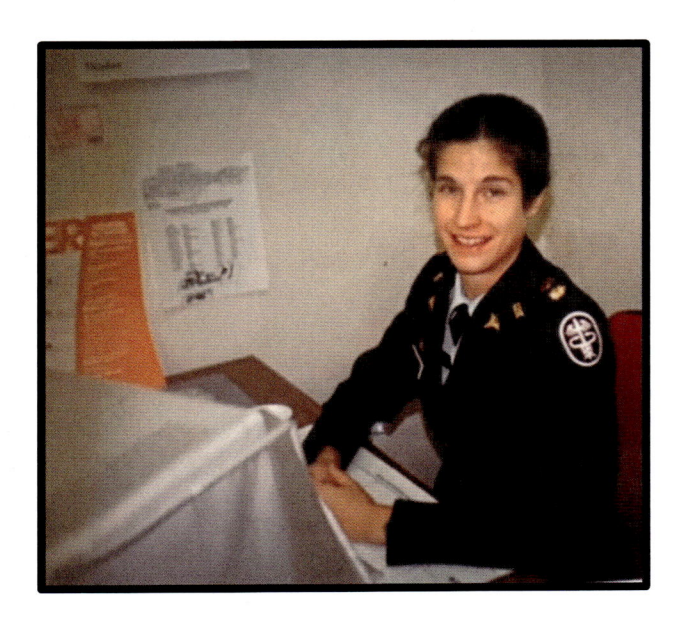

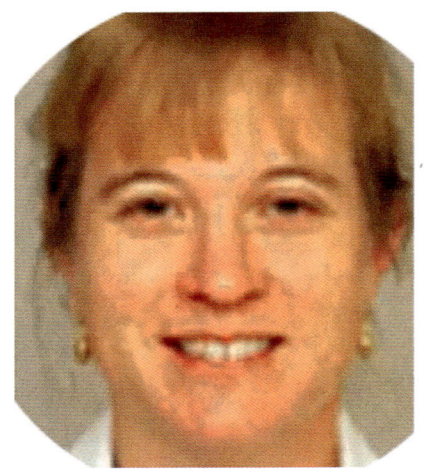

Leila Vieno Maria Siukola (Thurston)

was born in New Jersey. She graduated from Williams College (BA with honors, Chemistry, 1977). She received a MS (Material Science and Engineering) from the Stanford University School of Engineering (1978). She was a medical student at Tulane University School of Medicine (MD, 1983).

"I ended up attending medical school at Tulane in New Orleans. It gave me a chance to experience yet another part of the country. However, I strongly believe that if all I had seen of anesthesia was what I had seen in medical school, I would likely have been a surgeon. When we were getting ready to apply to residency programs, the Dean spoke with each of us, individually, to advise us on where to apply; when I said that I was going into anesthesia he said to me, "I'm sorry, I can't help you, nobody goes into anesthesia". I spoke to one of the surgeons with whom I had worked to ask whom I should seek out in the anesthesia department for advice. I was directed to 5 or 6 programs to which I should apply."

She interned (Rotating) at SCVMC (1983-1984) and did her Anesthesiology residency at Stanford (1984-1986).

"My initial introduction to the Department of Anesthesia at Stanford had been in 1978 via Jim Trudell's (Ellis Cohen's) lab. I had decided to drop out of my PhD program in the Department of Material Sciences in order to apply to medical school. I was looking for a short-term job at the same time that Dr Trudell (a running buddy of my advisor) was looking for someone with a chemistry background, who was good with instrumentation and only wanted a temporary job, it was a match made in heaven. I worked in that lab the year I applied to medical school and then came back to work on other research projects with Chuck Whitcher during my summers in medical school. At my interview for a residency at Stanford I still remember my interview suit and sitting in the office waiting my turn, a little on edge. However, the most memorable moment was when one of my interviewers (Dr Bunker?) asked, "Why isn't there a letter from Chuck Whitcher in your file?" I headed right for Chuck's office following that conversation."

Leila was on the Stanford faculty for a short time after training, and then worked intermittently at Stanford (1990, 1991). She worked as a staff anesthesiologist with TPMG – Santa Clara (1986-2020). For several years (1986-1991) she worked part-time as a clinical researcher for Nellcor. She retired from practice in 2020.

"I was fortunate to be one of the four people who were accepted into slots in the rotating internship that the Department had at SCVMC. I cannot imagine a better foundation for anesthesia. It gave an appreciation of various aspects of medicine and a broad experience with many types of patients and specialties. I have many memory snippets from that year: a page operator who worked hard until he got my name pronunciation correct, a young mother who was admitted in a diabetic coma, delivering a baby with undiagnosed gastroschisis, and watching my Attending's face fall when she realized that I had not over diagnosed bone cancer in a pediatric patient. I used a pocket slide rule to do calculations for my NICU patients (pocket calculators were expensive and disappeared, my slide rule was always where I left it)."

"The Pain Clinic rotation during residency was generally one contiguous month. Steve Fisk from Kaiser Santa Clara came to teach once a month in the Stanford clinic. One of my fellow residents was married to a surgical resident and was given permission to ask me if I was willing to split my pain clinic month so that he could have vacation at the same time as his wife. This resulted in my working with Dr. Fisk twice and then being offered a one-year position in his Department, just when I was about to start looking for a position in the area. My temporary position turned into 34 years, and I retired from Kaiser Santa Clara in 2020."

Leila enjoys reading, knitting and gardening and is active with the San Mateo County Rose Society and the San Jose Heritage Rose Garden.

Memories of Stanford:
- *The first two months of my residency years were also spent at Valley. I thought of it as a baptism by fire. It was a trauma center, had a very busy OR and labor and delivery suite. This was before pulse oximetry was standard of care, so there were 4 pulse oximeters for 8 operating rooms; who wanted to get one had to get in early or make a really good case to one of the residents who was to have one in their room. End-tidal gas monitoring was also not yet standard and SCVMC had either very little or no end-tidal gas monitoring. If you got a chance to lay down, it was on the couch in the anesthesia department lounge/office.*
- *The third month of my residency was my first at Stanford. It started on a weekend, and I felt like I had walked into a country club: I actually had a private call room and had time to spend in it. The OR's all had pulse oximeters and there was the mass spectrometer for end-tidal gas monitoring.*
- *Working on the Stanford campus broadened horizons even more. Specialization within the Department was more defined. Complex cases were more common. Patients came from around the world, frequently admitted the day prior to surgery. If my next day's patient(s) had not been admitted by the time my OR schedule was done, I would frequently go over to Maples pool, hand my pager to the lifeguard and swim laps in a lane close by, returning to the hospital following my workout.*
- *Among the variety of experiences that I recall are using an early version of automated record keeping and using a copper kettle machine. Going over to Hoover Pavilion to do anesthesia for cosmetic surgery tended to be an enjoyable change of pace. Working in the ICU alongside of Internal Medicine residents gave a broader perspective.*
- *We were always supposed to have our Attending present coming off of bypass. It was near the end of one of my months in the heart room and I made several attempts to reach my Attending, Dr Ream. Dr Stinson was the Attending surgeon and had witnessed my attempts. He said to me, "it's alright, I'll be your Attending".*
- *By contrast, Dr Larson was with you most of the time, always teaching. I remember one day we were in the OR, and he was asking me questions. After a while I hit my third "I don't know" and said "you must really think that I am stupid". Imagine my surprise when a week or two later one of my fellow residents let me know that Dr Larson had just complimented me.*
- *Three less than pleasant memories stand out in my mind. I recall being caught in a back and forth between Dr. Al Hackel and the pediatric surgeon one night; after several phone calls, I finally said that they had to talk with each other, as I was no longer going to be between them. On one of my ICU months, I had to call in a private specialist for a patient we were covering, and, of course, the specialist on call was the one that the surgeon did not want. My worst memory from residency was of a patient of mine having to be taken back to the OR and*

- *dying on the table; if I had done things differently, perhaps the outcome would have been different. I seriously thought about quitting my residency over this and must have mentioned it to someone; next thing I knew, Dr Sarnquist (acting head of the department) called me into his office and told me "You can't quit your residency over this". In some ways it was a blessing to have my first unexpected death occur while I was a resident.*
- *At one point, Dr Stanski was to be my evening Attending on OB. I put him into a bit of a tailspin when he asked me how long I had been doing this and I answered that it was my second month. He was much calmer when I clarified that it was my second month on OB, not my second month as a resident. I had spent very little time at the VA, so he did not remember me.*
- *I had been out for a few days with the "flu". I was feeling better and working with Dr Janet Wyner. I had been in the ladies' room and looked at myself in the mirror. I went out, looked at Janet and asked, "do I look jaundiced to you?" She took a good look at me and said "yes", so down to employee health I went. I remember thinking that I will be so angry at myself if it was Hep B as I was planning to get the immunization; it was Hep A. I missed 2-3 weeks and figured I would be making up the time later. When Dr. Fairley called me into his office near the end, I thought he was going to tell me how we would deal with the added time. Instead, he said that people have a right to be sick and since I hadn't ever been on probation, I would not have to make up the time.*
- *Possibly my favorite memory of the OR was in the last several weeks. Mike Rosenthal was my attending; he asked me "What is the MAC of forane (which was a relatively new drug)?" I must have given him a strange look, I certainly thought what kind of question that is to ask me. He said ,"No really, I don't know what the MAC of forane is".*
- *Ultimately, a couple of my residency rotations had a direct impact on my personal life. The first was our pediatric rotation at Oakland Children's Hospital. At the time, I had a friend who, with a friend had a 3-bedroom house in the Oakland hills, 10 minutes from the hospital. Rather than making the commute daily from Menlo Park, I stayed there; as a result, we became closer. This year, we will have been married for 35 years.*

John Henry Urbanowicz

was a Dartmouth College graduate (AB summa cum laude, Organic Chemistry, 1977). He received his MD from the University of Rochester, NY (1981). He interned and was a resident (Internal Medicine) at UCSF (1981-1983). He then completed his Anesthesiology residency at Stanford (1984-1986). He did a Fellowship (Cardiac Anesthesia) at the Cardiovascular Research Institute (CVRI) at UCSF (1986-1987). He served as an Acting Assistant Professor (Anesthesiology) at Stanford specializing in Pediatric Cardiac Anesthesia (1987-1989). After leaving the faculty he joined PAMF in 1989 and remained in that group until he retired (1989-2019). He was Chair of the PAMF Department of Anesthesia (1995-1997) and on the Clinical Anesthesia faculty at Stanford (1989-2002).

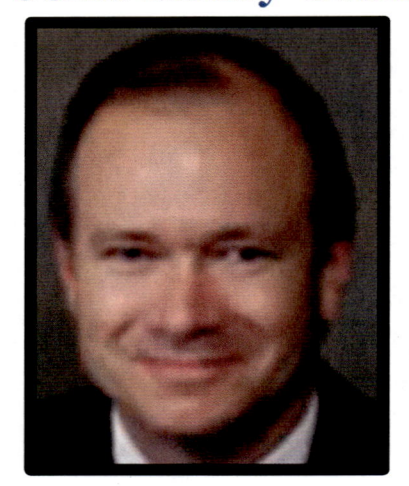

"I retired in 2019 after working at the Palo Alto Medical Clinic for 30 years. I now spend the majority of my time biking, hiking, flyfishing, reading and cooking."

Daniel Alan Waxer was born in Los Angeles. He attended USC (BS cum laude, Psychobiology, 1978). He was President and Founder of the Psychobiology Honor Society at USC (1977). He then was a Henry Luce Foundation Scholar at the Korea Health Development Institute, Seoul, Korea (1978-1979). He then obtained a MSEE degree (Electrical Engineering) working with Mark Yelderman on computer based OR monitoring while a medical student at Stanford (MD, 1983). He interned at SCVMC (1983-1984) and then did his Anesthesiology residency (1984-1986). He first worked in Redding, CA and later **in** Ventura, CA. He was Chair of the Department of Anesthesiology (1988-1990) and Chief of Staff at Redding Medical Center (1993-1994). He worked as an anesthesiologist at Community Memorial Hospital (2004-2016) and was Chair of Anesthesiology in Ventura (2009-2010) and President of the Ventura Anesthesia Medical Group (2012). Dan retired in 2017. He interests include motorcycles and piano.

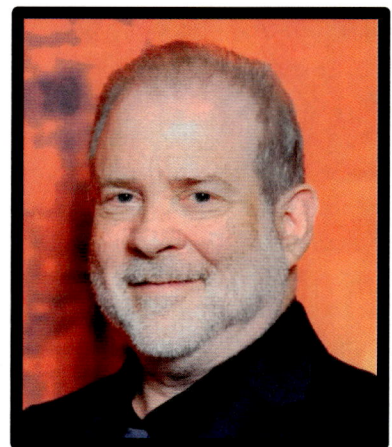

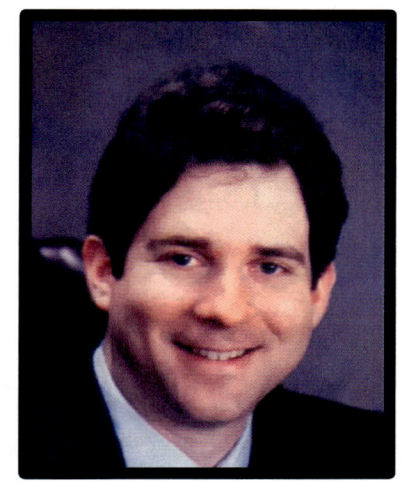

Interesting Anecdotes/Memories of Time at Stanford:
"I remember that when I began my residency, I heard of a tragic event occurring to another anesthesia resident of an unrecognized esophageal intubation. When my residency began cases were performed without routine pulse oximetry or capnography. This event, although not involving me directly, did significantly focus to never allow that to happen 'under my watch.' I wish I could explain it better, however it was an intense determination to avoid errors of a nature that could result in catastrophic outcome. I mention this now because looking back at the many tens of thousands of people I took care of I feel so lucky and blessed to somehow have 'gotten through it' without having to face that kind of terrible scenario. Yes, I have had people not make it and had other unfortunate outcomes. However, they were 'not unexpected' in that the circumstances were unfortunate and unrelated to anesthesia, or my actions (or inactions.) Somehow, that decision and determination in my first week of residency, stuck with me my entire career, and my 'wish' did come to pass, to essentially 'do no harm'. The message for the reader is, believe in yourself, be determined, and those intense decisions made with conviction, can in fact last a career. Somehow, it did for me. And I thank 'G-d', the 'Universe', or whatever 'High-Up' exists, for the help I received to honor my promise to myself, and to my patients.

Looking back, I could see at times unexpected synchronicities that occurred that worked to help me and my patient, at critical points, so I do believe there was help from 'Above.' Lorne Eltherington, my attending at the Pain Clinic once said to that he … "can use all the help I can get." I believe it is important to share openly, since we are all in the same 'boat' of having limited information, being imperfect, and at risk all the time of very bad events occurring. If I was to summarize how I believe I avoided 'bad' critical mistakes, it involved making, or finding ways to 'double check' myself as much as I could, and also, it was that I was generally skeptical of what was the 'actual environment' the patient was in, versus what I believed it was. In other words, I kept updating my inner (or mental) 'model' of what was 'going on' with more information as time went on to make sure my 'model' was still correct.

And that process never really ended, it kept going on throughout the entire case. Once in a while, I figured out that something significant was 'amiss' that I might have missed had I not been as a 'routine' skeptical. This continuous process of not being 'satisfied definitively' with the patients 'known state', I do think helped a lot to keep bad things from happening or spiraling out of control.

During my first ICU rotation on my first ICU overnight call shift, I remember the ICU Fellow 'checked-out' his 'step-down' patient to my care at the end of his day. I had never met the patient. All seemed to be in order, so there was nothing for me to do at the time. I went to sleep in the call room. My pager goes off at about 3 am. It is a nurse in the step-down unit taking care of this patient who I know almost nothing about. The nurse tells me: "Mrs X is sundowning, can I give her haldol?" (I had not heard of 'sundowning' before, so I asked her what she meant.) She was vague however, the impression was that the woman was 'confused'. I was tired and I wanted to go back to sleep, and the nurse gave me an 'easy out' if I just agreed to order haldol. However, something just did not feel quite right. It just did not add up. in my mind. I told the nurse, "no, don't give anything, I will come see her." When I got to the patient, I found a completely unresponsive elderly woman. It was a whole lot more than 'confused'. She was comatose! I quickly determined via the chart that her 'normal' state was awake and able to speak. I drew blood and sent off for stat labs. The stat glucose was something like 16. I hung D50 and after just a few minutes the woman woke up! Her not being diabetic gave no rational reason for her glucose to have been an issue. Except, she was comatose! I then had a mystery to solve. I had already asked what medications the woman had received, and the answer was only her "regular ranitidine 2ml IV." It did not add up. I asked to see the actual medication bottles that were used. (By this time, it was becoming 'political', the nurse and her supervisor were on my case. I remember the Charge Nurses saying, "Our nurses do not make mistakes, etc. , etc.") When I finally was able to examine the bottle. I looked very carefully at the bottle with the printed prescription label of "ranitidine", and I noticed that if one peeled off this label, underneath was a bottle of insulin! When the nurse had given 2 ml of what she thought was ranitidine, it was actually 200 units of regular insulin! Now, the mystery was solved, and I needed that, because I did not like the idea of 'things just happening'. No, I wanted to know how and what and why and also how we can help make sure it will not happen again. So, the 'upheaval' I made at that nursing unit, I hope helped prevent future 'events' or 'errors' like that one, that would be essentially fatal or grossly debilitating.

On that very same first ICU rotation call night, I diagnosed a pneumothorax on a post-CABG patient. A nurse called me about "low blood pressure" and wanting to "increase the inotropes". Here also, it did not feel right to just increase a drip, I needed to see what was going on. I examined the man, on a ventilator, and listened to him, and had a hunch maybe there is a pneumothorax (I had never diagnosed one before.) An x-ray confirmed a pneumothorax. I called the cardiac surgeon. He came in and I believe as my 'reward' he allowed me to place my first chest tube under his direct supervision, talking me through it. I appreciated that, especially since it was the middle of the night, and he took time out to spend a few minutes teaching me.

This call night was one of the highlights of my residency because it was when I knew (as opposed to hoped) I was 'cut-out' for the work I was doing and for succeeding at it. It was an important inflection point in my evolution from student to resident, resident to anesthesiologist. A few hours after these two events, we had morning ICU rounds with my attending Dr. Sladen and the other ICU residents and Fellows. I had two stories to tell. I sensed that Dr. Sladen was proud of his Stanford resident for 'coming through' perhaps more than expected and delivering for two patients who were at risk. I could feel Dr. Sladen's sense of satisfaction about that night, and that feeling was a wonderful feeling. It's like when you see a twinkle in someone's eye who you look up to and respect, who you want to learn from and emulate, like Dr. Sladen. At that moment that twinkle said more than words. It allowed me to know, on the inside, that things were right, and on course, and the course was true. Sometimes, 'twinkles' do last a lifetime..."

"Lorne Eltherington got a chuckle out of me, but also kept me totally focused at the same time. I was to perform my first cervical epidural steroid injection in a young woman, and just prior to placing the needle, I looked to him for any last words of advice. Lorne said, "Don't pith her." I will never forget that. It did take away some of the tension I was feeling at that moment because avoiding the risks was preeminent in my mind already. Also, I recall Jay Brodsky's humor and cheerfulness, and a warm smile. It was welcome relief from the otherwise intense seriousness, and mental focus during much of the days (at least for me.) I tended to be a bit serious, and the responsibility felt heavy, and having some humor and 'lightness', helped me in not feeling as overwhelmed as I otherwise might have."

Several other members of this residency class experienced difficulties with substance abuse and legal problems. Below is a newspaper article from the Los Angeles Times about two of our 1984-1986 residents, both working at South Valley Hospital in Gilroy, CA.

James Edward Pearson attended the University of Colorado School of Medicine (MD, 1982) and completed his Anesthesiology training at Stanford (1984-1986). He worked in Gilroy, CA. He subsequently had his medical license revoked and he spent time in prison for assorted felonies.

The Los Angeles Times – May 23, 1995

Medical Board Sues Administrator For Non-Disclosure : Hospitals: State Agency Brings Civil Action Against Official, Saying He Failed To Reveal Disciplinary Actions That Had Been Levied In Gilroy Against Two Physicians.

Making good on its promise to crack down on hospital administrators who withhold information about disciplinary actions against doctors, the state Medical Board filed its first-ever civil action Monday against the former head of a Gilroy hospital for failing to report actions against two physicians. The action was taken against the former CEO of South Valley Hospital in Gilroy. The Medical Board alleges he failed to notify the state, as required by law, that he and his hospital had disciplined two anesthesiologists then employed there. The Medical Board, charged with licensing and disciplining doctors, has suspended the licenses of the two physicians ...

"... The first physician was Dr. James Edward Pearson who is now in state prison for non-hospital related crimes. Dr. Pearson is serving a prison sentence for a series of felony convictions including sexual battery and rape. Prior to the convictions, complaints were made to the hospital beginning in 1991 about Pearson for allegedly demonstrating inappropriate anger and using foul language, the board said. Pearson was never formally suspended, but the board (the CEO) and a physician aid committee pressured Pearson to take time off and seek professional help and were under an obligation to report that to the state agency. Pearson left the hospital the day after being told to seek help and never returned, according to the board."

The other physician mentioned in the newspaper article was Dr. Lawrence Weiss.

"... (The second physician) ... Dr Lawrence Weiss was exhibiting "bizarre behavior" and subsequently was required to undergo routine drug testing. Although the tests failed to reveal drug use, the bizarre

behavior continued, the board said. The board quoted a nursing report that said on one occasion in 1991, Weiss, attempting to inject medication into an intravenous line before a surgery, repeatedly missed the line and instead injected the medication into bedding. Ballard met repeatedly with Weiss, who eventually was suspended in 1991, but the board was never informed, Arnett said. "We still haven't received proper notification," Arnett said Monday."

Lawrence Babbit Weiss received a degree (BS, Biochemistry, 1977) from Cornell University and his MD from Stanford (1982). He was an Anesthesiology resident (1984-1986). There was a concern, never proven, that drugs were involved in Dr. Weiss's erratic behavior. His license to practice medicine in California was subsequently cancelled. After leaving clinical medicine (1991) he worked in various roles within the biotechnology industry in natural products including chemistry, microbiology, pharmaceutical development, and product commercialization. He was the founder and Chief Scientific Officer (CSO) of CleanWell Company (2005-2014) and worked at AOBiome Therapeutics (CMO, 2014-2017). He is the founder and CSO of Symbiome and its CEO (2021-Present).

Substance abuse among anesthesiologists was a common problem during the 1980s. Two other members of this residency group lost their lives to drugs.

Dana Wolf Rosenberg (deceased) graduated from Duke University (MD, 1980) and completed his Anesthesiology residency (1984-1986). He married fellow Duke medical student Catherine deVries, who is now a renowned pediatric urologic surgeon at the University of Utah. Rosenberg passed away at his home from an overdose (1990).

Neil Francis Marley (deceased) was a graduate of the John Hopkins University School of Medicine (MD, 1981). He began his Stanford residency in Anesthesiology on July 1, 1984. He was placed on probation for substance abuse and voluntarily resigned from the program in November 1985. Sadly, he went to Atlanta and entered a rehabilitation program, but left before completing it. He died from shortly thereafter.

CHAPTER 3

H. BARRIE FAIRLEY
Department Chair (1985-1992)

In 1985 the renowned pioneer in respiratory physiology and critical care medicine, H. Barrie Fairley was recruited from UCSF to become the third Chair of the Stanford Department of Anesthesiology.

Henry Barrie Fairley was born in London in 1927 of Scottish parents – the only *sassenach* in the family at the time. His parents were high school sweethearts in Grangemouth, Scotland, and married there when his father returned from WWI. Fairley's father worked briefly in the Grangemouth office of an Edinburgh-based cargo shipping company, before moving to its Liverpool and then London offices, eventually managing the latter. His mother was a homemaker.

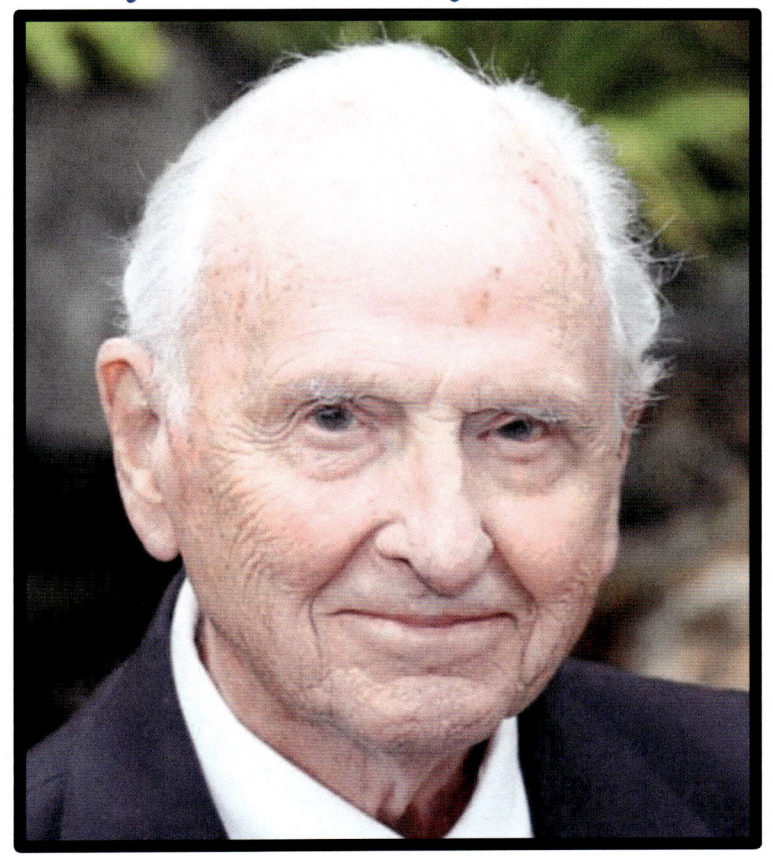

In those days, only 5% of the UK (and US) population had a university degree – the province of the wealthy and elite. The Fairley family didn't fall into either category. Nevertheless, despite the Depression, his parents struggled to ensure that Barrie had the education necessary to enter a profession. He attended private schools, first as a day student in London at Colet Court – St Paul's Preparatory School – then, with WWII looming, at a boarding school in Sussex at Ardingly College. In mid-1939 his family moved back from a few years living in Central London to their home in Orpington, Kent, a South-East London suburb. War was declared later that year.

"Subsequent war-related experiences while I was home from school on vacation included having a large proportion of the roof of our house blown off and the windows shattered one night during the London Blitz. My parents and I were in a reinforced concrete air raid shelter in the back garden, and we were unharmed. Later, while sitting for my 1st MB, BS exams in London

during raids in 1944, "flying bombs" fell nearby, and all the candidates had to shelter under their desks and work benches while items fell around them."

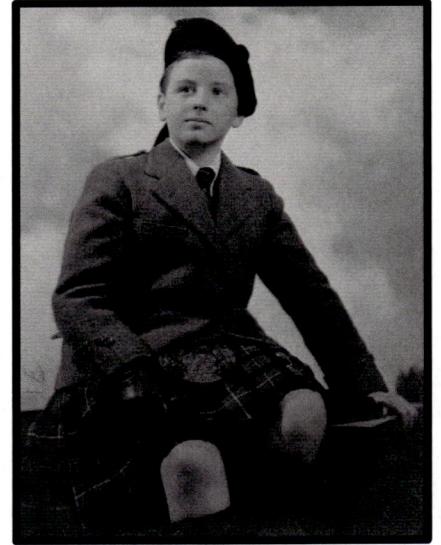

At age 15, Fairley passed the 'Oxford and Cambridge School Certificate' (the then universally accepted prerequisite in the UK for university admission) but stayed on at Ardingly another year, studying chemistry, physics, and biology as a preparation for medical school. On vacations from Ardingly, he was very active in the Boy Scouts, with his senior scout patrol installing Morrison air-raid shelters in people's homes. He was honored on the front page of the monthly *Scout* magazine by the UK's Chief Scout, Lord Rowallan, as the first in the organization to lead a patrol all of whom were King's Scouts (Eagle Scout equivalent) and had the 'Bushman's Thong', an award for outdoor activities.

1940

At that time there were 13 medical schools in the University of London. In 1943 Fairley was accepted to one of the smaller ones, Westminster Medical School, which the family GP had attended. Westminster's preclinical program was carried out at Kings College but, at 16 he was too young to enter and so completed the first year (chemistry, physics, and biology) at an affiliate – Chelsea Polytechnic, from which he passed the 1st MB, BS exam with the highest score in zoology among all candidates from the U. London medical schools. He then moved on to Kings College to study anatomy, physiology, pharmacology, and biochemistry for his 2nd MB, BS exam.

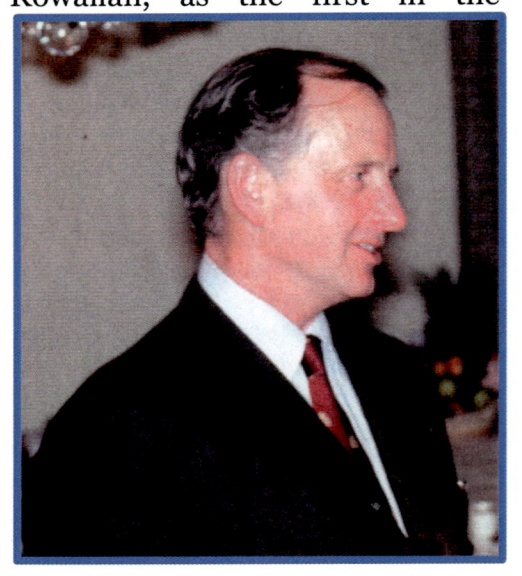

Fairley attending the annual "18 Club" dinner in London in 1980.

"In the UK the first degree in any faculty (school) is always a bachelor's degree. Hence "MB, BS" means Bachelor of Medicine, Bachelor of Surgery. It has three successive stages, each with a final exam as one moves on through the six-year program. An MD is a research-based postgraduate degree."

In 1946, at age 19, he began clinical studies at Westminster – with an all-male group of 18 contemporaries who, on graduation, would form the *18 Club* and meet at least

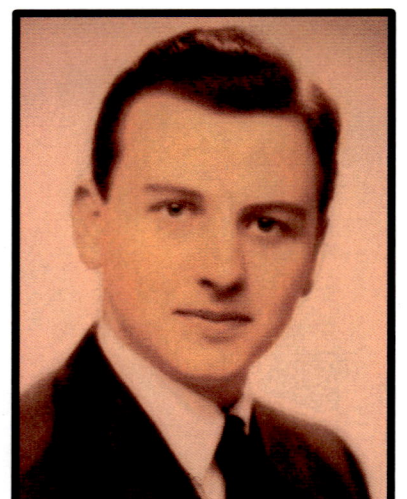

1947

40

annually through the rest of their lives (Fairley on occasional visits). At the time of this writing (2023) Fairley and a retired UK GP are the only two members remaining.

"At Chelsea Polytechnic, I learned fencing from Leonard Paul, a premier London teacher, and continued with the sport on the King's and then Westminster teams, becoming the captain of the latter including when they won the U. London intercollegiate championship. As was customary I was then named captain of the U. London team."

As it was wartime and doctors were required for the military, all medical degree courses were shortened by six months, with the result that Fairley passed the final MB, BS exam (the UK equivalent of an MD) in 1949, thereby "qualifying" for a license to practice medicine. However, as was common then, for practice he took another qualifying exam (this for the MRCS, LRCP degrees) that required six months less than the MB, BS. He passed. As a result, he became a house surgeon (surgical intern) at Westminster and took the final MB, BS exam while working in that position. This was on a firm (service) led by a famous thoracic surgeon, Clement Price Thomas, universally called CP and later knighted for performing a pneumonectomy for cancer (at Buckingham Palace) on King George VI.

"The term house surgeon, house anesthetist, etc., was used for trainees who lived in the hospital or medical school and were therefore available 24/7. My annual salary as a house surgeon was £450 (plus room and board)."

In his final year as a Westminster student, Fairley had won the Frederick Bird Prize in Obstetrics, Gynecology, Medicine, and Pathology, and decided to pursue a career as a gynecologist. In the UK, that would have required first obtaining the equivalent of surgical boards. There were none of today's specialty training programs and so one applied for a sequence of one or two-year registrar (resident) posts before taking the relevant specialty exam having read the related texts on one's own. That would be followed by a senior registrar job, usually of three years duration.

When Fairley finished his surgical internship, there were no surgical registrar posts open at Westminster, but there was a house anesthetist position available in their Department of Anesthesia. The leaders of that department, Ivan Magill and Geoffrey Organe enjoyed worldwide recognition. Fairley thought the experience gained might be useful in his planned Ob-Gyn career and so applied for the anaesthesia position and was accepted. In that first year, he administered 1,200 anesthetics (documented on Hollerith cards).

"As well as the technical aspects of anesthesia, I found the interactions with physicians across all surgical and some other specialties extremely enjoyable, both collegially and professionally. In addition, it provided a broad insight into the activities of the hospital's various departments. I also enjoyed the daily application of pharmacology and physiology knowledge to the choice of an anesthetic for patients with differing pathologies, and its delivery and monitoring, primitive as the latter was in those days. I changed my career plans although at the time I was not thinking about a career in academics, My goal was to become a versatile practitioner."

The required anesthesia training period in the US at that time was two years post internship, while it took about five or six years in the UK and five in Canada before becoming an independent practitioner. After a year as anesthesia junior registrar at Westminster and various other locums, then with two years of experience working in anesthesia, Fairley joined the Royal Air Force (RAF) with a three-year commission, as opposed to the two-year wartime National Service obligation. He rose to squadron leader in the RAF Medical Branch.

"I was 23 years old and married. There were benefits attached to being a "regular" as opposed to being drafted, including access to married accommodations, better pay, and a financial bonus on discharge that would be used to buy our first car, a Morris Minor convertible."

Fairley was posted to Germany from 1950-1952 at the British Air Force of Occupation specialty referral hospital in Rinteln, Westphalia. He finished his RAF career at a hospital in the UK. When the time came to leave military service in 1953, he considered three options – (a) continuing in the RAF, (b) getting back on the registrar ladder in the UK for at least three years and perhaps more, or (c) going overseas. With the last of these in mind, he wrote to the Canadian Anesthetists Society inquiring about opportunities in that country but did not hear back immediately.

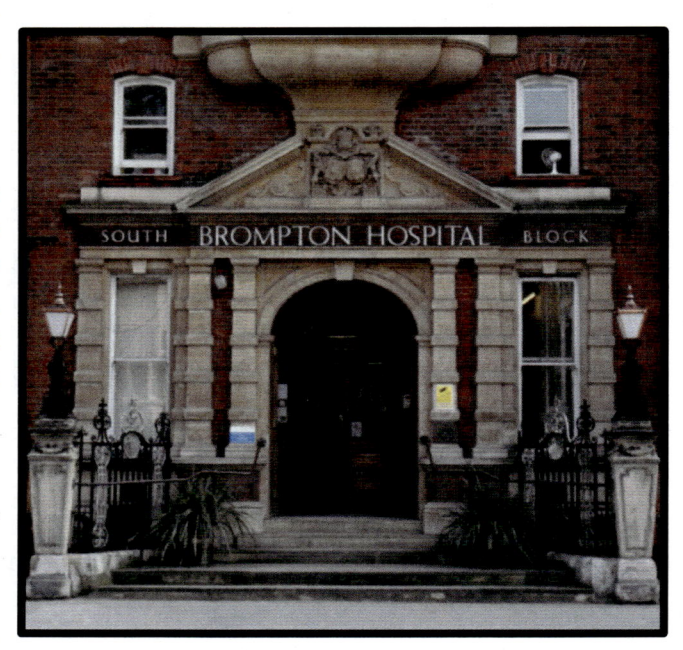

Meanwhile, the anesthesia chiefs at Westminster had arranged for Fairley to be appointed to the two-year registrar position at one of Britain's internationally acclaimed postgraduate specialty centers. All specialty centers were located in London. The Brompton Hospital was the one that dealt only with thoracic diseases – primarily pulmonary. There, he learned how to provide anesthesia for the full range of thoracic procedures. Among these were thoracoplasties (for tuberculosis) using multiple paravertebral blocks with light sedation, and the use of bronchial blockers placed through a bronchoscope. Cardiac surgery was in its infancy.

"One fateful day in 1954, I was called to the phone at the Brompton with Westminster's senior anesthetist Sir Ivan Magill on the line. He had received a letter from Toronto inquiring about me. There followed an offer to join the staff of the Toronto General Hospital (TGH) for a year, with the possibility of a permanent position."

So, now with six years of anesthesia experience and a subspecialty of Cardiothoracic anesthesia, yet still facing in the UK as many as three more years as a senior registrar, Fairley booked a berth on a transatlantic crossing and arrived in Toronto in May of 1955. His wife, Jean, who was a Westminster nurse, and their 2½ year-old daughter (born in the RAF hospital in Rinteln) joined him that Fall. He had developed a very positive opinion about their possible future as Canadians and was impressed with the medical environment. Fortunately, Jean liked Canada immediately.

Barrie had been allocated to work at TGH with the Chief of Cardiovascular Surgery, Wilfred Grant Bigelow. Bigelow was the first to demonstrate hypothermia for open heart surgery, and then continued with the introduction of the "heart-lung machine". During that hypothermia period Fairley and colleagues reported the phenomenon of rewarming acidosis [1] as well as other biochemical changes.[2]

In 1958, Fairley was asked by neurologist Richard Chambers, also from the UK, whether he could supervise the change at TGH from using the tank respirator ("iron lung") for respiratory failure to intermittent positive pressure (IPP) ventilation. Working with pulmonologist Colin Woolf and ENT surgeon Hugh Barber, they established the TGH Respiratory Unit in 1958. It would become Canada's first interdisciplinary ICU with Fairley as Director. While describing the four basic requirements of such units they reported their first 100 cases in 1959[3] and published a detailed report of their clinical management experiences a year later.[4]

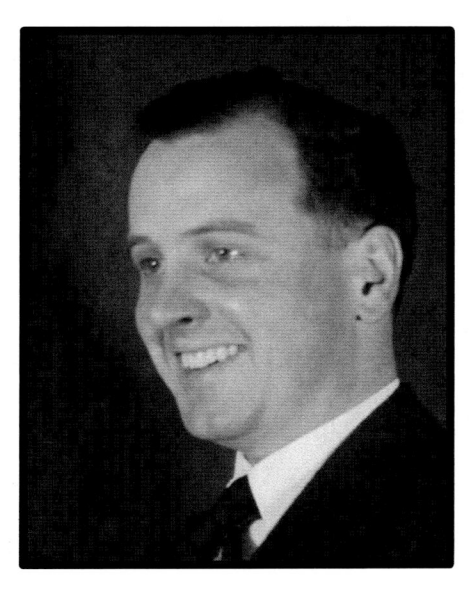

1957

Thereafter, Fairley investigated the physiology of mechanical ventilation and reported the results widely, as well as describing aspects of what is now ICU care. He subsequently received many invitations to be a visiting professor from centers in Canada and the US, as well as internationally.

In his early years at TGH he examined the function of mechanical ventilators in common use and discovered that the Bird ventilator that functioned from an oxygen source with the option to incorporate a in-line that was claimed to entrain air with a resulting 40% oxygen delivery, only function at that level if there was no downstream opposition. As the inspired pressure rose the entrained air decreased.[5] The ventilator was removed from the market. Another important issue at that time was accidental disconnection of a ventilator in an unconscious or paralyzed patient. With his laboratory technician, Fairley designed the first disconnect alarm.[6] That alarm was required for all patients receiving mechanical ventilation at TGH. A version of the alarm incorporating its features was subsequently incorporated in all ventilators being sold.

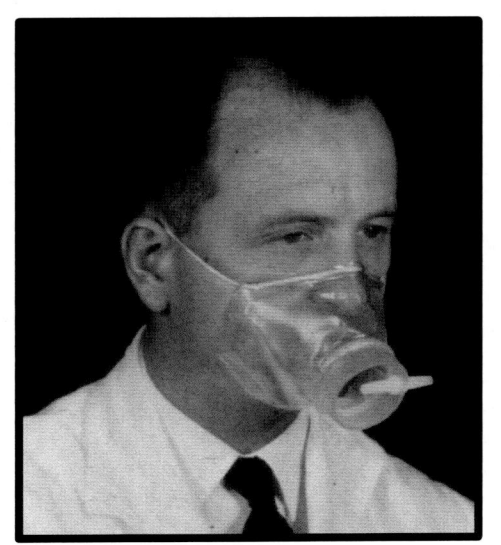

Wearing an oxygen mask that he designed

It was not until 1971 that the specialty of critical care medicine (CCM) became sufficiently common that the Society of Critical Care Medicine (SCCM) was formed, with Fairley as a founding member.

Other of Fairley's 'firsts' at the TGH were the organization of the Code Blue team and the details of the necessary equipment for resuscitation in all the hospital's wards (today's "crash carts"),[7] the introduction of blood gas measurements, developing a system of ambulance transportation to the hospital of patients requiring respiratory support, and the introduction of a Hyperbaric Medicine program at TGH with him as the Director.

Gradually, he was promoted up the University of Toronto academic ladder, becoming a full professor in 1968. He was now receiving invitations to move to other institutions. None was sufficiently attractive to consider a move, nor was he looking for one, until UCSF offered him a full professorship with the next tenured slot to become available. UCSF was one of the leading academic anesthesia programs in the US, with a level of expertise in respiratory physiology that was lacking in Toronto at that time.

Excerpted from: **Fairley HB. In at the start: recollections of the early days of critical care in Toronto. Can J Anesth (2018) 65, 1093–1099.**[6]

At TGH in the mid-1950s, patients requiring ventilation with a tank respirator were cared for in a side room off the corridor leading to one of the long, open medical wards. The nurse assigned to the patient's care would often be an "outsider" called in from an agency. On occasion, she would be unfamiliar with the other nursing personnel and the hospital's routines. It would have been unusual for the nurse to have seen a tank respirator before the assignment, or to understand even the basics of respiratory care management.

One day in 1957, a young neurologist Dr. Richard Chambers asked if I could help set up the type of care for paralyzed patients that he had experienced during his UK-based training. What followed was the establishment of TGH's "respiratory unit" in 1958, after caring for a few patients receiving intermittent positive pressure ventilation in side rooms, with untrained nurses. We recruited Dr. Colin Woolf, a South African respirologist who was the director of the pulmonary function laboratory, and Dr. Hugh Barber, an ear nose and throat specialist whom we met over emergency bronchoscopies to remove aspirated material from the lungs of patients in tank respirators. We would also require his skills to establish tracheostomy management protocols.

There was initial concern, particularly from internists who believed that intermittent negative pressure around the chest was essential for the maintenance of venous return and cardiac output. It didn't occur to them that their patients in the operating room were surviving intermittent positive ventilation during anesthesia, and they were unaware of the Scandinavian and UK experiences. When our recommendation for a specialized unit was presented to the TGH's Medical Board in December 1957, we were considered too junior to accomplish this. A "Respiratory Failure Committee," chaired by Dr. Bill Oille, an uninvolved senior cardiologist, was convened. Fortunately, he was very supportive and the board approved the four key principles for the management of patients with respiratory failure. They still remain the basics of any intensive care unit (ICU), and with the possible exception of the physician team composition, are taken as a "given" today. They were:

Patients would receive their care in a designated location.

Nursing care would be provided by permanent specially trained staff - perhaps the major factor in the later expansion to today's ICUs.

A neurologist, chest physician, anesthesiologist, and an ENT surgeon would oversee the unit, and a thoracic surgeon should be available for consultation - Dr. Griffith Pearson joined us for this purpose in the early 1960s.

Intermittent positive pressure ventilation would be the preferred method of respiratory support.

The first location for the unit was an unused operating room suite. We reported the results of our first 100 consecutive admissions in 1960 in paper that described respiratory support in a patient care setting other than the operating room. At this early stage of the unit's development, the survival rate in this group of patients with serious respiratory difficulty was 75%, which was a much better result than before.

In the following years, respiratory care units emerged around the world. It quickly became obvious that this arrangement could benefit a wider range of patients than those with respiratory paralysis and drug overdose. In our first 100 cases, we cared for patients with varying degrees of lung disease, and the postoperative care of surgical patients soon followed.

"Although UCSF's ICUs at two of their hospitals had Anesthesia leadership, related research was not strong, and they needed to add that component. In January 1969, my family departed Toronto in a blizzard, bound for San Francisco."

The UCSF department was one of only three institutions in the US at that time to have been awarded an NIH Anesthesia Clinical Training grant, designed to produce academically trained anesthesiologists for which there was a perceived national need.

At UCSF, John Severinghaus had identified the respiratory control center in the medulla and designed the carbon dioxide electrode as well as complete blood gas analysis equipment. He was a distinguished professor in the Department of Anesthesia as well as on the faculty of the Cardiovascular Research Institute (CVRI). Ted Eger, another anesthesia professor was the originator of the MAC (minimal alveolar concentration) measurement and an active investigator in the uptake and distribution of anesthetic agents.

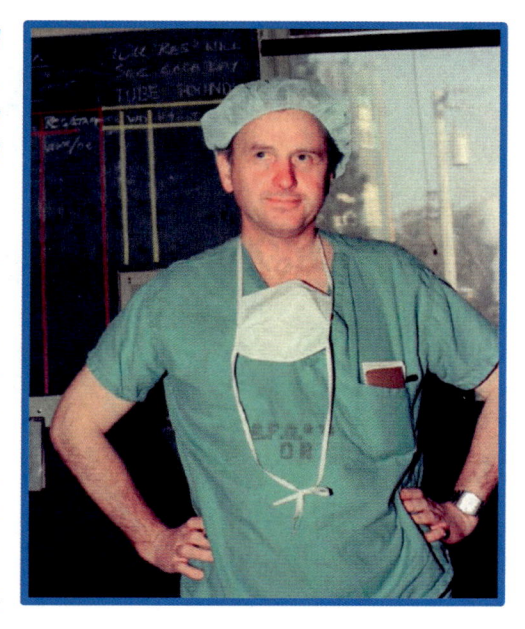

Severinghaus recommended Fairley to Julius Comroe, a pulmonary physiologist and Director of the UCSF-based CVRI. Fairley became one of the recipients of their NIH-funded Specialized Center of Research (SCOR) block grant. His portion of the grant involved the investigation as to whether mechanical ventilation for prolonged periods impaired subsequent lung function (it did not).

At UCSF while he applied for a California medical license, Fairley used his license reciprocity with Vermont to work as Chief of Service at the UCSF-affiliated San Francisco Veterans Administration Hospital (SF-VAH).

In subsequent years, Fairley became the UCSF Anesthesia Department's Vice-Chair for Clinical Affairs, particularly intensive care, and was also Chair of the Appointments and Promotions Committee advising the Chancellor of the four UCSF schools. During the Department Chair William "Bill" Hamilton's one year sabbatical at Oxford, Fairley served as the Acting Chair.

Phil Larson was the Department's Vice Chair at the time of Fairley's recruitment and was responsible for organizing medical student teaching during their anesthesia rotation at the Moffitt Hospital where he worked clinically as a cardiac anesthetist. When Larson moved to the San Francisco General Hospital (SFGH) as Chief of Service, Fairley (by now with a California license) moved to Moffitt Hospital and took Larson's cardiac anesthesia slot. Then, when Larson moved to Stanford in 1972, Fairley took over his position at SFGH, where he stayed until moving south to "the Farm" as Larson's successor as Stanford's Department of Anesthesia Chair in April 1985. He would once again be following in Larson's footsteps.

"On my arrival at Stanford, I was jokingly (?) asked by Phil Larson what job I would like next, because Phil could then apply for it."

During his final few years at UCSF, Fairley worked half-time as UCSF Associate Dean for SFGH, overseeing the contract with the City and County of San Francisco to provide medical care for the city's patients in return for the teaching and research possibilities. It was one of the leading county hospitals in the country.

Aided by Fellows who had just finished their residency in anesthesia, Fairley's most productive years were those at UCSF. He performed research on respiratory mechanics in acute pulmonary failure and his publications were numerous with over two thousand citations as of 2023. One paper, entitled '*The Optimum End-Expiratory Airway Pressure in Patients with Acute Pulmonary Failure*' was published in 1975 in the New England Journal of Medicine,[8] and has been cited hundreds of times. That article provided the foundation for protective lung ventilation strategies in ARDS. When the American Journal of Respiratory and Critical Care Medicine published a series entitled "*How it Really Happened*" it invited one leader best known from each key area of respiration research to describe how the work came about and the problems that had to be solved. The objective was to provide a source for new entrants to the field. Barrie Fairley was selected to represent Critical Care research and chose the New England Journal article as the basis for his contribution.[9] By the mid-1980s, Fairley had not applied to renew his last NIH grant since his focus was moving increasingly toward administration.

When Phil Larson's period as Chair at Stanford came to an end, there was a three-year interval before he was replaced. During that time John Bunker and Ellis Cohen served as Acting Chairs.

"A surgeon Bob Chase chaired the search committee to find a replacement for Dr. Larson. In the late 1970s, chairs for many West Coast anesthesia departments were being sought. There were at least five of us on the "short lists" for chairmanships. Larry Saidman (who later worked and retired from Stanford) went to UCSD, Ron Katz to USC, Tom Hornbein to the University of Washington, Ron Miller stayed at UCSF, and me. As I interviewed at each of these places, my focus was on the relationship between their Department of Anesthesia and the ICU. The answer at each place at that time was "none". Nor were they interested in there being one, particularly at the level in which I'd be interested. I remained as the only one of the short-listed group who was unappointed. Then the chair position opened at Stanford."

The final four candidates considered for the Stanford position were Michael Cousins, Ron Miller, David Longnecker, and Barrie Fairley. Ron Miller succeeded William Hamilton as Chair at UCSF, while Longnecker was considered still too junior to lead Stanford. Michael Cousins, the Chair of the Department of Anaesthesia and Intensive Care at Flinders Medical Centre, Adelaide, Australia, and an authority on pain management, was the search committee's first choice. Cousins had been an Acting Assistant Professor at Stanford from 1970-1974 and had collaborated on research studies with Richard Mazze at the PA-VAH.

"By coincidence, when Mike Cousins was appointed Chair at Flinders, he wanted to establish a presence in Critical Care. He negotiated a Co-Chair position with this in mind and offered it to me – but I declined."

Cousins initially accepted the Stanford job and was making plans to move, but then declined because his family did not want to leave Australia. Fairley was next candidate in line, and he was appointed Larson's successor.

"In accepting the offer of the Stanford Chair, one of the most attractive features was a very well-functioning clinical program in CCM led by Mike Rosenthal and three other anesthesiologists (Fred Mihm, Tom Feeley, and Rob Sladen). While not unique, this was a rarity. They did not need my input."

"One of the first events on joining the Stanford Department was a (postponed) party to celebrate 25 years since the move from San Francisco to Palo Alto in 1959."

Fairley discussed issues that concerned him with the recently appointed medical school Dean David Korn. Some were like those listed by Korn's predecessor, Dean Dominic Purpura, to Phil Larson when the latter stepped down. The major 'umbrella' item was non-university surgeons sharing the operating rooms at Stanford Hospital with faculty surgeons. Those non-faculty surgeons worked with the two or three independent private practice anesthesiology groups, who anesthetized many elective patients, but did not share the total around-the-clock coverage of all the out-of-hours surgical (and sub-specialty surgical) patients especially those with low-paying insurance or the indigent. The school's Department of Anesthesiology was therefore at a financial disadvantage. In addition, the overall control of the operating rooms was in the hands of the nursing staff. The goals of the medical school and its academic faculty were not a priority with the hospital administration.

"This was exactly the opposite of what I had experienced at UCSF, where there was one Department of Anesthesia that provided the anesthesia care for all surgeons' patients, whether university faculty or private practitioners. Thus, the total income from anesthesia services was available for all the university department's purposes. Very telling with respect to the Stanford hospital and medical school's priorities was the fact that the University's President chose to receive his medical care from the private side of the house."

Other issued included:
- Inequities in faculty salary distribution.
- Unclear ground rules as to faculty clinical time and the prerequisites for promotion.
- In interviews with various surgery leaders in the recruitment process, several had complained of the effects of faculty moonlighting on-call at night at private hospitals, in contravention of the Faculty Practice Program and university rules.

"This made out-of-hours procedures likely to run late more difficult to schedule, but of course moonlighting was an attempted solution on the part of members of the department to respond to their low salary scale."

- Although there were two self-supporting basic scientists in the Stanford Anesthesia Department (Jim Trudell, Joan Kendig), there were no physician anesthesiologists

at Stanford with a NIH research grant. The grant-supported physician research was largely being done at the PA-VAH and, other than the space allocated to the two basic scientists, there was minimal lab space in the department at Stanford.
- The salary levels compared unfavorably with those of the nearest competition – UCSF - and were perhaps a third or less of the estimated incomes of those in the private groups working in the same operating suites. There was a syphoning off of the reimbursements from a large proportion of the highest payers for anesthesia care at Stanford to the private groups.

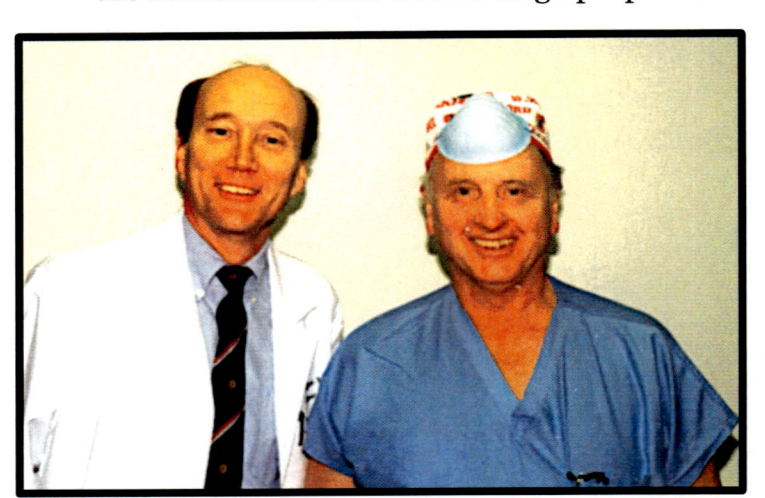

John Brock-Utne with Barrie Fairley

At an early Anesthesia faculty meeting after starting his appointment, Fairley laid out his plans for reimbursement, work hours, and promotion. Those rules would be applied evenly to all faculty. First, the expectation would be that there would be a full five-day work week. Any freeing of individuals from clinical duties would be to provide time for them to conduct their academic program as opposed to pursuing outside personal interests. Second, with the assumption that everyone was therefore fully engaged, salaries would be equal across the board for any given academic rank and years in a position. Promotions would depend on academic productivity and require, broadly speaking, national recognition for the associate level, and international recognition to become a full professor.

"Administratively, one of my first moves was to purchase the then relatively new IBM PCs to replace the staff's typewriters and the paper and pencil ledgers in the business office. This was also the period when the Internet and email were developing."

An early decision was to bring in an outside reviewer of the department's research program. One of the results was the appointment of Richard Mazze as Vice-Chair for Research.

A problem that Fairley experienced at UCSF was that of narcotic addiction among anesthesia residents. This also existed at Stanford and nationally. He developed a program to deal with this at the same time as being appointed Chair of the hospital's Physician Wellness Committee.

Major events in the following years included:
- The move to the new hospital addition (300 Pasteur Drive) with the transformation of the old office space in the Grant Building to laboratories.
- The planning of the layout of faculty and administrative offices plus a Department library and meeting space above the operating rooms in the new hospital addition.

- The move of Frank Sarnquist from the PA-VAH faculty to become the first Medical Director of the Stanford Hospital operating rooms. That position was eventually shared by a surgeon appointed from among the private groups.
- The change in the length of the American Board of Anesthesiology (ABA) residency requirement from two to three years, a very worthwhile decision given the increasing complexity and diversity of the anesthesiologist's repertoire.
- The introduction of the requirement that appointment to the Voluntary faculty would be limited to those with an ongoing anesthesia practice elsewhere.
- The first-time designation of Stanford as a Level 1 Regional Trauma Center.
- The opening of the Lucile Packard Children's Hospital. When the pediatric cardiac surgery group came from Children's Hospital in San Francisco, Stanford Hospital (not the medical school) subsidized their anesthesiologist's income, portending what would become necessary on a broader basis later.
- The start of a liver transplant program.
- The building of a new Stanford Pain Management Center clinic in the Boswell Building that housed other out-patient clinics, and expansion of the pain management program. Lorne Eltherington left for private practice. The pain faculty included Darrel Tanelian and Bill Forrest. Tanelian's research program was boosted by the addition of Bruce MacIver. Bill Brose returned after spending 1988/1989 at Flinders University working with Michael Cousins to join the pain group. The group was supplemented by the addition of a pediatrician anesthesiologist, Yen Chi Lin, who was a skilled acupuncturist.
- With the advent of the trauma center and an increase in obstetric deliveries, the start of in-house faculty calls at nights and on weekends, to be shared by faculty anesthesiologists from the PA-VAH as well as Stanford. Other than the Emergency Department we were the first department to have in-house faculty around the clock. There was salary allocated for this and, therefore, faculty could trade off their on-call time together with that reimbursement. Call obligations would cease for those at or beyond 65 years of age.

"A major but gradual trend that had started before my arrival was the delay of admission of patients requiring even major surgery until the morning of surgery, emphasizing the importance of specialized preoperative assessment prior to arrival. All Stanford patients were already being assessed by nurse practitioners a few days preoperatively in an area adjacent to the OR suite, but now faculty availability for consultation was scheduled. It was not until Don Stanski's time that one of the former residents, Stephen Fischer organized this country's first pre-anesthesia clinic."

During the years 1985-1992 there were many faculty achievements worthy of mention.

For example, David Gaba's development at the PA-VAH of medical simulation along the lines of flight simulators was special. His work has since been copied in multiple disciplines world-wide.

Mervyn Maze moved his research program from the PA-VAH to the UK when he was appointed Professor and Department Head at Westminster Medical School - Fairley's alma mater that became the Imperial College of Medicine London.

Among our postgraduate Fellows at the PA-VAH Steven Shafer was developing a career in pharmacokinetics and pharmacodynamics with his mentor Donald Stanski. Another Fellow, Ron Pearl (CCM) would subsequently become a highly successful Chair of the Department.

"After arriving, Ron Pearl was my very first new appointee to the faculty."

The daily clinical workload at Stanford was orchestrated by Jay Brodsky, who allocated faculty and residents to the various ORs and other locations requiring anesthesiology support. Among his key recruitments were John Brock-Utne from Durbin, South Africa, as a full Professor, resulting in a significant increase in clinical investigation in the Stanford ORs.

John Brock-Utne: I was recruited from South Africa. Barrie said he would support my moving costs. I presented him with the bill after arriving at Stanford. He looked at the bill and said, "I will pay half and then both you and I are going to be equally unhappy".

Richard Jaffe and Alex Macario, both of whom would go on to make significant contributions to the Department were recruited from our residency program, as were Emily Ratner, and Rona Giffard who would later become Vice-Chair of Research.

At the medical school level, Barrie Fairley initiated a monthly dinner meeting that was attended by all department Chairs (but not the Dean) to discuss shared administrative problems. He was Chair of the medical school's Faculty Practice Committee and collections were a major concern among every department leader.

Despite the Dean's encouragement to stay, Fairley's decision not to apply to renew his appointment as chair in 1992 related in large part to the adverse trend of the department's finances. The increasing patient load around the clock, with many of those patients having poor or no insurance coverage, compared unfavorably with the private anesthesia groups' patients. This was exacerbated by the limited financial support for the department by the hospital for care of the low-paying patients. Dean Korn brought in an outside committee to analyze the issue but, while agreeing that there were problems, they were unable to make actionable recommendations. The introduction of a new tax by the Dean on the practice income of those departments without out-patient clinics had added to the problem. This was primarily to bolster the financial health of departments with outpatient clinics, a poorly reimbursed activity. However, it had a devastating effect on the Department of Anesthesia's finances and, paradoxically, anesthesiologists would now be boosting surgeons' incomes.

At the Dean's request, Fairley stayed on the faculty for two more years after stepping down to help with the transition of the new Chair Don Stanski. Frank Sarnquist was the acting chair during that interval. Then, in accordance with his long-term plan, Fairley retired from anesthesia "square wave" (flat out to zero) and went on to other pursuits. Starting in 1992 with three months at Spanish-language immersion schools in Costa Rica and Mexico while on sabbatical leave; he subsequently attended a total of nine schools in seven countries. He returned to school at San Jose State University, where he acquired BA and MA degrees in Spanish and Latin American History. His bilingual master's thesis was on the "anesthetics" used by the Incas 400 years before anesthesia was officially discovered. A summary of the findings was published in the Spanish society's journal.[10]

In 1986 an anonymous donor established the annual 'H. Barrie Fairley Excellence in Teaching Award' for the Stanford anesthesiologist deemed by our residents to be the best teacher on the faculty. In recognition of his many contributions, Fairley also received a Lifetime Achievement Award from the American Society of Critical Medicine in 2001. UCSF sponsors an annual 'H. Barrie Fairley Seminar in Intensive Respiratory Care'.

As a gesture of gratitude for the springboard they provided for his career, Fairley also made a generous contribution to the University of Toronto to endow the 'H. Barrie Fairley Professorship in Critical Care'. In 2020 Robert Fowler, the inaugural H. Barrie Fairley Professor at the university and Chair of the Canadian Critical Care Trials Group, proposed that a portion of the endowment investment be used to support the university's junior critical care faculty. The 'H. Barrie Fairley's Scholar Competition' was created. Funds are provided for a specific program of research for as many as three assistant professors during the first year of their appointment. Barrie Fairley's legacy of excellence in research continues in Toronto.

In 2015, following his wife's death the previous year, Barrie Fairley moved to retirement facility - Vi at La Jolla Village in the San Diego area where his daughter and grandchildren live.

"In my remaining years I shall always be grateful for the opportunity to work at one of the country's foremost universities (Stanford), and for the associations I made along the way."

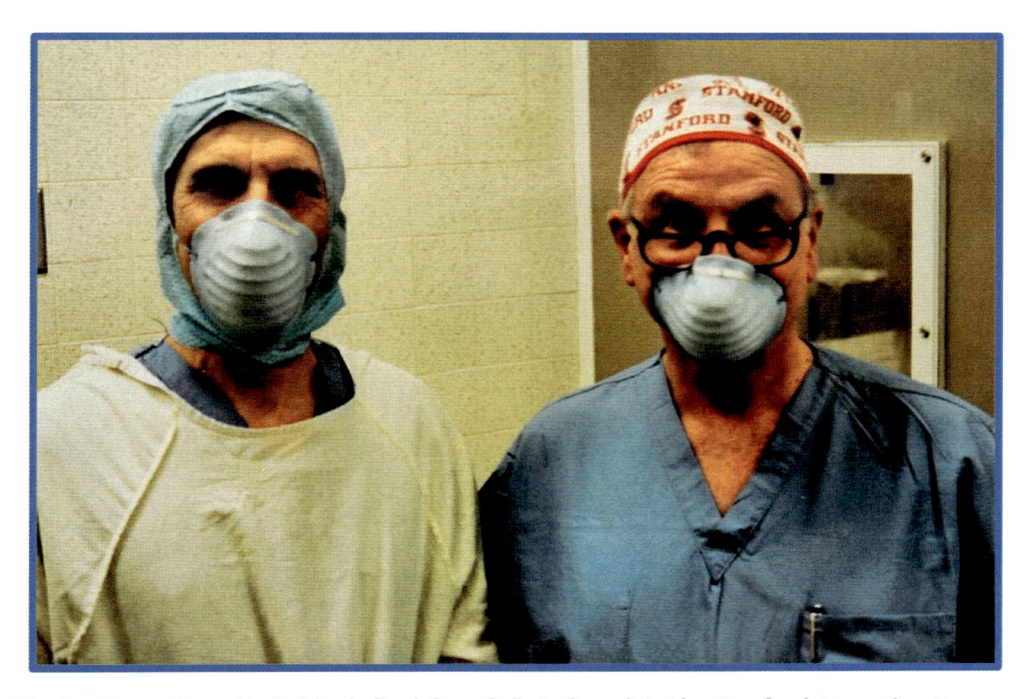

With Stanley Samuels on Dr. Fairley's final day of clinical work in the Stanford Operating Rooms

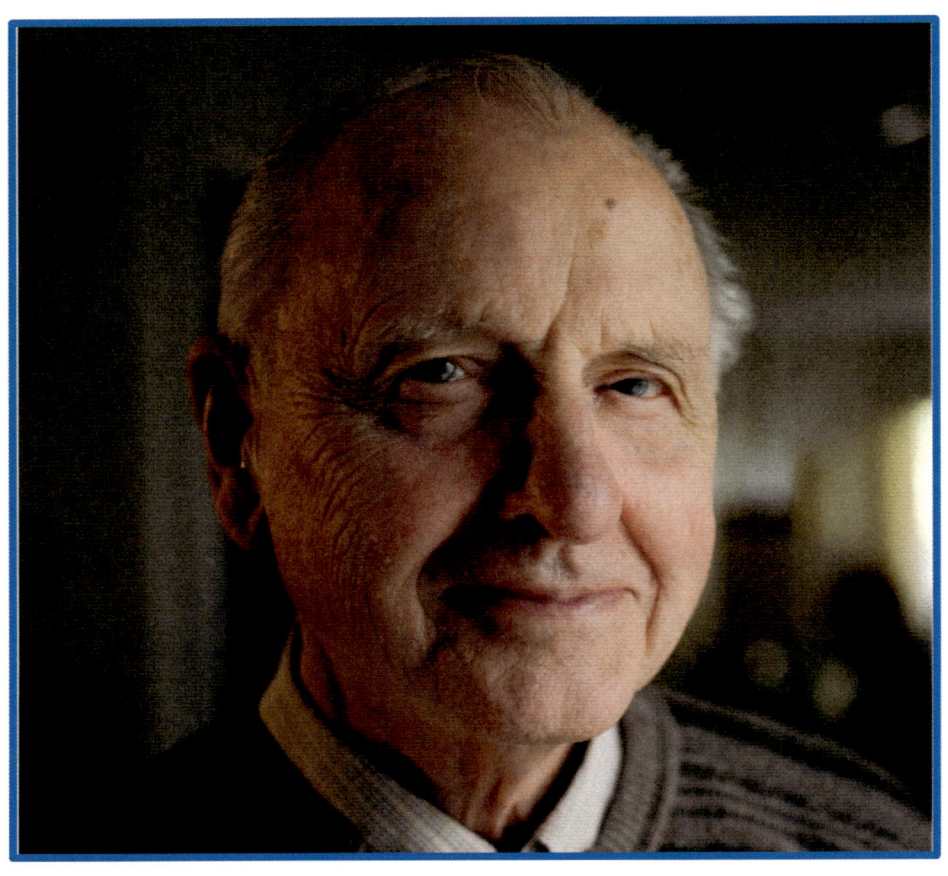

2010

REFERENCES

1. Fairley HB, Waddell WG, Bigelow WG. Hypothermia for cardiovascular surgery: acidosis in the rewarming period. Br J Anaesth (1957) 29:310-318.
2. Waddell WG, Fairley HB, Bigelow WG. Improved management of clinical hypothermia based upon related biochemical studies. Ann Surg (1957) 146:542-559.
3. Barber HO, Chambers RA, Fairley HB, Woolf CR. A respiratory unit: the Toronto General Hospital unit for the treatment of severe respiratory insufficiency. Can Med Assoc J (1959) 81:97-101.
4. Fairley HB, Chambers RA. The management of the patient with respiratory insufficiency. Can Anaesth Soc J (1960) 7:447-490.
5. Fairley HB, Britt BA. The adequacy of the air-mix control of ventilators operated from an oxygen source. Can Med Assoc J (1964) 90:1394-1396.
6. Lamont A, Fairley HB. A pressure-sensitive ventilator alarm. Anesthesiology (1965) 26:359-361.
7. Fairley HB, Wigle ED. Hospital facilities for the management of acute cardiorespiratory failure. Can Med Assoc J (1964) 90:376-377.
8. Suter PM, Fairley HB, Isenberg MD. The optimum end-expiratory airway pressure in patients with acute pulmonary failure. NEJM (1975) 292:284-289.
9. Fairley HB. Ventilating the acutely injured lung. Am J Resp Crit Care Med (2001) 163:1049-1050.
10. Fairley HB. La "anestesia" en el imperio incaico. Rev Esp Anestesiol Reanim (2007) 54:556-562.

Former residents contributing to this book were asked about memories of their residency at Stanford. Many fondly recalled working with Dr. Fairley.

- **Joe Andressen**: *My first day in the OR was with Dr. Fairley! As the new incoming Department Chair, he came on the scene with much fanfare; with a broad smile and distinctive white OR shoes he skillfully guided me through my first anesthetic. Several weeks later I took care of a young man with renal failure. Immediately after induction, the patient's EKG went from sinus rhythm to asystole. A Code Blue was called, and CPR began immediately. I stood above and aside the patient and administered chest compressions as the room filled with a dozen staff. Dr. Fairley entered the room and looking over the situation called out with a half-hearted smile, "Dr. Andresen, does this happen often when you administer anesthesia?" Fortunately, our efforts paid off and the resuscitation was successful, and the patient went home several days later.*
- **John Cooper**: *H.B. Fairley – What a guy! Barrie showed me how to comport calmly, like a gentleman, but remain rock hard, steadfast, and principled under pressures from surgeons bent on their particular care plans, needs and timelines.*
- **Linda Mignano**: *I was on my own one day in the Stanford OR taking care of a young man who had extreme needle phobia. It took me a while to cajole him into letting me place a local anesthetic for an IV using the absolute tiniest gauge needle and all the tricks in the book to place it painlessly. He admitted it didn't hurt, but he still was on the verge of panic over a small cannula. Right then, Dr. Barrie Fairley walked into the room. I don't know where I got the idea, but I introduced Dr. Fairley to the patient, as the Chief of the Department of Anesthesia, who had come just for him, to place his IV, and as the top anesthesiologist, he was the best at placing IV's of anyone in the whole Stanford University Hospital. I also told him that Dr. Fairley would get it in the first try! Of course, he told me I shouldn't ever say that to the patient, but I would have none of that. Instead, I handed him the cannula, told him to challenge himself, and took the IV tubing and sedation in hand while I distracted the patient. He had it in no time, but the look on his face was unforgettable: he looked like a little league baseball player who just surprised himself by hitting his first home run.*
- **David Fitzgerald**: *I ended up in physician leadership after Stanford. At one point nearly 500 anesthesiologists and eighty facilities were under my direction. Barrie Fairley, for me, was an ideal leader. He was honest, transparent, and always accountable for his decisions, and his mistakes. Very different style to subsequent leaders. Often, I would ask myself what Barrie would do in this situation with my leadership challenges.*
- **Emily Ratner**: *Barrie Fairley – "Always have a plan B."*
- **Richard Snyder**: *When I started residency at Stanford, the Department Chief was H. Barrie Fairley, an experienced clinician leader. I remember him as having the look, accent, and mannerisms of Anthony Hopkins. I may have his words not exact, but my memory is of all the new residents were in the auditorium and Dr. Fairley told us, "I'm sure you're all familiar with the Kafka short story, 'the Cockroach'." In terms of the hierarchy, you are now all cockroaches. Furthermore, punctuality is expected. If you are late or don't show up, I will only accept a note from your coroner." I realize that these days these words might not be acceptable, but at the time, they were oddly comforting as we all knew that we were in a place that prioritized excellence and integrity. I remember Dr. Fairley as a fair, compassionate, and funny clinician leader.*

- <u>Michael Mellethin</u>: *I never knew the Chief of Anesthesia at UCLA, but Dr. Barrie Fairley made it a point to be my attending my very first day at Stanford. I'll never forget his interest and kindness.*
- <u>Bill Longton</u>: *Barrie Fairley "a good surgeon deserves a good anesthesiologist ... a bad surgeon needs one".*
- <u>Martha Cox Ho</u>: *My first year in anesthesia was also Dr. Barrie Fairley's last before retiring. I remember lengthy discussions with him about anesthesia principles and history, of course, but also was so impressed at how he methodically set himself up for success in retirement by carefully cultivating interests outside of medicine. Lessons in anesthesia, lessons in life.*
- <u>Beemeth Robles</u>: *Great memories from Stanford. So many opportunities and blessed to have had my experiences. My "fondest" memory was when during my second year, I decided to bring music to the OR. On this particular day, I was working with my Chairman, Barrie Fairley ... A great mentor... staring at my sound system while looking over his glasses at me he said, "great music, great sound. Music is a distraction." That was the last time I took music to the OR and I have never missed it.*
- <u>Adam Rubinstein</u>: *H. Barrie Fairley's distillation of anesthesia – "you're doing fine as long as the blood is going round and round and the lungs are going up and down" – truer words have never been spoken.*
- <u>Russell Allan</u>: *I remember Dr. Fairley saving an airway with a retrograde wire but not before popping his knuckles, pulling up his scrub pants, and turning his OR cap sideways!*
- <u>Jeff Clayton</u>: *"Never push potent poisons into passive paralyzed patients" and "Just do the right thing" —— Dr. H.B. Fairley*
- <u>Rick Mantin</u>: *I was in the Operating Room one day with H. Barrie Fairley as my attending, and he challenged me intellectually if we really needed to keep anesthetized patients paralyzed and mechanically ventilated. I vividly remember him lamenting that modern (1992) anesthesia was turning into "Pumping Potent Poisons into Paralyzed Patients." To this day, I often choose to let some of my anesthetized patients remain unparalyzed and breathing spontaneously when appropriate, even under GETA and especially towards the end of a case.*
- <u>Kayvan Ariani</u>: *I remember Dr. Fairly quizzing me during cases on a variety of topics. He once asked me what the units were of something rather obscure. I told him multiple times that I didn't know, but he pressed on. So, I took the bait and blurted out an answer to his question. I immediately regretted my decision as he guffawed in disapproving astonishment at my wrong answer. The following week, however, we had another case together and he began showing me respiratory flow/volume curves, drawing them out for me. The night before the case I happened to have been reading the chapter in Nunn's Applied Respiratory Physiology on this topic. I noticed the flow/volume curve he had drawn was slightly wrong ... and I corrected him on this. He looked at me in glowing, approving astonishment that I had known this detail. Even though I told him that I had just read about this the night before, he was so thrilled that I knew this that he was still bringing it up an hour later in the case, shaking his head in amazement. I must admit that the redemption felt good!"*

- <u>John Loftus</u>: *A quick anecdote involves Dr. Barrie Fairley, who was Chair of the Department of Anesthesiology during my time at Stanford. I was working furiously on a submission to the IRB for the first clinical study Dr. Cohen and I put together, and we were coming up to the deadline. I ran down to the OR as to obtain Dr. Fairley's signature as he was putting on his shoe covers to begin his on-call coverage that evening. He calmly, and respectfully stated that he never took care of administrative work when he was taking care of patients. I was certain the submission would be late, and our research delayed three months. Dr. Fairley signed the IRB proposal the next morning after a long, agonizing night for me. And he made a quick call and it was accepted for consideration in that IRB cycle. Later in my career, I was appointed as Physician-in-Chief at the Kaiser Permanente Oakland Medical Center with 1200 physicians and 4000 support staff under my responsibility. My first morning in the OR setting up for a CABG on a patient with an EF of 17%, one of the chiefs of a surgical department came in to my OR and started discussing some of her departmental needs. Dr. Fairley's wisdom immediately came to mind, and I asked her to talk to me that evening after my clinical work. Thank you Dr. Fairly.*

CHAPTER 4
1985

The year 1985 began with creation of the Internet's Domain Name System. On March 15th, **symbolics.com** was registered as the first Internet domain name. Michael Jordan was named NBA Rookie of the Year and the film *Back to the Future* was released. The Super Mario Bros game was introduced for the Nintendo gaming system and Microsoft Windows 1.0 was also released. Both enjoyed immediate success. Less successful was Coca-Cola changing its formula and releasing 'New Coke'. The response was overwhelmingly negative, and original Coca-Cola returned to the market in less than three months.

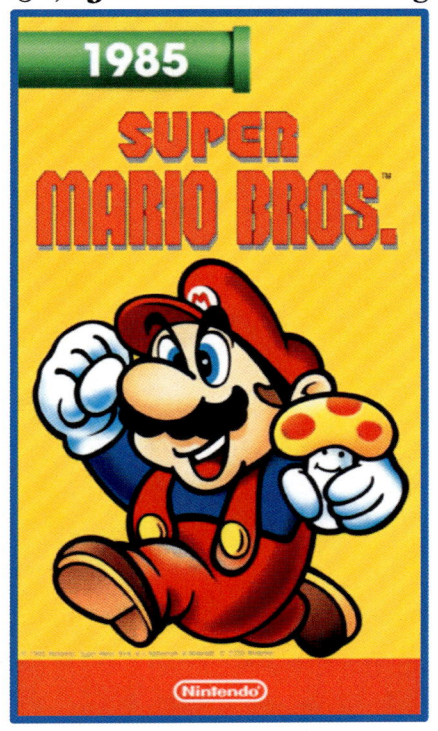

The first *Rock In Rio* (Brazil) concert was held drawing an audience of 1.5 million fans. Forty artists gathered to record '*We Are The World*' for African famine relief. The *Live Aid* concert for famine relief was also held simultaneously in London and Philadelphia and was broadcast worldwide. In Embu das Artes, Brazil, forty years after the end of WW2, American, Brazilian, and West German forensic pathologists exhumed the remains of Josef Mengele, the physician notorious for Nazi human experimentation on inmates of Auschwitz concentration. The mystery of his whereabouts was finally solved! The wreck of the Titanic was also located in 1985.

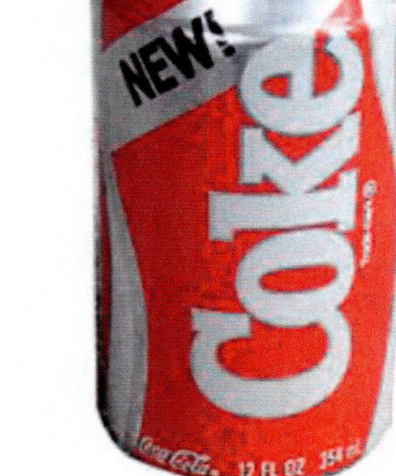

The International Physicians For the Prevention of Nuclear War (IPPNW) organization won the Nobel Peace Prize for, what else but the '*prevention of nuclear war*'. In Louisville, Kentucky, William Schroeder became the first artificial heart patient to physically leave a hospital after he spent a total of 15 minutes outside before returning to his ward. In 1985 the *Anesthesia Patient Safety Foundation* (APSF) was founded by the ASA.

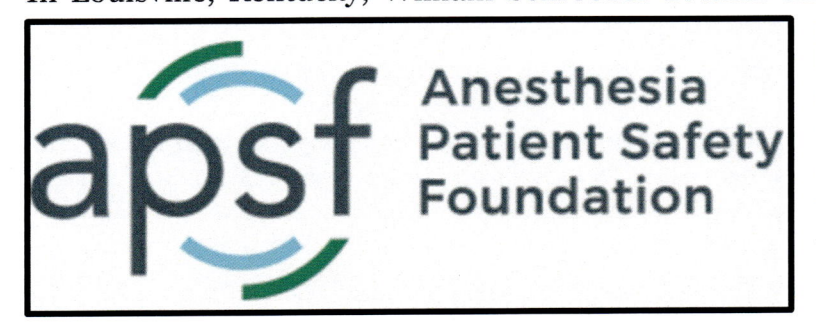

Leslie Comer Andes attended Ohio State University (OSU) as an undergraduate (Bsc Agr, 1976) and then OSU College of Medicine (MD, 1983). She interned at Riverside Medical Center, OH (1984), did her residency in Anesthesiology (1985-1987) at Stanford, followed by a Fellowship (Neuroanesthesia) at UCSF (1987-1988). She worked as a free-lance anesthesiologist in the SF Bay Area for several years (1987-1994), then at Marin General Hospital doing mostly OB Anesthesia (1994-2001). She took a couple of years off to travel (2001-2004) then returned to Stanford for another Fellowship (OB Anesthesia) (2004-2005). In 2005 she took a job in Phoenix with Aubrey Mazze's Valley Anesthesiology Consultants.

"Many thanks to Sheila Cohen and Ed Riley for taking me as an OB Anesthesia Fellow. In 2005 I took a job in Phoenix with Valley Anesthesiology Consultants. Thanks Aubrey Maze and Dean Smith, with assist from Jay Brodsky! I ended up working primarily at Barrow Neurological Institute doing mostly intracranial cases (aneurysms and AVM's). Very lucky to work with the excellent surgeons and anesthesia colleagues at BNI. While there I wrote two of the neurosurgical chapters in Larry Chu and Andrea Fuller's 'Manual of Clinical Anesthesiology, 1st edition'. I am quite sure Andi and Larry were tearing their hair out over how late I was getting them done! Working at BNI was often a 12–14-hour day, with little energy left for projects like this."

Along with former Stanford anesthesia resident Charles Tadlock, Dr. Andes co-edited a "question and answer" book on physiology. She was appointed to the CSA's Impaired Physicians Committee by Dr. Tom Feeley, who was CSA President that year. She was one of the original authors along with Jerry Matsumura of the CSA's *'Curriculum on Impaired Physicians'*, which became the basis for the ASA's work on Impaired Physicians/Physician Health and Well-Being.

"My interest in this developed after several residents and attendings that I knew at both Stanford and UCSF had drug issues, a couple of which led to fatal or near-fatal overdoses. Education on this within our specialty seemed long overdue."

Interesting Anecdotes/Memories of Time at Stanford:

- *Ron Pearl was the Chief Resident when I was a second year. I had my only high spinal while working together at the VAH one day during my third month of residency! He showed me how to put an IV in the EJ. A learning opportunity all around.*
- *Jay Brodsky was my advisor during residency. I remember him being very supportive, and dressing down one of the ER docs when I got called to a trauma alert one time and the ER doc was unhappy about something.*
- *Phil Larson told me that I didn't ask enough questions, and I have tried to take that to heart ever since.*
- *Overall, I can't imagine a better place to have trained, and it definitely prepared me for the work I've done over the last >30 years. I spent 9 months out of the 2 year residency at SVCMC ("Valley"), and very much enjoyed working there as most of the attendings were somewhat more hands off, and the cases were typical county problems that I liked dealing with (trauma, etc). My time at Stanford Hospital was also inspiring and I am still in awe of the knowledge base of the attendings.*

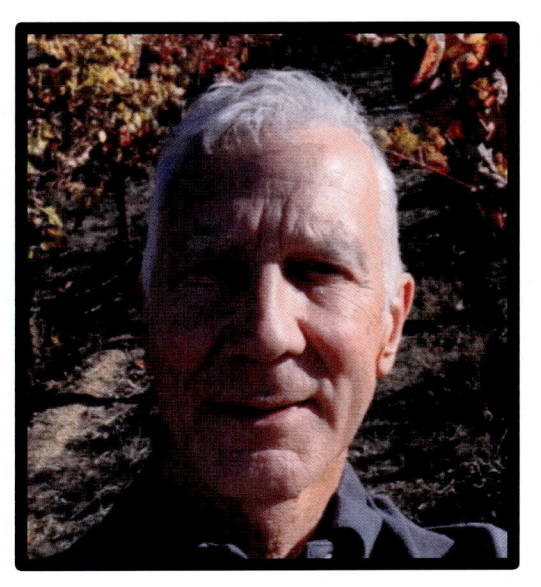

Joseph Stanley Andresen was born at Mills Memorial Hospital in San Mateo. He was an undergraduate at Berkeley (AB, Genetics, 1978). He received his MD from UCSF (1982). He interned and completed a residency (Internal Medicine) at UCD (1982-1985) and a residency (Anesthesiology) at Stanford (1985-1987). From 1987 through 1989 he did freelance work at Marin General Hospital, John Muir Hospital in Walnut Creek, St. Mary's Hospital, South San Francisco, and Providence Hospital, Oakland. He worked at El Camino Hospital in Mt. View, CA (1989-2004) and then Washington Hospital, Fremont, CA (2004-2017) following the infamous exchange of anesthesiologists at both hospitals. (see below)

California Healthline Daily Edition

Summaries of health policy coverage from major news organizations

WEDNESDAY, NOV 24 2004

Hospital Replaces Anesthesiology Group After Health Insurance Contract Dispute

El Camino Hospital in Mountain View on Monday replaced Northern California Anesthesia Associates, a 19-member physician group, with a new group of anesthesiologists because of a disagreement with NCAA over health insurance contracts. El Camino officials say NCAA physicians initiated the disagreement by saying they would refuse to provide anesthesia for elective surgeries. However, the physician group says hospital officials tried to require it to sign the same health insurance contracts as the hospital. NCAA says the contracts' reimbursement rates do not cover the cost of care. As a result, the physician group has set its own rates and billed patients for the amount not covered by their health insurance. Hospital spokesperson Judy Twitchell said that El Camino has received "numerous complaints" from patients regarding the doctors' billing practices. The anesthesiologists say they have received only one patient complaint. El Camino officials gave the doctors until Friday to provide services at the contract rates, but they refused to do so, according to the Mercury News. NCAA doctors said they would perform only emergency anesthesiology after Friday's deadline.

    NCAA spokesperson Noah Griffin said the doctors expected to work alongside a new group of anesthesiologists while negotiations continued, adding that the physician group had not anticipated being escorted from the hospital by security and local police officers. Dr. Paul Goehner, an NCAA anesthesiologist, said the doctors feel that El Camino CEO Lee Domanico acted inappropriately when he asked to see the anesthesiologists' billing records and tried to become involved in-patient care issues and the doctors' financial performance. El Camino board member Wes Alles said the hospital wanted a greater role in how the doctors bill patients and generally operate, according to the Mercury News. Twitchell said, "It's about business principles and how we want to operate the hospital." She added that the hospital believed NCAA physicians' rates were higher than rates of other anesthesiology groups in the area.

Eight anesthesiologists from Washington Hospital Healthcare System in Fremont on Monday replaced NCAA physicians, after the Washington Hospital physicians "abruptly left" their previous positions, the Mercury News reports Nancy Farber, CEO of Washington Healthcare, said, "We were very disappointed with Fremont Anesthesia Consultants for moving forward in this manner, abandoning without notice those patients who were scheduled for surgery and in need of their services. "Some El Camino surgeons postponed or moved operations to other facilities so they would not have to work with a group of anesthesiologists that was unfamiliar with their casework. However, El Camino officials said 13 of the 17 procedures scheduled for Monday were performed as planned.

Andresen was the editor of the Santa Clara and Monterey County Medical Society Bulletin (2006-2016), and medical editor of SCOPE at El Camino Hospital (1996-2004). He has worked for the Accreditation Association for Ambulatory Health Care (AAAHC) as a surveyor (2005-Present). Starting in 2017 he has been with PAMF serving as Medical Director of their San Carlos Surgery Center (2017-Present).

"Retirement: No immediate plans. I have the good fortune of a loving family with our daughter and son both living in the Bay Area. Current position offers a work/life balance that took me three decades to find. Working with a diverse and collaborative group of colleagues is truly a gift."

"As a contrast to time in the OR, I cherish the outdoors whether sailing competitively in the UK and Europe or learning to start a vineyard on rural land in the Russian River Valley."

As for memories and anecdotes ... All of those listed below were either mentors or influenced my development as a young physician and budding anesthesiologist in a profound way. A few memorable moments and memories:

- *Stanley Samuels: Stanley Samuels was truly our North Star in the neuro room. His gentle encouragement and distinctive accent are something I remember to this day.*
- *Ron Pearl: The King of pulmonary hypertension research and always available for new and old residents alike. Dr. Pearl's long tenure as Department Chief spoke to not only his research accomplishments but ability to balance the many challenges of running a clinical and teaching program. My favorite memory of Ron was during the San Diego ASA convention where we had access to San Diego Padres baseball stadium. I took a photo of Ron in the dugout holding the phone as he was about to send in the relief pitcher! During the COVID pandemic, we corresponded frequently as he shared Stanford Hospitals experience and how we could best keep our staff and patients safe in those first months and year.*

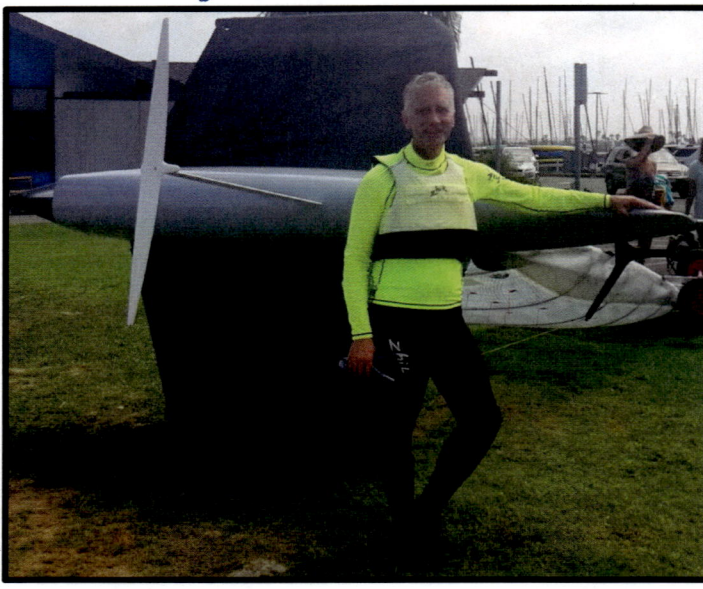

"The challenge to rise above the water on this foiling Moth sailboat!"

- *Sheila Cohen: The true "Godmother" of OB anesthesia during my time at Stanford. Learning not to panic when hearing "stat C-section" and receiving the gratitude of a labor patient from an epidural well done were pearls she shared. And when Maria, my wife was induced for the birth of our daughter, Dr. Cohen made a timely appearance facilitating a joyous labor experience for which we are eternally grateful.*
- *Jay Brodsky: It was my privilege to present a chest case at Stanford Anesthesia Grand Rounds where Jay was the Attending physician - an innovative combination of regional and general anesthesia to improve patient outcomes and post-op comfort!*
- *Kevin Fish, Jeff Bader, Dick Mazze, Mervin Maze, Ed Yhap and Frank Sarnquist: The true gentleman of Palo Alto VA anesthesia services. Each with their own perspectives who willing shared their knowledge and guidance through my training time.*
- *Dave Gaba: The father of simulator training which now is the gold standard for training medical students and residents in the OR, ER, clinics. I never suspected that I would become a star videoed in that early OR simulator when multiple unexpected mishaps caused me to spring into action. Dr. Gaba used this example in his lectures to demonstrate the importance and value in simulator training to improve patient safety and physician performance. I'm still waiting for my royalties from my cameo appearance!*
- *There are many others (Janet Wyner, Rob Sladen, Carter Cherry ...) that come to mind as I reflect on my time as an anesthesia resident at Stanford. All of these individuals and experiences shaped me to become the competent and confident new graduate first entering practice in 1988 and the physician I have matured and become over the past three decades through today.*

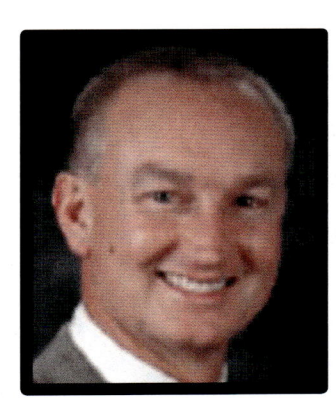

Edward Robert Baer graduated from UCSD (MD, 1979). He attended Stanford for medical school (MD, 1983), interned (Internal Medicine) at Stanford (1983-1984) and then completed his Anesthesiology residency (1985-1987). Following residency, he was a Fellow (CCM) at Stanford (1987-1988). He has worked in the AAMG in Palo Alto for his entire career.

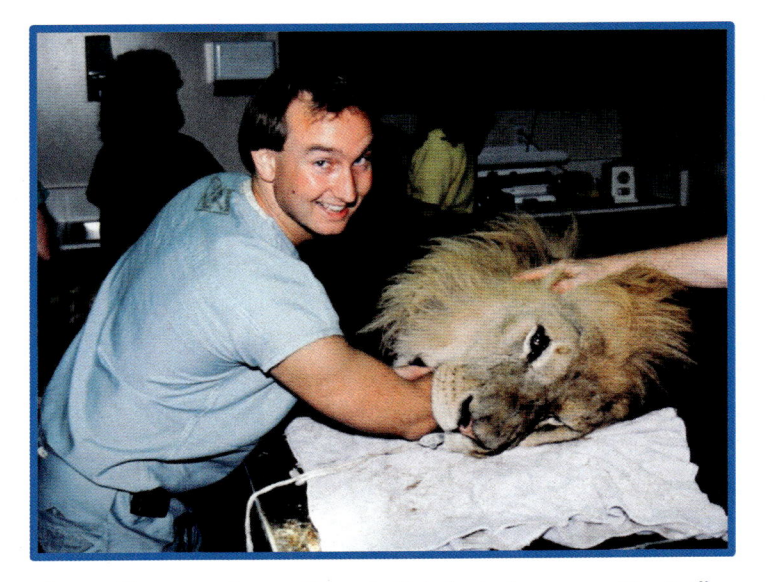

"Dr. Mihm taught me how to intubate larger patients."

William George Brose was born in Oakland. He was an undergraduate at Stanford (BS, Chemistry, 1980) and then attended the University of Kansas Medical School (MD, 1984). He interned (Internal Medicine) at SCVMC (1985) and completed his residency in Anesthesiology (1985-1987). He was Chief Resident his final year. He did a Fellowship (Obstetrical Anesthesia) (1988). He was appointed a Physician Specialist (1988) and then Assistant Professor (Anesthesiology) in 1988.

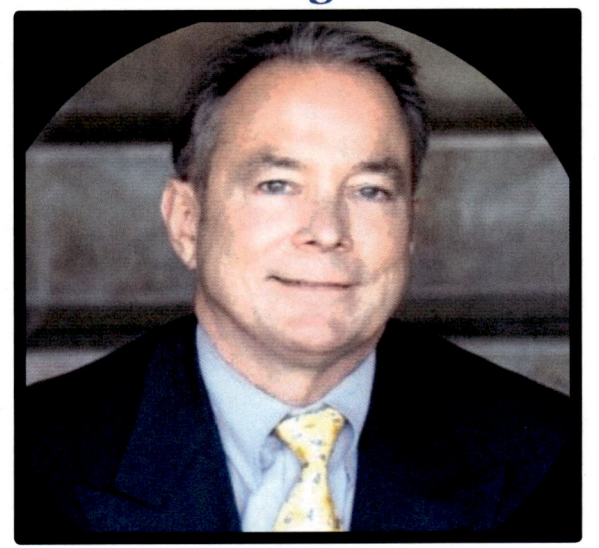

The following year he did a second Fellowship (Pain Medicine) at Flinders Medical Centre, Adelaide, Australia (1989). He trained with Michael Cousins as a Clinical Research Fellow. He returned to Stanford (1989) where he was appointed Medical Director of Pain Management Services (1989-1997). He was promoted to Associate Professor before taking a leave in 1997.

Bill was the Chairman and CEO of HELP Pain Medicine Network (1997-2018). They created and operationalized clinical content, policy, procedure, and process for Interdisciplinary Pain Rehabilitation for the first and largest Pain Medical Network in California, before closing in 2018. He is the owner of William G Brose, MD Inc, Danville (2015-Present), a medico-legal firm consulting for physician defense in Medical Board of California wrongful prescribing matters. He was also CMO of Opioid Management Strategies and Solutions (OPOS) Inc., San Mateo, CA (2018-2021).

Bill Brose is board certified by the ABA in Anesthesiology and Pain Medicine. He is currently a Clinical Professor of Anesthesia, Perioperative and Pain Medicine, Stanford University (2021-Present).

"I'm the happy father of 6 kids and 6 grandkids, still alpine skiing and loving my wife/life."

Interesting Anecdotes/Memories of Time at Stanford: "Starting the Modern Stanford Pain Medicine program with focus on interdisciplinary service delivery with creation of outpatient clinic, inpatient acute and chronic services, Inpatient Interdisciplinary Pain Program and subsequent research program focused on pharmacokinetic and pharmacodynamic modelling of opioids for use in clinical pain treatment. I was followed by Dr. Ray Gaeta who led the program for a subsequent decade until the position was assumed by current Director Sean Mackey who has grown the research program to #1 in the country in terms of funding and clinical programs, to have offerings at all of the current Stanford satellite locations. It was the real Wild West with the time from innovation to treatment measured in seconds to minutes including expansion of epidural and intraspinal medication trials, IV lidocaine infusions, PCA and increasing interventional treatments to compliment the foundations of interdisciplinary care. We take all of these for granted today at Stanford, but 35 years ago none of this existed and it was through the hard work and innovation of a few that these unique and differentiating services were created."

John Robert Cooper

John Robert Cooper was born in Burbank, CA. He was an undergraduate at Stanford (AB, 1978) and then attended UCSD (MD, 1983). He interned (Primary Care/Internal Medicine) at UCSF (1983-1984). He then completed his Anesthesiology training at Stanford (1985-1987). He was the Chief Resident his final year. He was on the Stanford voluntary Clinical Faculty (1987-2004) and served on the Department's Anesthesia Care Review Committee (1988-1996).

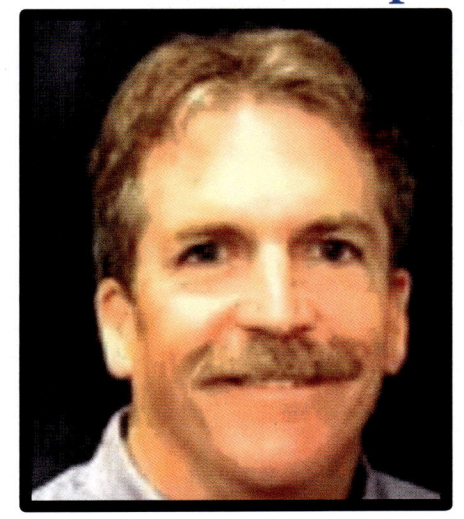

John Cooper worked as a staff anesthesiologist at PAMF his entire clinical career (1987-2022), and was Chair of their Department of Anesthesiology (1992-1998). John was also Medical Director at PAMF's SurgeCenter of Palo Alto (2000-2012). He currently is Medical Director of PAMF's Outcomes Information and Co-director of Quality, Surgical Services (PAMF) (2012-Present).

The PAMF Outcomes Information Program is a scalable and automated program designed to report on longitudinal safety and efficacy outcomes following office visits and hospitalizations (all cause) and discrete medical interventions such as surgery. PAMF Surgical Services is engaged in transparency and public reporting of quality and safety outcomes to promote improvement and patient satisfaction. It makes those outcomes readily available to providers and patients and other end-user stakeholders. The goal is to learn to understand and leverage PAMF's own big data for the benefit of patients, providers, and other stakeholders.

"My retirement plans … when they throw me out or I can no longer identify my car keys as being such."

John Cooper was a diving physician and Medical Consultant to the Monterey Bay Aquarium (1985-2005). He is a life-time swimming enthusiast and continues to swim 3-4 times per week.

"There have been many outside interests over the years. Recently I have become very interested in the neuroscience of consciousness and human cognition and have helped edit and bring to print a book written by a former Stanford Biology Professor and mentor, Chuck Baxter, titled "Natural History of Cognition – Mind over Matter". This has dovetailed very nicely with a current interest in neural networks, deep learning and artificial intelligence especially as applied to understanding human cognition as well as aiding in my efforts at PAMF to gather data and report on the effectiveness and safety we render to our surgical and non-surgical patients."

"When not noodling around in the literature of consciousness or pursuing the data that matter to PAMF's patients and providers I enjoy hanging with my wife, family, and friends, "head-first" surfing (aka boogie boarding), hiking, biking, reading, and running wild with a small pack of grandchildren."

I am grateful to many of the faculty, including but not limited to those mentioned below. I've tried to encapsulate the unique core of what I learned from each and what I often think about when I recall those days and the wonderful contributions to my education as a clinician and a professional:

- *Frank Sarnquist: I had the luxury of spending my entire first two weeks of residency working 1:1 with Frank at PA-VAH. I believe I fully imprinted on him then and I guess you could say I was one of his lucky ducklings. I know I feel that way as I picked up so many, many good habits and approaches from him.*
- *Jay Brodsky: I learned so many things from this fellow, but I think especially of the critical thinking that Jay, almost joyously, would apply to my proposed care plans as he pointed out the glaring holes lying therein. This little voice over my shoulder has stayed with me through the years and during many of the tougher clinical situations I have been challenged with.*
- *Stanley Samuels: I am grateful to Stanley for showing me that the practice of anesthesia could (and SHOULD) not only be competent but FUN. Thank you, Stan!*
- *Al Hackel: Al interviewed me as a residency applicant. Luckily his paperwork was lost in the process, and I snuck in. Thanks, Al, for terrible paperwork. I'll always remember that late night he taught me the use of the whiskey nipple on a take-back, full stomach neonate who had recently undergone a lower back, large nevus excision and was now in our care for exploration of an expanding hematoma. (And I always thought that small bottle of whiskey on the pediatric cart was for the Attendings!!!)*
- *C. Philip Larson: From Phil I think I learned a wonderful way of critical thinking that included his generous help preparing me for oral boards as well as a really great way to approach the wave of medical and scientific literature we confront daily. The latter has benefited me my entire career and is something I've sought to share with colleagues and students when opportunity arises.*
- *Norman Shumway: He was not Anesthesia faculty but wow, along with a few other Stanford surgeons, taught me a lot. For instance, how to actually look at a patient at the bedside and not the numbers scrolling across a screen and, of course, "all bleeding stops!".*
- *Then there was the gaggle of residents which Stanford trained and educated who then joined me in practice and with whom I've become friends and from whom I learned an enormous amount about life, politics, and clinical practice. I am grateful to have been surrounded by so many smart people throughout my career, especially - Steve Merlone, Tom Gaston, John Urbanowicz, Janet Wyner, Dick Hunter, Scott Rudy, Anne Evans, Patricia Curtis, Chris Cartwright, and Paul Eckinger.*

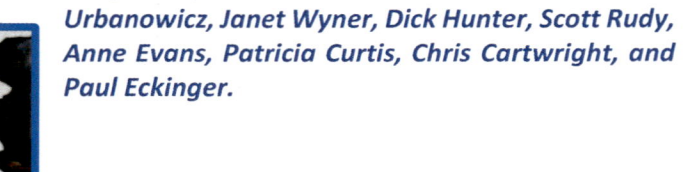

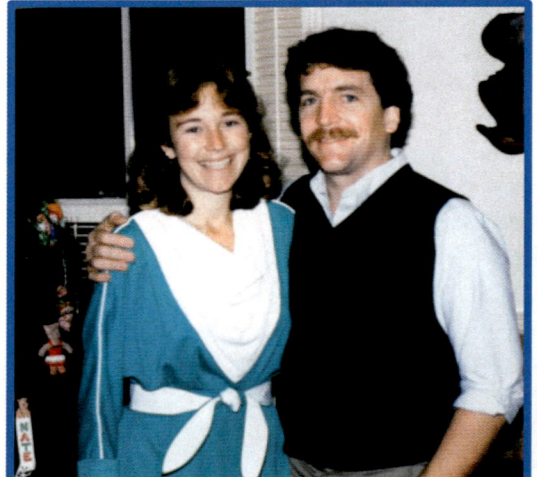

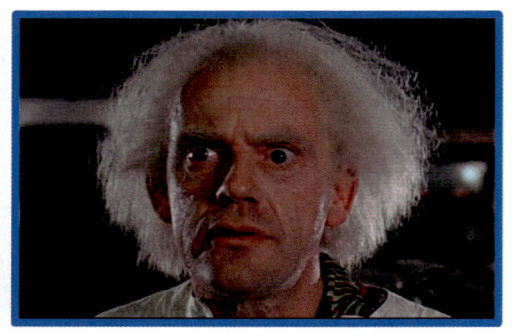

THEN **NOW**

Stephen Paul Fischer received his medical degree from UCSF (MD, 1980). After interning (Internal Medicine) at UCSD (1981) he completed residencies in Internal Medicine (1982-1985) and Anesthesiology (1985-1987) both at Stanford.

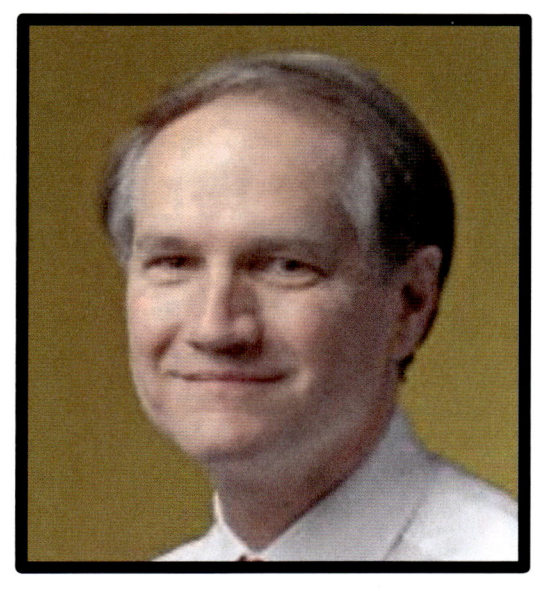

In 1993 Chair Donald Stanski asked Fischer to organize an anesthesia clinic with the goal of enhancing preoperative assessments and patient preparation to reduce the number of surgeries that were being delayed or cancelled. With his background in Internal Medicine and Anesthesiology Fischer was ideally suited to develop such a clinic. Stephen Fischer is credited with being the first person to implement a comprehensive preoperative assessment clinic in the United States. Fischer envisioned a "one-stop experience" where all tests, evaluations, and information a patient needed prior to anesthesia could be concentrated in one centralized location. As Medical Director he created 'The Stanford Model', a clinic with exam rooms, a space for patient education, admitting personnel, phlebotomy and EKG services, and a comfortable waiting area (1993). It was initially located in the back of the Anesthesia work room but expanded in size once the hospital administration recognized its value. Fischer was invited to lecture and present grand rounds at 26 hospitals across the country on *"The Stanford Model: How to Develop a Preoperative Anesthesia Clinic"* (1996-1998) He published a description of his experience with creating the clinic in Anesthesiology.

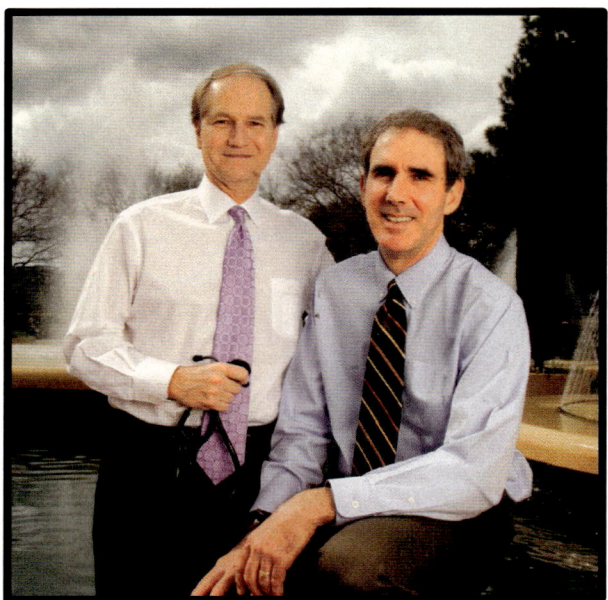

(Fischer SP. Development and effectiveness of an anesthesia preoperative evaluation clinic in a teaching hospital. Anesthesiology (1996) 85:196-206.)

The Stanford Model: Specific problems and concerns were presented, along with the methods Stanford chose to approach these issues. The resulting Anesthesia Preoperative Evaluation Clinic (APEC) provides a comprehensive service for referring physicians and their presurgical patients. All consultations, physical evaluations, educational resources, laboratory and electrocardiographic services, and hospital admissions and registration are available in one centralized location.

Stephen Fischer is now an emeritus Associate Professor of Anesthesia but remains active as Director of the clinic he created 30+ years ago.

"The Clinic has recently moved to 900 Blake Wilber and not one anesthesiologist, surgeon, or anyone has dropped in for candy and conversation. Oh, but I now have a window!!!"

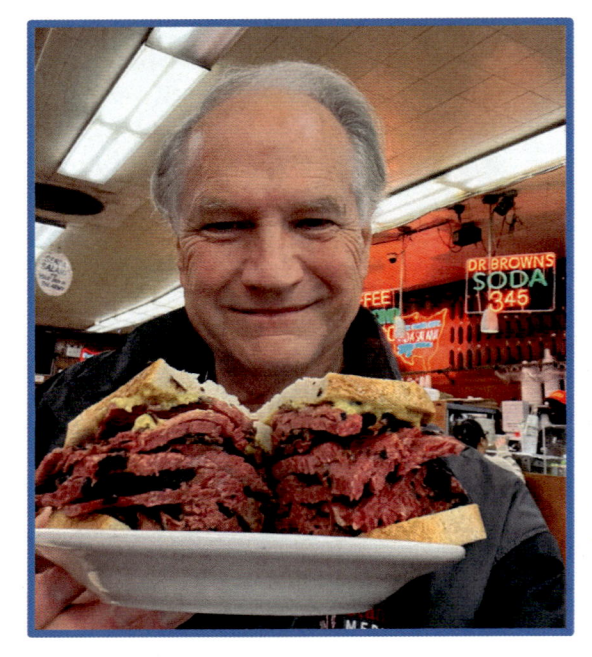

"My most memorable anecdote at Stanford was a trip to the New York PGA meeting in the mid-90s for presentations with Jay Brodsky. On free time, Jay wanted to hunt all the unique, underground record stores in Greenwich Village for Leonard Cohen bootleg records. Who is Leonard Cohen??? But even more amazing was for a guy from New York City (actually the Bronx) he didn't know the best pastrami sandwich in the world was at Katz's Deli, on Houston Street in lower Manhattan which first opened its doors in 1889. We bribed our way in and used hard cash $$$ to get a 6-inch sandwich of mouthwatering, delicious pastrami, which to this day I can see that big Jay smile as bits of pastrami and deli mustard covered his face and fingers. Super fantastic!!!

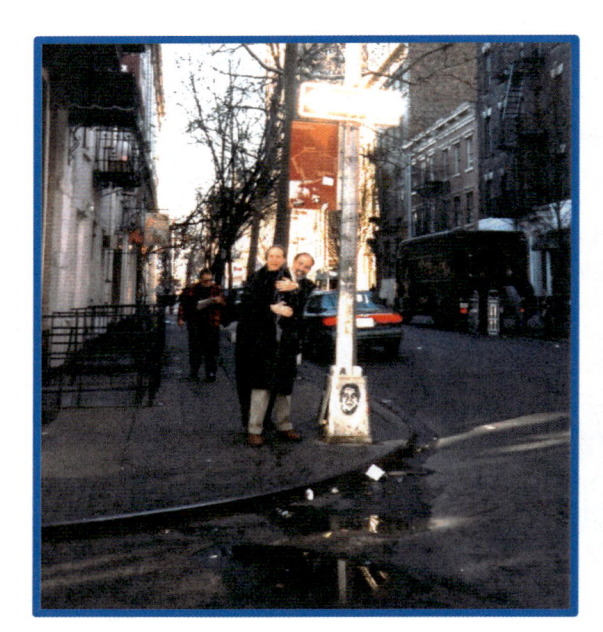

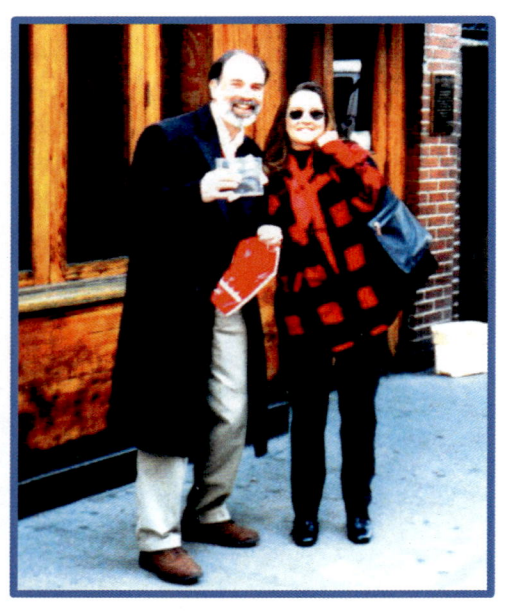

(L) Stephen Fischer and Jay Brodsky in Greenwich Village, NYC (1997). (R) Jay and wife Ana celebrating scoring an illegal Leonard Cohen bootleg CD thanks to Stephen.

Robert Mathew Hansen was born in Jersey City, NJ. He was an undergraduate at Brown University (BA, Mathematical Economics, 1973) and has a degree (MBA, Health Care Management) from the Boston University School of Management (1973-1975). He was an assistant to the Administrator at University Hospital, Boston (1974-1977). He attended the Boston University School of Medicine (MD, 1977-1981). He was an intern and resident (Internal Medicine) at UCSF (1981-1983) and completed a Fellowship (CCM) at UCSF (1983-1984). He then worked as an ER physician at Valley Memorial Hospital, Livermore, CA (1984-1985) before training in Anesthesiology at Stanford (1985-1987). He was Managing Partner at Redding Anesthesia Associates Medical Group (1987-2022). He was on the active medical staff at Shasta Regional Medical Center, Redding, CA until he retired from practice (1987- June, 2022).

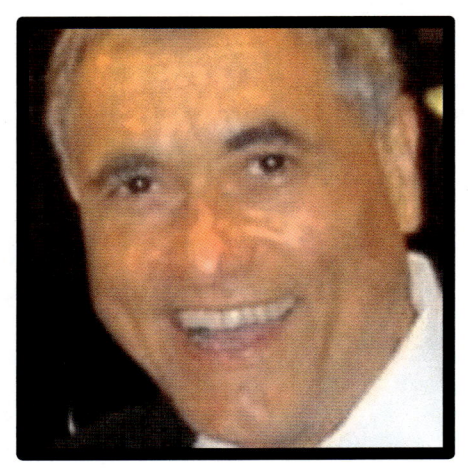

Bob was a member of the Boston and the Massachusetts State Emergency Medicine Committees and helped develop the "point of entry" plan for the Boston EMS system while working as a hospital administrator for University Hospital, Boston, before medical school. That hospital merged with Boston City Hospital to form the present Boston Hospital. He was Director and then Chairman of the Board of Shasta Regional Medical Center (2004-2006). He was a member of the Board of Directors and then President of Board of Physicians For Excellence in Redding CA (2005-2006). The organization was the mechanism for physician participation in the co-management and co-ownership of Redding Medical Center.

His current interests include the effects of lifestyle (nutrition, exercise, sleep, stress reduction) on health and health care policy. He launched a blog in 2013 that discusses evolutionary health, nutrition, exercise, and health policy (http://practical-evolutionary-health.com).

"My early interest in health care policy started with a health economics class at Brown. That led me to pursue a degree in Health Care Management. While finishing graduate school at night and working full time as an administrator at University Hospital, Boston, I experienced a life changing event when my father, mother, and sister were hospitalized within a few weeks of each other with serious illnesses. I spent many hours on weekends driving from Boston to NJ and NY to negotiate the health care system as a patient advocate for my family. That led me to apply to medical school with a desire to shape health care policy in some meaningful way. But the allure and satisfaction of clinical medicine has kept me occupied since then. I am finally coming full circle and have launched this blog about health, nutrition, and lifestyle from an evolutionary perspective, including comments on health policy along the way."

Dr. Hansen is on the Board of Directors of Physicians for Ancestral Health (2019-Present). Hansen has lectured at the fourth International Evolutionary Health Conference held in September 2023 on the topic of Cardiovascular Risk Assessment.

Ancestral health incorporates the best practices of traditional societies with modern medicine to prevent and treat chronic disease using lifestyle interventions. This includes (but is not limited to) nutrition, physical activity, restorative sleep, sunshine, positive social interactions, stress management, and a sense of greater purpose and meaning in life. Physicians for Ancestral Health is a non-profit organization whose mission is to educate and promote awareness about Ancestral Health within the medical community worldwide, as well as the general public at large. By doing this, we hope to help create a community where both doctors and individuals are empowered to focus on long-term health rather than just the treatment of disease. We seek solid scientific evidence for all healing practices, ancestral and modern, natural, and pharmaceutical. All sources of evidence, from case studies to epidemiology to randomized clinical trials, should contribute to our judgment as physicians about the interventions that will most benefit our patients.

Bob Hansen writes, "I just finished writing a paper (primary author) with 3 colleagues as a rebuttal to the Eat Lancet agenda. The topic will be along the lines of eliminating meat from the human diet will not improve human or planetary health. It covers regenerative agriculture integrated with eco-friendly animal husbandry to store carbon, regenerate biomass in soil, conserve water and eliminate toxic agro-chemicals while improving human health. One credible estimate suggests that if all planetary agriculture was converted to no-till, cover crop, crop rotation system with mulch, manure and compost replacing fossil-based fertilizer, eliminating the need for toxic pesticides, we could sequester 30% of the annual GHG carbon emissions in soil (biomass), improve crop yield per acre, decrease input costs including diesel fuel, and enhance crop resilience. The paper discusses controlled trials supporting the consumption of meat for human health, the significant downside of eliminating meat especially in low-income countries, and the negative environmental and human health effects of grain production and consumption."

Hansen is also a jazz pianist. He played with the now defunct StraightAhead Big Band and StraightAhead Combo. He is currently a member of the Shasta College Jazz Band and Combo. He was Chairman for Fundraising and Grants on the Redding Symphony Board of Directors (1991-1996). As a member of the board and Chairman of three committees he wrote multiple grants and organized fundraising, also chaired Budget and Artistic Committees. He is on the board of directors and Treasurer of the Redding Performing Arts Society (2023-Present).

"Great memories of faculty especially Jay Brodsky, Sheila Cohen, and Stan Samuels, the three most influential faculty who helped shape me as a clinician. Sheila gave my wife Kathie a labor epidural for the birth of our son Bobby and resuscitated Bobby who had cord wrapped 3 times around his neck. Bobby attended Princeton along with both children of Joe Andresen, another Stanford Anesthesia Alum."

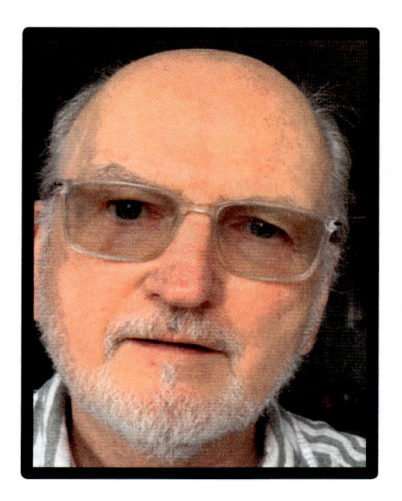

Karel "Karl" Merlin Kretzschmar was born in England where he received degrees (BSc, MSc, Physics) and a PhD (Muscle Physiology). He then attended medical school at UCSF (MD 1982). He did his internship and a residency (Pediatrics) at UCSF (1982-1984) and a residency (Anesthesiology) at Stanford (1985-1987). Immediately after completing training, he was appointed the head of perinatal anesthesiology at Mount Zion Hospital in San Francisco. When Mount Zion became part of UCSF, he was offered a position at UCSF but chose to become a partner at Santa Rosa Medical Center. Later, he was Chief at Kaiser Permanente - Richmond. He is now retired.

George Ichung Lee graduated from UCSF (MD, 1983) He interned at Northwestern University (Internal Medicine, 1983-1984) and was a Stanford resident in Anesthesiology (1985-1987).

Donald Miller Mason Jr was born in San Francisco. He attended Berkeley for his undergraduate education (BS Phi Beta Kappa, Electrical Engineering and Computer Science, 1979). He worked as a Staff Scientist for the Division of Biology and Medicine at the Lawrence Berkeley Laboratory doing research on algorithms for reconstructive tomography for SPECT (1980).

A SPECT (single-photon emission computerized tomography) scan is a type of imaging test that uses a radioactive substance and a special camera to create 3D pictures.

He received his medical education at Stanford (MD, 1983). He was an intern (1983-1984) and started a residency in Internal Medicine (1984-1985) at Stanford, then switched and completed a 2-year Anesthesiology residency (1985-1987). He then resumed and completed his Internal Medicine residency (6 month, 1987) followed by a CCM Fellowship (6 months, 1989) at Stanford. During that time, he worked as Critical Care Transport physician for Stanford University Hospital (1985-1989) under the supervision of Ronald G. Pearl.

Following his training he worked as an anesthesiologist and Director of Continuing Medical Education for the now defunct Valley Anesthesiologists Medical Group, Inc. at SCVMC. He then worked as an anesthesiologist and CCM specialist at various locations in California, Washington, Montana, and Wyoming (1991-1993). In 1993 he began working in Las Vegas, NV (1993-2011), and then in Reno with Associated Anesthesiologists of Reno (2011-2016) (renamed Mednax (2016-2020) and then acquired by North American Partners in Anesthesia (2020)). He was the Medical Director of the Intensive Care Unit (2017-2021) and a member of the Medical Executive Committee (2019-2021) at Northern Nevada Medical Center, Sparks, NV. He was on the board of directors at Incline Village Community Hospital, Incline Village, NV (2013-2022).

Dr. Mason has served as the President and Chairman of the Board of Integrated Medical Management, Inc, Las Vegas (1996-2006, 2010-2011), as Director and Secretary

(2006-2010) and Vice-President (2011-2017) of Integrated Medical Management Inc. It is an anesthesiology billing and practice management company (renamed US Anesthesia Partners, USAP). Don had an appointment as Clinical Instructor (Anesthesiology) at Stanford (1989-1995). He currently works for the Veterans Health Administration in the Department of Surgery at VA Sierra Nevada Health Care System, Reno, NV (2019-Present).

He has been active as a volunteer anesthesiologist on numerous medical missions (1988-1997).

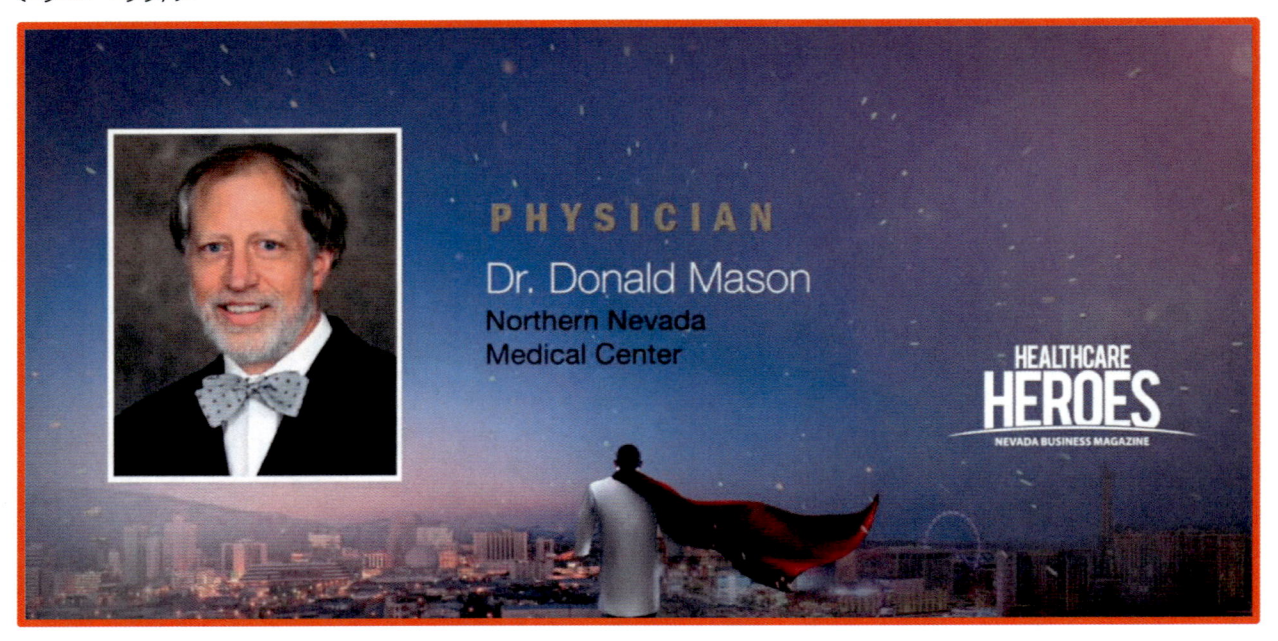

"Apart from the current Chief of Anesthesia (Brian Bateman) who I have not yet met, I worked under every anesthesia Chair at Stanford since the Department relocated in 1960 from SF to Palo Alto. I worked with Phil Larson as a medical student doing school rotations, and then with Drs. Bunker, Cohen, Fairley, Stanski, and Pearl as either a resident or Fellow. I regard my time with the Department warmly and am most respectful and thankful for all I learned there from the many faculty."

"I do recall a patient that neither I, you (Jay Brodsky), or Mark Schulman could intubate for a David Schurman redo THA. You performed a tetracaine + neo spinal and told Dave he had four hours to finish the procedure. At hour four I was alone and performing a halothane mask anesthetic (no LMA in those days). The procedure went on for at least 2 more hours."

Ira Scott Segal attended the University of Wisconsin - Madison as an undergraduate (BS, Biochemistry, 1980). He is a graduate of the University of Minnesota Medical School (MD, 1984). He spent a Transitional internship at Hennepin County Medical Center (1984-1985), and then his residency (Anesthesiology) at Stanford (1985-1987). He did a Fellowship with Mervyn Maze at the PA-VAH publishing 10 research papers. He returned to Minnesota and is now retired.

Interesting Anecdotes/Memories of Time at Stanford:

- *As a third-year medical student, during an ASA sponsored anesthesiology preceptorship in 1983, I formulated a goal to help invent an anesthetic that had a greater respiratory and cardiac therapeutic index with a knowable cellular mechanism of action. With a small cadre and Mervyn Maze, as the principal investigator, dexmedetomidine was invented during my Fellowship at Stanford University. Very early during our investigations we recognized dexmedetomidine's unique potential to improve the status quo in multiple ways. Although we thought of it as a prototype at that time, it remains the only CNS alpha2-adrenergic receptor agonist for human clinical use. Dexmedetomidine use continues to evolve; recently the FDA approved it for sublingual treatment of acute agitation in schizophrenia and bipolar disorders and two new synthetic pathways have been discovered.*
- *Mervyn and I also investigated CNS catecholamine modulation of the anesthetic state, how G-protein function changes during anesthesia, invented a drosophila model to study cellular and molecular mechanisms of anesthetics, and performed human studies with a CNS alpha2 adrenergic receptor agonist.*

Gwendolyn "Gwen" Marie Stritter was born at Fort Bragg, NC. She graduated from Stanford (MD, 1984). She interned at the University of Washington (1985) and then and was a resident (Anesthesiology) at Stanford (1985-1989). She served as the Director of the Kaiser San Jose Pain Medicine Clinic (1990-2000). She is board certified in Anesthesiology and Pain Medicine (1996-2016).

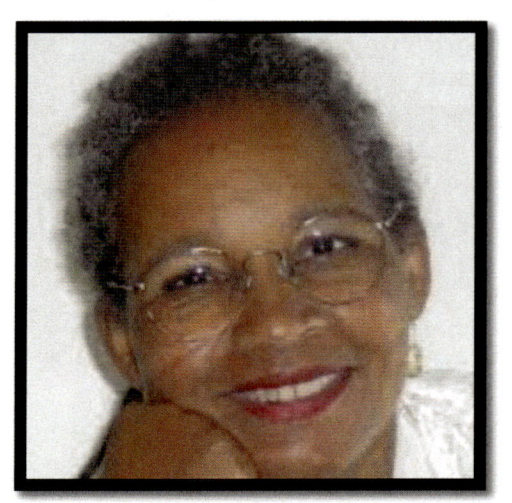

In the late 1990's a shift in California medical economics resulted in more patients but less resources at her pain clinic. Looking at other practices, she saw that these belt-tightening changes were not restricted to just one hospital group. After much thought, she made the decision to leave anesthesia practice behind and to train in the nascent field of Medical Advocacy. She subsequently studied with Dr. Mark Renneker for 12 months as she honed her advocacy skills and then opened her own private advocacy practice, Stritter Medical Consulting (2000-2013).

What is a medical advocate? A medical advocate aims "for truly optimal, comprehensive, no stone left unturned, pull-out-all-the-stops health care". Physician medical advocates:

- *do all those things for their patients that doctors do for themselves or their loved ones when faced with a serious or life-threatening illness.*
- *often act as a personal medical navigator*

She works by putting patients in charge of their own cases by:
- *Helping them learn everything they can about their condition.*
- *Doing intensive case-specific research and then reporting back to them in language they can understand.*
- *Helping them assemble the best medical team - often by locating and arranging referral to local, national or international experts.*
- *Helping them manage their doctor-patient relationships so they can direct their physicians more effectively.*
- *Helping them understand and choose between the various treatment options; acting as a sounding board for new treatment ideas.*
- *Helping them integrate <u>evidenced-based</u> complementary and alternative treatment approaches into their treatment plan.*
- *Helping them cut through clinic/hospital/insurance red tape.*

Sadly, complications from breast cancer treatment put an end to her medical advocacy practice in 2013. However, she was able to use her pain management training to set up one of the first opioid-free double mastectomies done in the Bay Area (2013). She had no opioids during surgery or in the post-op period.

She served as Executive Director of People-Powered Research (2013-2020), a grass-roots organization that aimed to crowd-source data on the efficacy of natural compounds/methods used concurrently with conventional cancer treatment, with an eye towards finding candidates for formal clinical trials. She has appeared on radio, lectured, and has written many articles on medical advocacy. She also co-authored the chapter on medical advocacy in the textbook '*Patient Advocacy for Healthcare Quality: Strategies for Achieving Patient-Centered Care*' (2007).

She is currently mostly retired but still finds time to mentor physicians who have clinical advocacy practices. She is based in Portola Valley, CA.

Interesting Anecdotes/Memories: There were three activities that I loved and will never forget:
- *Dr. Mihm invited me to the San Francisco Zoo where I was able to intubate a lion!*
- *I thoroughly enjoyed the "bucket runs" for the heart transplant service. Getting transported in Lear jets and helicopters was quite exciting.*

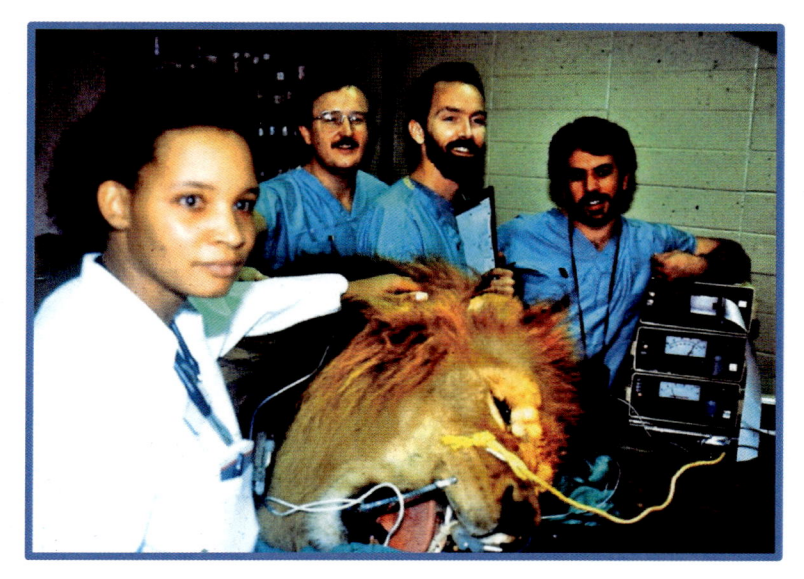

- I really enjoyed helping to write the protocols to start the Stanford Hospital Acute Pain Service in the late 1980's. It was a rocky start until we figured out the difficulties inherent in permitting the pain resident to take call from home.

"There was also a 1985 SCVMC case that I will never forget: An awake patient on low dose IV pressors presented for emergent laparotomy. The patient crashed during my low-dose etomidate-containing rapid sequence induction. The central line (that had been previously placed in ER) had stopped working. Fortunately, the situation was immediately rectified, the patient quickly resuscitated, and the procedure completed without further complications. Subsequent presentation at M&M rounds resulted in strong criticism for giving the low-dose etomidate – the consensus was that I should have given muscle relaxant only for the induction because the patient was on pressors. As you might guess, I felt terrible about my clinical "misjudgment". Fast forward about 3 years, an ER doc presented a striking talk at the annual ASA conference. He discussed how, after presenting for emergent surgery (s/p GSW in the ER parking lot) with some hemodynamic instability, he was given only muscle relaxants for induction and much of his surgery. He discussed in graphic and excruciating detail how surgery without anesthesia felt, his subsequent severe PTSD, and ended his talk by begging the audience to remember his case and to consider alternatives to muscle relaxant-only induction and maintenance in cases of awake patients with some hemodynamic instability."

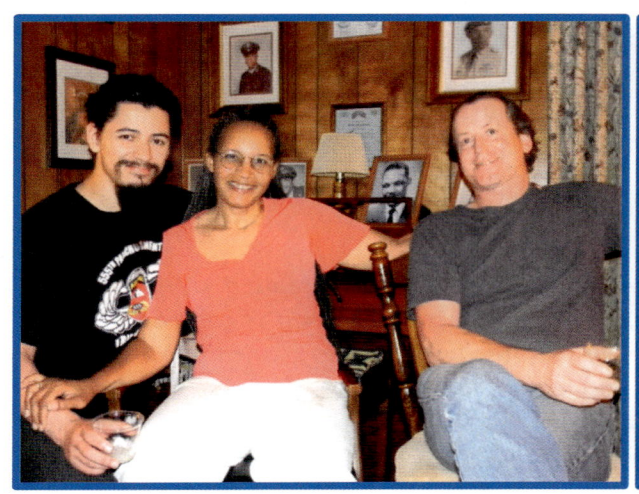

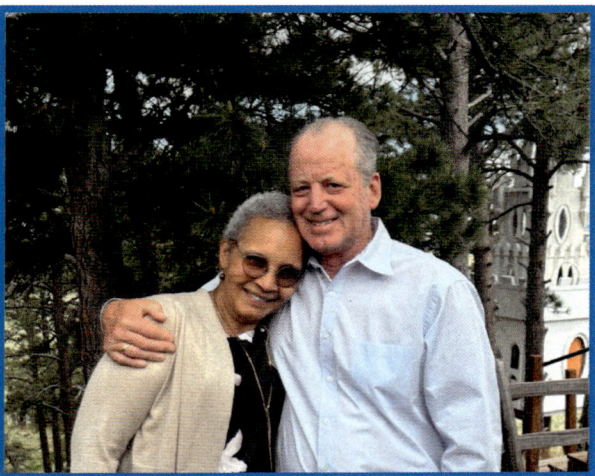

Darrell Lee Tanelian studied at Marquette and Stanford University (BS, Neurobiology, 1975). He did research at Woods Hole Oceanographic Institution (1978) and studied neural systems and behavior for postgraduate work in Marine Biology at Stanford University (1977-1979). He received a PhD (Neuroscience) (1979-1983) and his medical degree (MD, 1984) from Stanford. He interned (Internal Medicine) at Stanford (1984-1985) followed by his Anesthesiology residency (1985-1987), and then a Fellowship (Pain Management). He earned a MBA (Finance) from Southern Methodist University - Cox School of Business (1997-1999).

Following his Pain Fellowship, he was appointed to the faculty as an Assistant Professor (Anesthesiology) working on the Pain Service (1988-1992). He helped develop an ACME accredited Pain Fellowship Program at Stanford. He also established a basic science research laboratory and created the pain research program. He was awarded the Parker B. Francis Investigatorship in Anesthesiology Award for studying the effects of tissue injury on nociceptor physiology and pharmacology. He was funded by an American Cancer Society grant for work on "cancer pain - peripheral sensory mechanisms". He developed of a silicon laser microprobe for controlled sensory nerve stimulation at the Beckman Laser Institute.

Dr. Tanelian was appointed Professor (Anesthesiology) at the University of Texas - Southwestern Medical Center (1992-1999). He developed, directed, and managed The Eugene McDermott Center for Pain Management and Pain Fellowship Program and The Pain Neuroscience Basic Research Center. He also directed the Zale Lipsy University Hospital Inpatient and Post-Operative Pain Program. He was awarded the Jane and Bill Browning, Jr., Chair in Medical Science at UT -Southwestern Medical Center.

Dr. Tanellian is the Founder, former owner and President of HealthConnexin (2004). HealthConnexin is a health services, wellness, and fitness company which empowers consumers regarding their healthcare and provides services and products for consumers as well as healthcare providers directed at education, monitoring, restoration of health and prevention of disease.

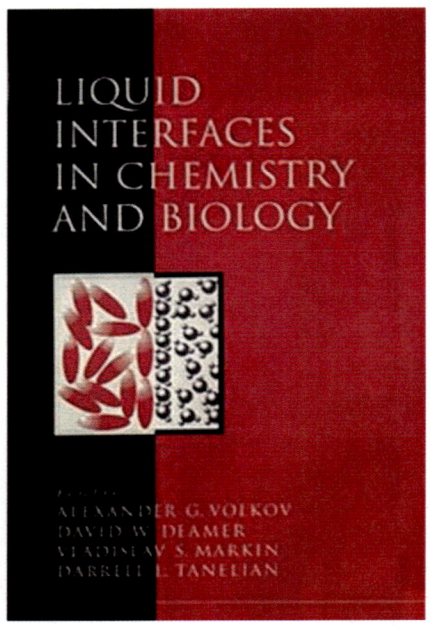

What are Connexins? Connexins (gap junction proteins) are structurally related transmembrane proteins that assemble to form vertebrate gap junctions. Each gap junction is composed of two hemichannels, or connexons, which consist of homo- or heterohexameric arrays of connexins, and the connexon in one plasma membrane docks end-to-end with a connexon in the membrane of a closely opposed cell. The hemichannel is made of six connexin subunits, each of which consist of four transmembrane segments. Gap junctions are essential for many physiological processes, such as the coordinated depolarization of cardiac muscle, proper embryonic development, and the conducted response in microvasculature. Connexins also have non-channel dependent functions relating to cytoskeleton and cell migration. Mutations in connexin-encoding genes can lead to functional and developmental abnormalities.

Book summary: Get ready for an extraordinary new health concept Molecular Fitness, a state of optimal wellness literally from the inside out! The Connexin Connection is based on over a decade of disease prevention research by Darrell L. Tanelian, M.D., Ph.D., and his synthesis of more than five thousand published scientific papers on connexins. This book associates the beginning of multi-cellular life, 600 million years ago, with the advent of the connexin molecule. Today, this molecule is largely responsible for our body's intercellular communication and provides us with the first unified scientific explanation of illness and wellness. The Connexin Connection identifies the critical factors in our diet and our lifestyle that enhance connexin function to help us to perform our best mentally and physically and enable us to live healthier longer. Dr. Darrell L. Tanelian, M.D., Ph.D. a world-renowned authority on the role of nutrition and lifestyle in optimizing molecular function advocates keeping the connexin molecules in our bodies OPEN and CONNECTED. The path to optimal wellness begins with this book.

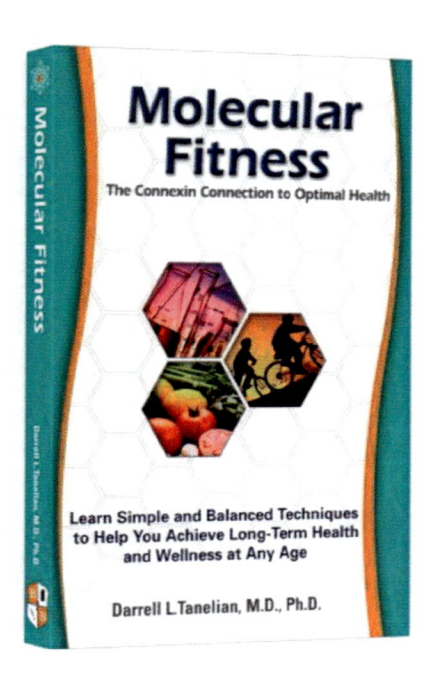

Amanda Dawn Tucker obtained a medical degree from the University of Leeds School of Medicine, UK (1976). She received post-graduate certifications in Obstetrics and Gynecology and Children's Health. She spent one year training in Emergency Medicine and another in Pediatric and General Surgery before she left the UK for further postgraduate training. She was an Anesthesiology resident at Stanford (1985-1987). She also trained at Harvard in Pediatric Cardiology and Pediatric Intensive Care. At some point her resume states that she also trained in "Anti-Aging Medicine".

Dr. Tucker was part of the Federal Disaster Medical Alert Team (1987) and was a Life Flight Physician at Stanford for two years. She has been active as a physician-in-charge of patient transports to neonatal and pediatric critical care facilities on several critical care transport teams at Boston Children's Hospital, the Hospital for Sick Children, Toronto, and a Mountain Rescue Physician for Parks Canada in Lake Louise, Canada.

She had worked in Honolulu but filed for bankruptcy in 2014. Her last practice location was in Longmont, CO, with another office in Aspen, CO. She has been involved in legal difficulties in Colorado concerning public housing.

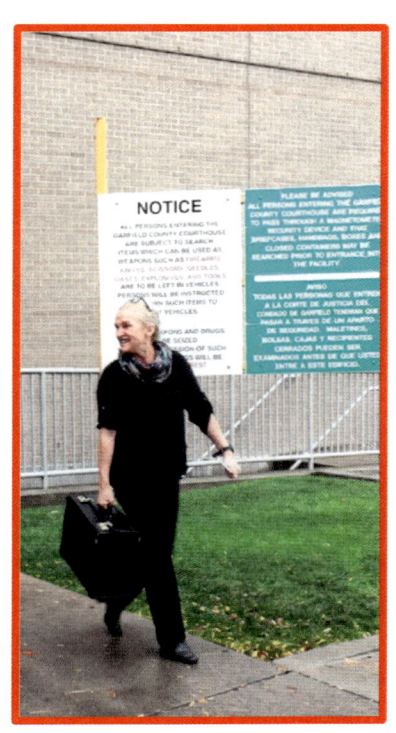

Amanda Tucker leaving the courthouse during her eviction trial.

The ASPEN TIMES (April 2007)
A doctor has filed court papers that the housing authority's bid to kick her out of her Ritz-Carlton Club affordable housing unit is an "invalid attempt to enact rent control." Dr. Amanda Tucker, whom the Aspen/Pitken County Housing Authority sued in Match 2006 continues to live in the deed-restricted townhouse. The housing authority claims that Tucker, an anesthesiologist, did not complete an application in order for her to qualify for ownership of the Category 3 housing unit, which puts a $91,000 cap on yearly earnings for owners. At the time Tucker bought the Ritz-Carlton unit, she owned seven pieces of real estate in Hawaii.

Theodore "Ted" Henry Tuschka

was born in Fresno. He attended high school in Beirut, Lebanon, then graduated from USC (BA, Physics, 1969-1973). He obtained a MS degree (Chemistry) at California State University – Fresno, followed by a PhD (Organic Chemistry) at UCSB (1976-1980). He then attended the Keck School of Medicine/USC (MD, 1984). He did an internship (Transitional) at USC/LAC Medical Center (1984-1985) and then his residency (Anesthesiology) at Stanford (1985-1988). He did a Fellowship (Research) with Jim Trudell at Stanford (1987-1988) and was a Clinical Instructor (Anesthesiology) (1988-1989). He has practiced his entire career at Community Memorial Hospital, Ventura, CA, (1990-Present).

Ted enjoys backpacking, off road driving, hot rod cars, scuba, jogging and firearms. He and his wife now live on a ranch in Idaho, but he still continues to work about one week a month in Ventura.

Story time:
- *I was in the OR with Transplant surgeon and subsequent US Senator from Tennessee Bill Frist MD. The room is filled with about 10 cardiac surgeons from South America who are observing. As we were warming the patient Frist looks up at the group and stated with an elegant Southern drawl, "When this thing takes its first beat it'll bring a tear to your eye".*
- *The Cardiac team was on a midnight harvest by helicopter. We landed on the roof and our boys dissected the heart and retired to the lounge for coffee while I babysat. A team from St Elsewhere opened the belly and began dissecting the kidneys. Things were going well until the guy whacked the renal vein, the belly filled with blood and the heart went flat. I informed our surgeon that things were going downhill, and he said he wanted to see the heart eject once before we took it. I shoved a bag of blood down the cordis and saw one full ejection. Then cross clamp, cardioplegia, and 20 minutes later we are in the chopper heading home.*
- *Guy got into a fight with his wife, and he became our cardiac donor. She left but when she came back the next morning for her clothes to go to work, he jumped out of the rafters with a rope around his neck hanging himself as she opened the garage door. At that time, we had to transport the heart-lung donors back to Stanford before harvest. As the jet turned at the end of the runway the light streamed through the window and the donor started blinking. The surgeon agreed that the light was bothering his eyes, so I taped them closed and initiated muscle relaxation.*
- *Every morning at 6 am I tried to break 100 mph on the Los Altos Hills 280 on-ramp to Stanford with my 1980 Corvette. One morning I had a late case, so I went in at 9 am. Low and behold my 100-mph entrance was 10 cars ahead of a CHP and he lit up like a Christmas tree. To avoid jail for speed > 100 mph, I accelerated to 160 mph and the CHP disappeared in my rearview mirror. I exited US 280 at the curving Page Mill off ramp and parked in the middle of the SUH parking lot. Entering the hospital like a Viet Cong on patrol I never heard about it again.*

- *On a helicopter pick up to SCVMC at night, as we were landing in a parking lot the copilot opens door and steps out on the runner. When I asked him what he was doing he said, "Looking for phone lines".*
- *Interplast: We arrived at Leonardo Martinez Hospital in San Pedro Sula Honduras late on a wet afternoon. As our bus came down the hill, we could see the hospital parking lot was filled with tents, campfires, and people. They had been coming out of the jungle with their cleft lipped babies to meet us. The next morning, we started work - one OR, two operating tables and no anesthesia machines. Anesthesia was an O2 tank to an isoflurane vaporizer filled with halothane delivered through a Mapleson D. Monitoring was a precordial stethoscope, manual blood pressure cuff and no EKG or SaO2. By the late morning, we were getting nauseated from halothane being vented directly into the room. This was addressed with a large diameter tube to exhaust both circuits out the window. When I went to lunch, I observed three guys on the bench outside the window inhaling from our exhaust system hose and handing it back and forth. I walked by a woman on a gurney who had needed a C-section with the feet of a dead baby protruding from her vagina. Later that day I intubated a man who had been hit in the face with a machete. Nothing looked familiar, just bumps where the teeth should have been. I realized the machete had split between his upper lip and nose. I was looking at the tops of the molars in his maxillary sinus. Removing the laryngoscope and moving down one revealed the larynx. I guess we operated on about 100 kids.*

Unfortunately, Dr. Tuschka has experienced his own legal problems. He was found guilty of actually showing concern for his operating room staff's safety managing an untreated HIV+ patient.

AORN (May 2013)
California Court Rules Action Unethical And Discriminatory

When anesthesiologist Theodore Tuschka, MD, learned the patient he was about to wheel into the OR was HIV-positive, he canceled the case over concerns for his safety and the well-being of the operating room staff. A California judge has called his fears unreasonable and in violation of state law that protects all citizens from unlawful discrimination.

The patient arrived at Community Memorial Hospital in Ventura for hernia repair surgery in February 2009 and was placed in a curtained pre-op bay. Court records show she gave a pre-op nurse a list of her medications, signed a hospital consent form, and discreetly told the nurse that she was HIV-positive. The nurse, apparently unfazed, started the IV. A few minutes later, Dr. Tuschka approached the bedside and reviewed the patient's chart. According to court records, he quickly and loudly announced that the patient was HIV-positive, commented that her chart contained no information on her viral load or T-cell count, and asked if she was on anti-retroviral (ARV) medications. The patient said she was not, having been instructed by her immunologist 2 months earlier to stop taking the medications after experiencing unwanted side-effects.

Dr. Tuschka left to call the surgeon, who was fully aware of her patient's condition. He testified that the surgeon agreed with his assessment to cancel the case because the patient's viral load was unknown. According to the court records, Dr. Tuschka returned to the patient, telling her he wanted "to keep himself safe, and the people that he works with safe." He wrote the following in the patient's chart: "Patient with HIV positive off medications two months. Suggest workup by treating physician documenting viral loads and infectious status. Hopefully patient will be on meds or have documented nonviremic state for the safety of the operating room personnel."

The notation turned out to be a smoking gun, according to court documents, which say it fully corroborates the patient's testimony that staff safety was Dr. Tuschka's sole reason for cancelling the case. In court, Dr. Tuschka claimed he canceled the case to protect the patient — experts testified the patient was at increased risk for infection because she had stopped taking her ARVs, and if the mesh the surgeon planned to use to repair the defect became infected, it would be harder to treat in an HIV-positive patient — but admitted his documentation did not reflect that concern.

Dr. Tuschka's canceling of the case and conduct toward the patient was insensitive and possibly unethical, note court documents, which cite the AMA's code of ethics: "A physician may not ethically refuse to treat a patient whose condition is within the physician's current realm of competence solely because the patient is seropositive for HIV. His actions also violated a California law that broadly prohibits discrimination based on, among many factors, disability, and medical condition. The court ruled "a person with HIV is disabled as a matter of law" and, in this case, "an HIV-positive patient was denied medically necessary surgery because an anesthesiologist unreasonably feared for his own safety and that of the operating room staff."

"Dr. Tuschka did not discriminate on anyone because of his or her HIV status," says his personal attorney, John Hunter. "Even [the patient's] infectious disease doctors testified that her health and safety were best served to postpone surgery until she was back on her regular medications." Mr. Hunter says Dr. Tuschka's defense team will petition the Supreme Court of California to review the case. "The appellate court took a hard look at the actions and basically jumped to the conclusion that [Dr. Tuschka] unlawfully discriminated against the patient based on her disability," says the patient's attorney.

> **California Civil Rights Department**
> April 17, 2013
>
> Maureen K. v. Tuschka (CA2/6 B236150 4/17/13) Unruh Act/HIV Disability Discrimination
>
> The Unruh Civil Rights Act provides a comprehensive statutory scheme to protect all persons from unlawful discrimination. A medical doctor is not immune from the broad sweep of the Act. The irony here is that appellant was in need of surgery to repair an umbilical hernia, and turned to the medical profession for help. She was turned away minutes before surgery because of a disability - she was HIV-positive. The surgery was abruptly canceled in the hospital's pre-operative room by the anesthesiologist, respondent Dr. Theodore Tuschka, after he learned from appellant's chart that she was HIV-positive and was not taking anti-retroviral (ARV) medications. Respondent refused to go forward with the surgery because of his concern for his own safety and that of the operating room staff.
>
> As we shall explain, the trial court prejudicially erred by submitting the issue of whether appellant was disabled to the jury. A person with HIV is disabled as a matter of law. Here there is an additional reason why appellant is disabled as a matter of law: respondent "regarded or treated" her as a person with a disability.
>
> Appellant's complaint against respondent alleges causes of action for disability discrimination in violation of the Unruh Civil Rights Act (Civ. Code, § 51, et seq.) and violation of the Confidentiality of Medical Information Act (CMIA) (§ 56, et seq.). She appeals from the judgment entered in respondent's favor after the trial court granted his motion for summary adjudication of the CMIA claim and the jury found that she is not disabled within the meaning of the Unruh Civil Rights Act.
>
> The Legislature has determined that a person with HIV is disabled as a matter of law within the meaning of the Unruh Civil Rights Act. This is not a question for the jury. As a consequence, we reverse the judgment as to this cause of action. However, the trial court correctly granted respondent's motion for summary adjudication of the cause of action for violation of the CMIA because respondent did not disclose any individually identifying medical information.
>
> http://www.courts.ca.gov/opinions/documents/B236150.PDF

Court's Conclusion: An HIV patient's viral load or T-cell count is not determinative of operating room safety, as long as reasonable universal precautions are taken. No medical doctor should have liability for refusing to perform a procedure that he or she believes will harm the patient. That is not what happened here. Here, an HIV-positive patient was denied medically necessary surgery because an anesthesiologist unreasonably feared for his own safety and that of the operating room staff. The denial was based on her HIV-positive status and was a violation of the Unruh Civil Rights Act.

Kelly Louis Crawford graduated from the John Hopkins University School of Medicine (MD, 1978). He completed a residency (Internal Medicine) at Stanford (1978-1981). He began an Anesthesiology residency in January 1985 but resigned from the program in December 1985 for "unresolved allegations of improper behavior". Crawford subsequently worked in Kaiser Permanente - San Jose practicing Internal Medicine.

CHAPTER 5
1986

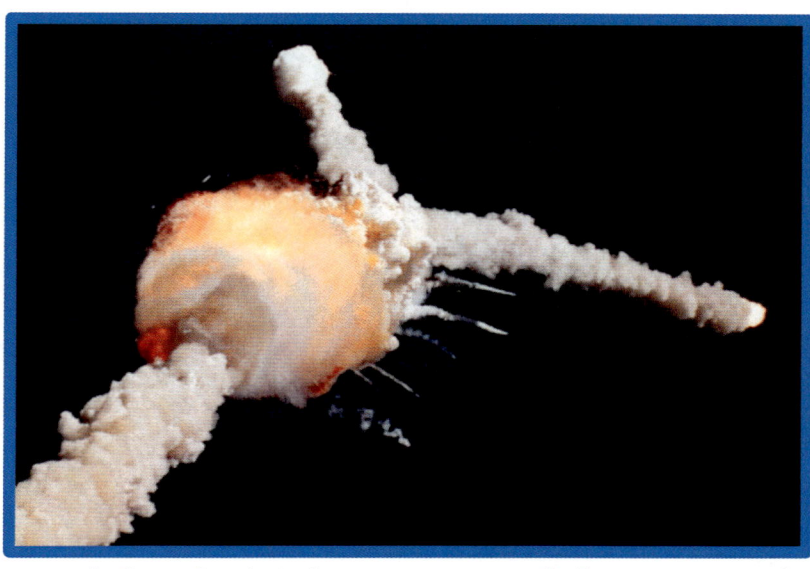

Several major disasters occurred during 1986. The Soviet nuclear reactor at Chernobyl exploded on April 26th causing the release of radioactive material contaminating most of Europe. It remains the world's worst nuclear accident. In the USA the Space Shuttle Challenger disintegrated 73 seconds after launching, killing all seven astronauts on board. In the UK the first case of Bovine Spongiform Encephalopathy (BSE), more commonly known as *Mad Cow Disease*, was discovered in November. BSE was linked to Creutzfeldt-Jakob disease in humans who consumed infected meat and relatives. Millions of cattle were culled to stop the epidemic, which didn't officially end until 1998.

On more positive notes the Oprah Winfrey Show debuted on national television on September 8th. The NBC television network introduced its famous peacock logo. The original *Top Gun* film starring Tom Cruise premiered that year, as did Andrew Lloyd Webber's *Phantom of the Opera*. Future 'non-Hall of Famer' Barry Bonds made his MLB debut for the Pittsburgh Pirates, and on September 7th, 1986, the Cleveland Browns became the first NFL team in history to have a play reviewed by instant replay.

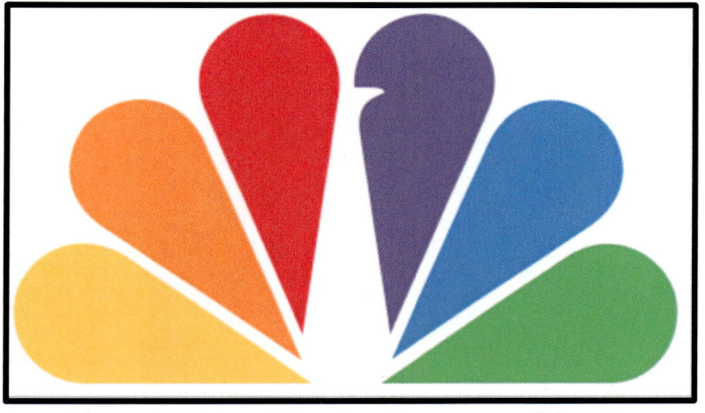

Smoking was banned on all public transport in the United States including trains, planes, and automobiles. A new Federal holiday honoring Martin Luther King Jr. was created.

In December the first heart + lung + liver transplant was

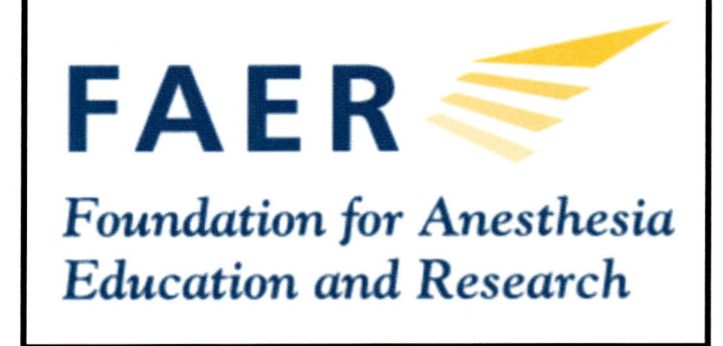

performed - but not at Stanford. The historic procedure occurred at Papworth Hospital in Cambridge, England.

The ASA approved the first medical standard-of-care statement for basic intraoperative monitoring, subsequently publishing its evidence-based *'Practice Parameters and Standards, Guidelines, and Statements'. The ASA also created the Foundation for Anesthesia Education and Research (FAER) with* William K. Hamilton of UCSF as its first president (1986-1989). Future FAER presidents affiliated with Stanford included Donald R. Stanski (1993), Patricia A. Kapur (1994), and Myer H. Rosenthal (2001-2002). The length of an Anesthesiology training was increased from two to three years for the residents starting in 1986.

Bradford William Beebe (deceased) was born in 1954.

He grew up in the Bay Area attending Los Altos High School. He received his MD from the George Washington University School of Medicine (MD, 1981) and did an Anesthesiology residency at Stanford (1986-1989). He practiced for a short period of time locally, and sadly passed away June 1993.

David Norman Buckley was born in Vancouver,

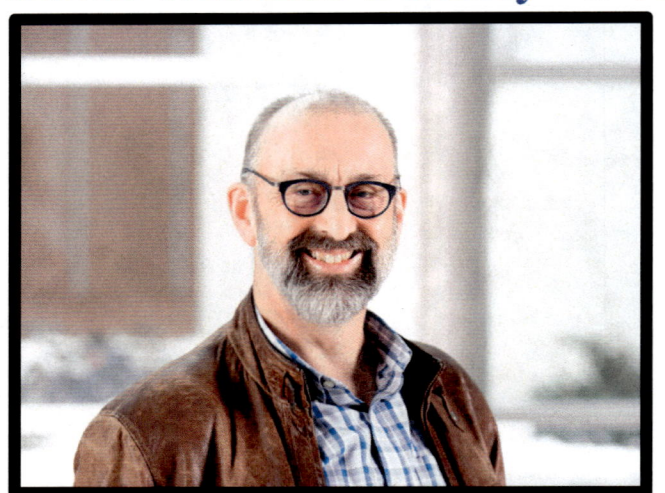

British Columbia, Canada. After obtaining his undergraduate degree (BA, Psychology, 1977) he graduated from the Faculty of Health Sciences, McMaster University, Hamilton, Ontario, Canada (1982). He interned (1983) and began his anesthesia residency at McMaster (1983-1986) and completed a Canadian required additional year of anesthesia training at Stanford (1986-1987). He returned to McMaster University for a Fellowship (Pain Management).

"I had looked forward to working in the Chronic Pain Clinic as part of my year at Stanford, with Director Lorne Eltherington. I was more than delighted upon arriving to discover that the renowned Michael Cousins was a Visiting Professor for that year so I also got to work with him and learn from him to my great pleasure. Years later I was able to 'return the favour' when I nominated him for an honorary degree at McMaster University Faculty of Health Sciences and he was awarded this degree in the presence of his friend and colleague Phil Bridenbaugh."

Norm Buckley was a faculty member in the Department of Anesthesia at G. DeGroote School of Medicine, McMaster University since 1988. His interests were acute and chronic pain management. He held the positions of Operating Room Director, Chief of Anesthesia (Chedoke-McMaster) and Deputy Chief (Hamilton Health Sciences Corporation). He led the development of the acute post-operative pain service for adult and pediatric patients, the pediatric sedation services, and was the initial Director of the Pain Management Centre at the Hamilton General Hospital (2000-2014).

In 2017 Dr. Buckley completed 13 years as Chair of the Department of Anesthesia (2004-2017). He established the Michael G. DeGroote National Pain Centre and was Scientific Director of the Michael G. DeGroote Institute for Pain Research and Care. He was principal investigator for the *Chronic Pain Network*, a Canadian Institute Health Research initiative to establish a national pain research network. It is now called *Knowledge Mobilization Network*. He also served as founding Chief Scientific Officer (CSO) of the Centre of Excellence for Chronic Pain in Veterans (2019-2022).

He was a member of the Canadian Center on Substance Use and Addiction (CCSA) National Advisory Council '*First Do No Harm: Responding to Canada's Prescription Drug Crisis*' (2013) and on the Expert Advisory Council member for the Canadian Pain Task Force (2019-21).

He retired from the McMaster faculty in 2018, and from its affiliated hospitals (Hamilton Health Sciences, St Joseph's Hospital) in 2024. He is Professor Emeritus in the Department of Anesthesia, Michael G. DeGroote School of Medicine, McMaster University. He lists "musician" as his major outside interest.

"I play in the Weston Silver Band, a British Brass band based in the Greater Toronto Area and recognized for its history (over 100 years) and successes in international competition (the North American Brass Band Association."

"I experienced the impact of being at Stanford when I attended one of the regular journal club meetings and we discussed 'halothane hepatitis'. The discussant for those rounds was John Bunker, former Chair at Stanford and Chair of the National Halothane Study conducted in the early 1960s. His presence offered a remarkable insight into the issues at hand and the importance of careful epidemiological analysis of problems of this sort."

Norman Buckley has the distinction of being the only former resident, to our knowledge, of being the answer to the $400 double-jeopardy question "what is pain?"

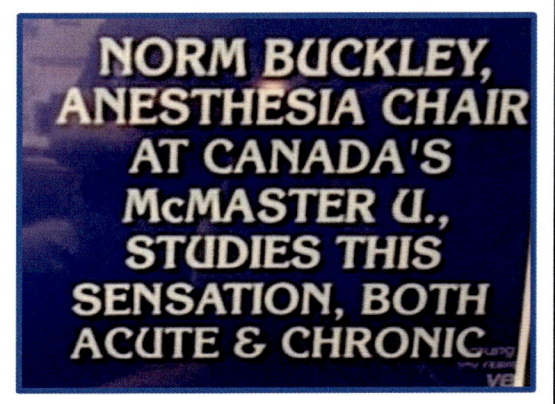

My dad is a Jeopardy clue

Celebrated McMaster professor gets Jeopardy spotlight
Feb. 12, 2016

By The Hamilton Spectator
'What is pain?'

That was the right answer on the TV game show Jeopardy Thursday night, pushing a celebrated McMaster professor into the spotlight. In an episode of College Jeopardy, under the category 'Doctors Within Borders,' players were given the answer: "Norm Buckley, anesthesia chair at Canada's McMaster University, studies this sensation, both acute and chronic." Contestant Sarah Dubnik gave the correct response.

Buckley, director of the Michael G. DeGroote Institute for Pain Research and Care, professor and chair of the Department of Anesthesia of the Michael G. DeGroote School of Medicine, is known around the world for his research and clinical work that focuses on pain. According to the McMaster daily news, the Jeopardy question came as a surprise to Buckley.

Sadly, we recently learnt that Sandra Chaplan has passed away.

Sandra Reading Chaplan (Eggers) (deceased) attended Yale University (BA, Literature, 1977) and Weill Cornell Medical College (MD, 1980-1984). She was an Anesthesiology resident (1986-1989) and Chief Resident during her final year. Following residency, she did a Fellowship (Pain Management at Stanford (1989-1990). She was on our faculty for 3 years before leaving for UCSD in 1993 as a training grant Fellow to work with Tony Yaksh.

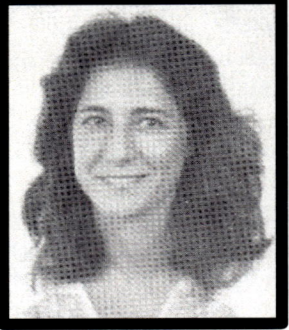

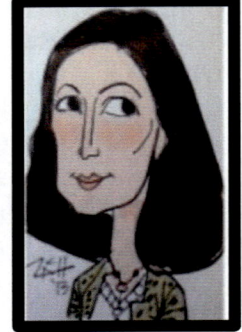

During her time at UCSD she published 14 papers which largely focused on neuraxial drug action. She was among the first to systematically study the action of intrathecal Ca++ channel antagonist SNX111 (later known as ziconotide). Her collaboration at UCSD with David Luo led to the identification of the upregulation of dorsal root ganglion alpha$_2$ delta calcium channel subunit and its correlation with allodynia in nerve injury. Perhaps her publication of greatest interest was her seminal paper describing assessment of tactile threshold in rodents using the classic up down testing method. That paper to date has received over 5,800 citations and that number continues to grow, reflecting its significant impact upon preclinical threshold evaluation.

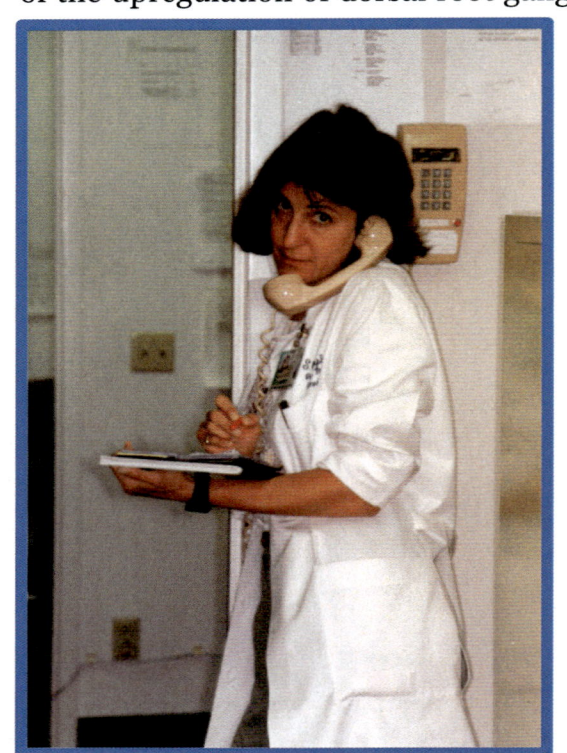

Sandy later worked in the pharmaceutical industry for Janssen Research & Development, LLC, San Diego, as Global Clinical Lead - Wave Early Development Unit. She was Director Clinical Research and then Senior Director, Neuroscience External Innovation and Biology Team Leader (Pain and Related Disorders) for Johnson & Johnson. During her research career, she displayed a continued high level of activity in both the academic venue and in the pharmaceutical industry with more than 87 papers accumulating over 10,000 citations.

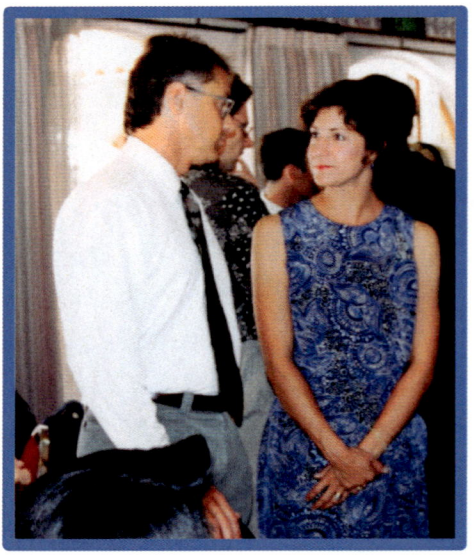

Sandra Chaplan and husband

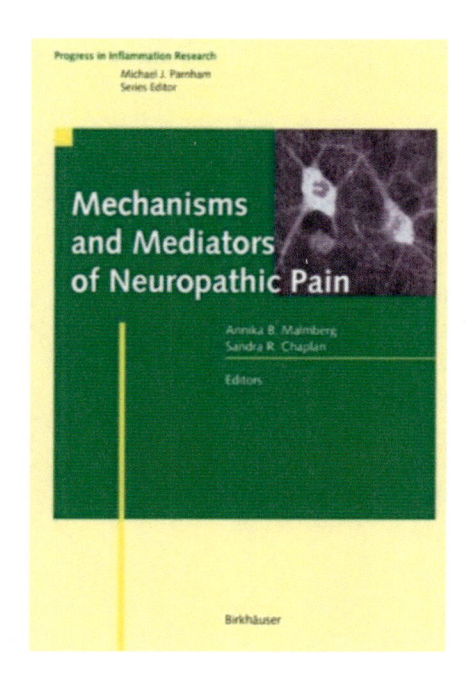

Ray Holladay Engstrom did his undergraduate work at Brigham Young University (BS, Chemistry, 1981) and then earned his medical degree at UCI (MD, 1985). He interned and completed his Anesthesiology training at Stanford (1985-1989). He was briefly on our faculty as a Clinical Assistant Professor covering Pediatric Cardiac Surgery (1989-1990). He and fellow resident David Fitzgerald left Stanford and joined the private practice group Anesthesia Consultants of Costa Contra, Inc (1990). That group merged with another from Mount Diablo Hospital and became Medical Anesthesia Consultants (MAC). (In 2013 MAC was sold and renamed MAC Sheridan. In 2017 MAC Sheridan was sold to Envision Physician Services.) Ray was Director of Cardiac Anesthesia at San Ramon Regional Medical Center (1990-2004), at John Muir Health (2004-2006), and for Stanford Health Care Tri Valley, ValleyCare Health System (2006-2023). He retired from clinical practice in 2023.

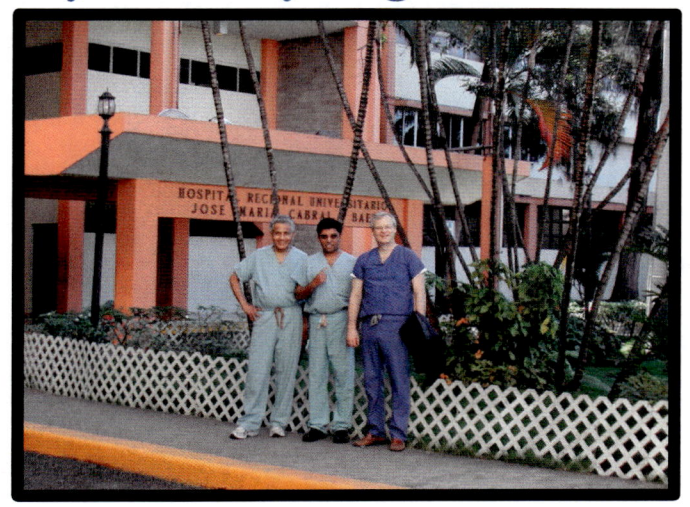

"This past year I retired from clinical practice when our group which had been bought out by private equity dissolved. I was Director of Cardiac Anesthesia at Tri-Valley Stanford at the time working with Drs. Longoria and Marie Currie. We were hoping that the anesthesia department at Tri Stanford would merge with the Stanford anesthesia group, but the hospital brought in another national anesthesia company to staff it."

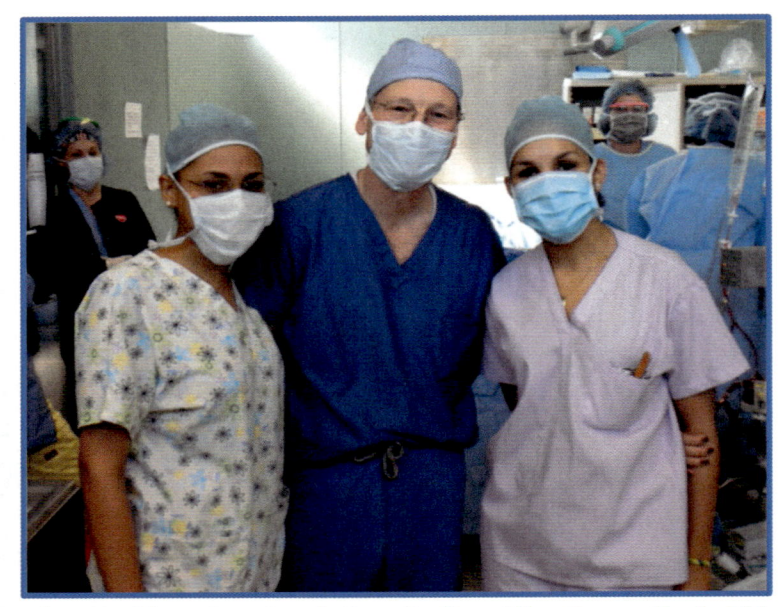

"I was part of the Stanford resident class that started in 1986. There were 4 of us that had a combined internship and residency that began in 1985 - Robert Kaye, Steve Marlowe, George Wakerlin, and me. The 1986 class also included David Fitzgerald, Rona Gifford, Richard Jaffe, Kristi Peterson, Sandra Chaplan, Marilyn Roper, to name a few. We were the first anesthesia residency class to complete a residency that included a CA_3 year. David Fitzgerald and I spent our CA_3 year doing Cardiac Anesthesia with an emphasis on Pediatric Cardiac Anesthesia. The cardiac anesthesia faculty at the time included Bruce Bollen, John Urbanowicz, Ellen Finch, Gordon Haddow, Ron Pearl, Tom Feeley, Allen Ream, Kevin Fish and others. The Peds anesthesia attendings included Mike Champeau, Larry Feld, Al Hackel, to name a few.

After Dave and I finished there was a departure of a number of faculty. John Urbanowicz left for private practice at Sequoia Hospital in Redwood City. Ellen was married to the cardiac surgeon Stewart Jamieson who had left for a brief period to go to UCSD. Allen Ream retired around that time. Bruce Bollen left for the University of Iowa. On the Peds side Larry Feld left for private practice at CPMC and Mike Champeau stayed in Palo Alto in private practice with the AAMG. John Cooper joined the PAMF.

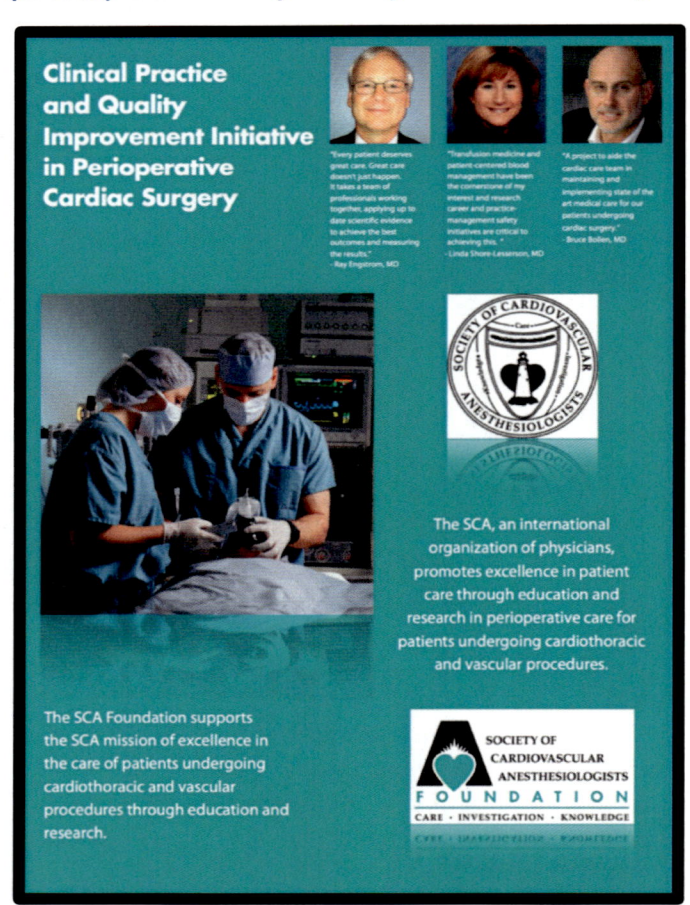

Following residency Dave accepted a clinical appointment on the Stanford faculty to help Vaughn Starnes develop his pediatric cardiac surgery program. Vaughn had returned from a Peds Cardiac Surgery Fellowship at Great Ormand Street, London. I had accepted a Fellowship and clinical appointment at Penn State to work with David Larach in peds cardiac anesthesia. At the last minute, Dr. Fairley talked with Penn State and worked out for me to stay at Stanford as clinical faculty helping Dave staff Vaughn Starnes' cases. Robert Moynihan was recruited from Boston Children's Hospital to round out the peds cardiac anesthesia group.

While Dave, Bob and I were covering the peds cardiac surgery cases we had several

CA₃ residents that spent 6 months at a time on the service. These included John Archer (who went on to train in Peds anesthesia at CHOP), Pat Curtis (who married Larry Siegel) and Ed Bertaccini (who joined the PA-VAH ICU group). We had Talmage Egan (current Chair of Anesthesia at University of Utah) doing pharmacokinetic studies with Don Stanski. He would come into our room to draw samples to study the pharmacokinetics of sufenta on neonates on CPB.

Richard Jaffe, Rona Giffard, and Kristi Peterson stayed on at Stanford. Kristi married Bill Decampli another Stanford Cardiac Surgery Fellow. Bill briefly joined Niels Young at Oakland Children's Hospital but eventually left for the Deborah Heart and Lung Institute in Pennsylvania and Kristi left to go with him. Sandra Chaplan who was one of the Stanford Chief Residents in 1989 left and pursued a research career in San Diego.

Dave Fitzgerald, Robert Moynihan, and I covered all of Vaughn Starnes' pediatric cases until he left for USC/LA Children's Hospital. Around the time Vaughn was leaving, Bob Moynihan left to join the CASE anesthesia group in Sacramento, Dave Fitzgerald left for private practice in Walnut Creek joining the AACCI group that was the forerunner of Medical Anesthesia Consultants (MAC), the group Arne Brock-Utne joined later. I left several months later in 1990 to join the same practice. Stanford worked out a temporary plan to staff Vaughn cases by having the three of us return for a week at a time to cover his program. This arrangement lasted for several years until they recruited Greg Hammer.

Dave Fitzgerald would go on to become President of Medical Anesthesia Consultants (MAC) for over 20 years and stewarded it into the largest private practice group in the Bay Area. At its height it had over 120 anesthesiologists. I founded the Cardiac Anesthesia subgroup within MAC that grew to 6 TEE certified cardiac anesthesiologists covering 4 East Bay hospitals. Bob Kaye finished a Peds Fellowship at CHOP and went on to have a successful career at the Daughter of the King's Children Hospital in Virginia. Steve Marlowe went into private practice in Santa Rosa and George Wakerlin, after completing an ICU fellowship at Stanford joined Kaiser in Fairfield.

Bruce Bollen has remained a close friend and mentor of mine over the years. Bruce has been a driving force within the Society of Cardiac Anesthesiologists (SCA). He and I submitted in 2012 a proposal to the SCA for a project entitled 'Continuous Practice improvement (CPI)'. It was subsequently approved by the board of directors and is now a significant effort by the SCA. The CPI group has published several guideline papers over the last several years. I have attached the original proposal. We also held fundraising in San Francisco to jump start the effort. Bruce was presented with the Lifetime achievement award by the SCA in Toronto during the April 2024 Annual Meeting.

COMPREHENSIVE VALUE BASED QUALITY MANAGEMENT PROGRAM IN PERIOPERATIVE CARDIAC SURGICAL CARE

PROPOSAL TO SOCIETY OF CARDIOVASCULAR ANESTHSIOLOGISTS AND FOUNDATION

AUGUST, 2012

SUBMITTED BY PROJECT MANAGEMENT GROUP

RAY ENGSTROM, MD
BRUCE BOLLEN, MD
STAN SHERNAN, MD
NANETTE SCHWANN, MD
MURALI DHARAN, MD

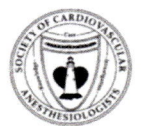

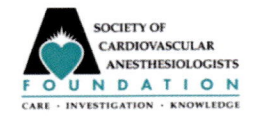

SOCIETY OF CARDIOVASCULAR ANESTHESIOLOGISTS
FOUNDATION
CARE · INVESTIGATION · KNOWLEDGE

Like many of our former residents, Ray has been active in medical missions to under-developed countries. He has used his expertise in cardiac anesthesia to help with mitral valve replacement procedures in the Dominican Republic.

"In 2010 I got involved with the Heart to Heart Mission run by Dr. Bob Piscato in Fort Myer Florida. From 2010 until 2020 we took our heart team from John Muir/San Ramon and spent 10 days once a year to Santiago Dominican Republic. During the 10 days we would do 10-12 mitral valve replacements for end stage mitral valve stenosis from rheumatic heart disease. We would bring donated supplies for the week. I got a used Acuson echocardiography machine with 2 TEE probes donated to the program. During those trips we completed over 100 mitral valve replacements."

David Curtis Fitzgerald

was born in St. Louis, MO. He attended UCSD (BA, Biomedical Engineering, 1980) and then the University of Arizona College of Medicine (MD, 1984). He interned (Internal Medicine) at UCLA and then completed his residency (Anesthesiology) at Stanford (1986-1989). Following residency, he did a 9-month Fellowship (Cardiac Anesthesia) at Stanford. He was appointed an Acting Assistant Professor (Anesthesiology) (1989-1990), then Assistant Professor (1990-1993).

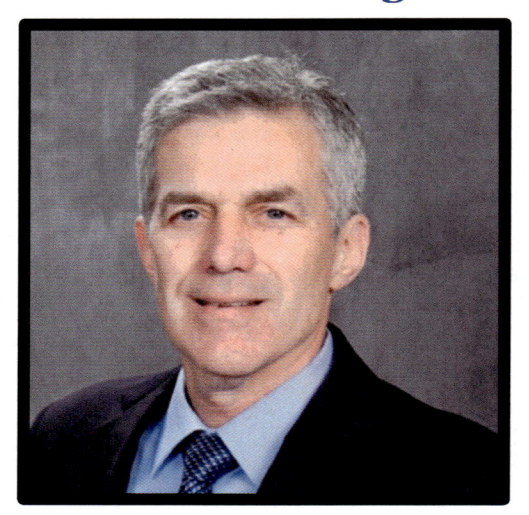

"Stanford residency in the late eighties was the real deal. Great experience, great teaching and groundbreaking clinical experience and research. There really are not many things in life that meet all expectations. Stand out items: I chose the Stanford anesthesia residency because I had an interest in cardiac anesthesia. In the second year of my residency, Tom Feeley called me into his office and said that pediatric cardiac surgeon Paul Ebert abruptly retired from UCSF. Norm Shumway saw Ebert's retirement as an opportunity for Stanford to become the premier center for pediatric cardiac surgery. Shumway called up his protégé, Vaughn Starnes (in the middle of his Fellowship at Great Ormond Street) to head up the new program. Tom Feeley said that the anesthesia department had to quickly provide a high level of pediatric cardiac anesthesia to support Starnes. He said they could no longer rotate residents through cardiac surgery for a one-month rotation as they had done in the past for adults. He asked if I would work exclusively during my third year of residency in the heart room to help get the pediatric cardiac surgery program going. My attendings were Ellen Finch and John Urbanowicz, both clinically outstanding, but with little pediatric cardiac anesthesia experience. Starnes was also clinically outstanding but hadn't finished his foreshortened Fellowship in pediatric cardiac surgery. Starnes would routinely be on the phone to London with his teachers at GOS in the early mornings before cases asking for advice. A challenging and fascinating couple of years. Ray Engstrom joined the team that year. Somehow, we all figured it out, and provided excellent care. We performed many hypoplastic left heart repairs, pediatric heart and heart-lung transplants, and the first living related lung lobe transplant from a parent to their child."

He continued as a Clinical Assistant Professor (1993-1997). After leaving Stanford David had the same career path as fellow resident Ray Engstrom. They both worked for the Medical Anesthesia Consultants (MAC) group (later Envision Physician Services). David was an Executive Vice-President at Envision. He continues to work part time in private practice as an anesthesiologist in the SF East Bay.

"The Stanford routine for transporting cardiac surgery to the ICU (with the infamous ramp that caused hypotension) was with an old-fashioned manometer "to watch the BP bounce". Well, that didn't work for 3 kg infants. John Urbanowicz was able to get the 'pink ladies' who ran the gift shop to buy us the first actual digital transport monitor."

"Working with the two new 'attendafellows', Steve Shafer and Larry Siegel was a pleasure. Both were incredibly smart and energized when they came to Stanford. I learned a lot from both".

Finally, "When the place gets desperate, the desperate get placed" (Jay Brodsky). I probably used that quote hundreds of times (with citation, of course) throughout the years".

Teresa Chun Flory (deceased) graduated from (MD, 1984), did her internship (Transitional) at Stanford (1984-1985), and her residency (1986-1987). She worked for the PAMF.

Rona Greenberg Giffard

graduated from UC Berkeley (AB Biochemistry with honors, Phi Beta Kappa, 1974). After graduation she was in the NIH Medical Scientist Training Program (1978-1984) receiving a PhD (Structural Biology) from Stanford University (1983) and an MD from the Stanford School of Medicine (1985). She interned (Internal Medicine) at Kaiser - Santa Clara (1985-1986). After completed a residency (1986-1989) she was a Fellow (Anesthesia-Neuroscience). She was appointed an Assistant Professor (Anesthesiology) (1990-1997), was promoted to Associate Professor with tenure (1997-2004), and then full Professor (2004). She was also a Professor of Neurosurgery (by courtesy). In 2018 she retired as Professor of Anesthesiology, Emerita, in the Department of Anesthesiology, Perioperative and Pain Medicine.

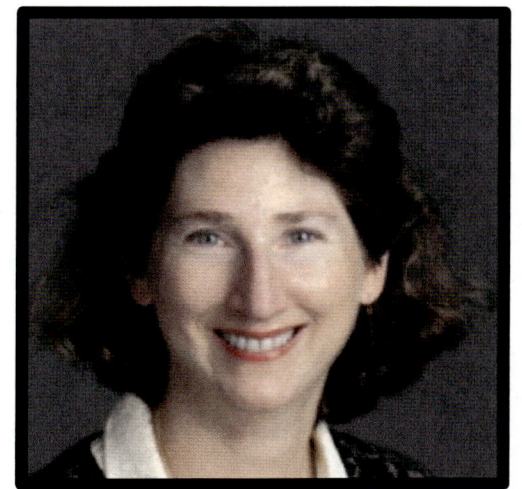

Rona was Vice-Chair for Research in the Department (1999-2012). She was a member of the Faculty of the Neurosciences PhD Program (1992-2018), a member of the Faculty of the Neonatology and Developmental Biology Program (1992-2018), a faculty member of the Program in Molecular and Genetic Medicine (1992-2018), a member of the Faculty of the Cell Biology Program (1993-2018) and a member of Bio-X (1998-2018) - all at the Stanford University School of Medicine

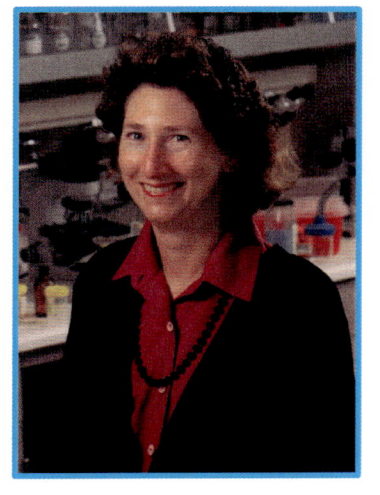

She was a representative on the medical school's Faculty Senate and was Chair of their Steering Committee. She was also Chair of the School of Medicine's Appointments and Promotions Committee and held other important positions at the medical school.

In addition to the ASA, CSA and IARS, she was a member of the American Association for the Advancement of Science, the American Society for Cell Biology, the Association of University Anesthesiologists, the Association for Women in Science, the Society for Cerebral Blood Flow and Metabolism, the Society for Neuroscience, and the New York Academy of Sciences. She served on several journal editorial boards and has been very active mentoring women in medicine and scientists in anesthesiology. Helping young anesthesiologists get academic jobs and set up their labs was one of the highlights of her time at Stanford.

Dr. Giffard published 140 peer-reviewed papers in prestigious journals. Her research was continuously funded by the NIH for 28 years, and she received grants from other agencies and associations. She studied the cellular consequences of brain injury, especially ischemic injury, using primary cultures of neurons and astrocytes from mice, as well as employing rodent models of stroke. She has a special interest in cellular resilience and ways to increase brain cell stress tolerance.

Dr. Giffard has been a Visiting Professor and invited speaker at dozens of venues. Among her many honors and awards are the Department's Ellis Cohen Achievement Award (2009), the Bugher Award from American Heart Association (2000-2004), the IARS Frontiers in Anesthesia Research Award (1998-2003), and the Ellen Weaver Award from the Association for Women in Science, Northern California Chapters (1997).

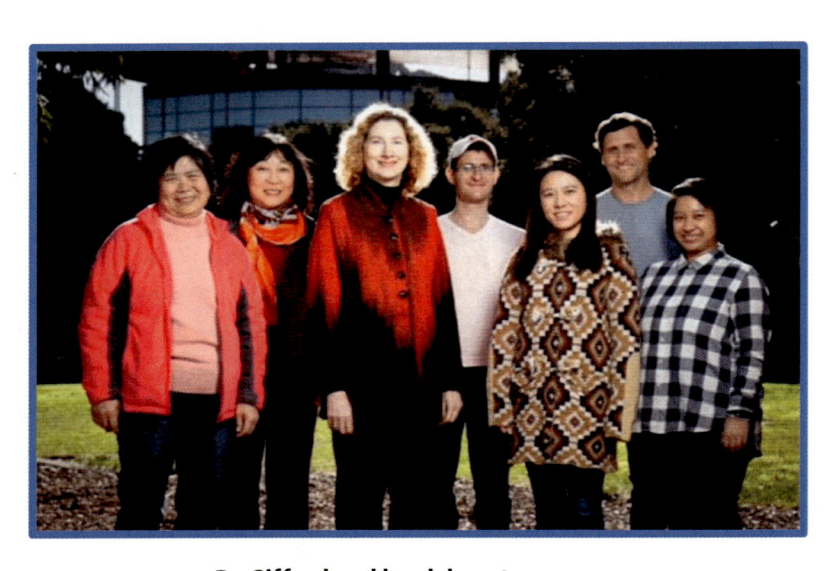

Dr.Giffard and her laboratory group

Malcolm Warrington Howard is a graduate of the University of Virginia (MD, 1979). He completed a CA3 year of training at Stanford (7/1/86-6/30/87). He worked in the local Palo Alto area.

Robert Paul Kaye was born in Queens, NYC. He attended Northeastern University (BS, Pharmacy, 1980) and received his medical degree from SUNY - Buffalo (MD, 1985). He interned at SCVMC (1985). He was an Anesthesiology resident (1986-1989) at Stanford, followed by a Fellowship (Pediatric Anesthesia) at Children's Hospital of Philadelphia (1989-1990). He worked at Children's Hospital of the King's Daughters, Norfolk, VA (1990-2008). He then worked at Joe DiMaggio Children's Hospital, Hollywood, FL (2008-2015) before returning to California as an Associate Professor (Anesthesiology) in the UCD Department of Anesthesiology & Pain Medicine at UCD Children's Hospital, Sacramento (2015-2022). He retired in July 2022.

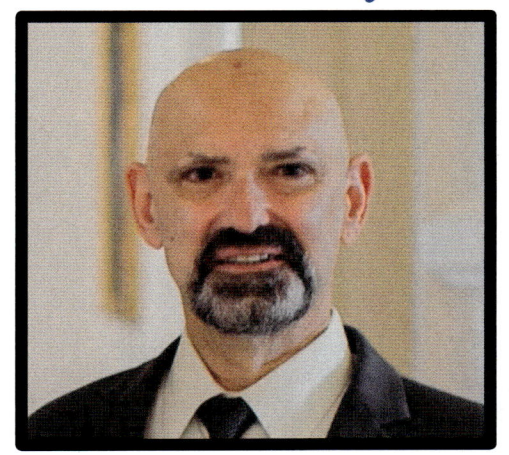

He enjoys underwater photography. He is qualified as a Mindfulness Meditation Teacher by the Center for Mindfulness at the U. Mass Medical School to teach the Mindfulness-Based Stress Reduction course.

Mindfulness is a practice of present moment awareness. Mindfulness increases ability to see things as they arise clearly without judgment. Mindfulness facilitates both focusing and widening our attention as we become aware of ourselves and the world around us. The "goal" is to be more fully present in our lives.

"I feel that I received excellent training in the Stanford Anesthesia Program. I also had a really nice time! I was always treated with kindness and respect."

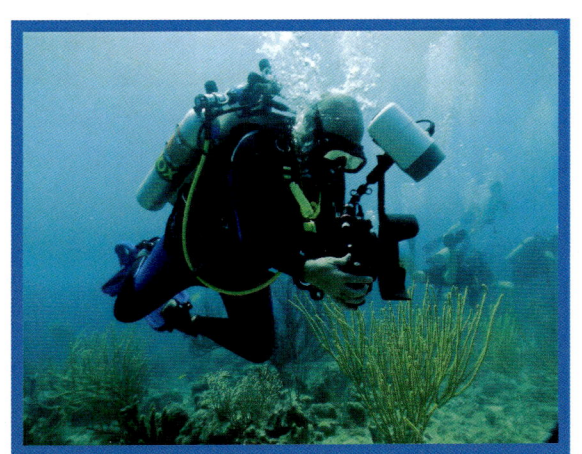

Steve Laurence Marlowe worked at Syntex Research, Palo Alto before attending George Washington University School of Medicine (MD, 1985). He interned and completed his Anesthesiology residency at Stanford. Marlowe worked in Santa Rosa, CA, affiliated with multiple hospitals in the area including Santa Rosa Memorial Hospital, Petaluma Valley Hospital, and Queen of the Valley Medical Center, Napa, CA.

Kristi Lyn Peterson (Decampli) was born in Minneapolis, MN. She attended the University of Minnesota (BS, 1979) and Medical School (MD, 1985). She interned (Rotating) at Hennepin Country Hospital. (1985-1986). She completed her Stanford residency (1986-1989) followed by a Fellowship (Cardiac anesthesia) at PA-VAH (1989-1990). She was then appointed to the faculty as an Assistant Professor (Anesthesiology) in the Medical Center Line doing adult and pediatric cardiac anesthesia at Stanford University Hospital (1990-1997). She left Stanford for the Children's Hospital of Philadelphia as an Assistant Professor (Anesthesiology) at the University of Pennsylvania (1998-2002). She retired from clinical practice in 2002.

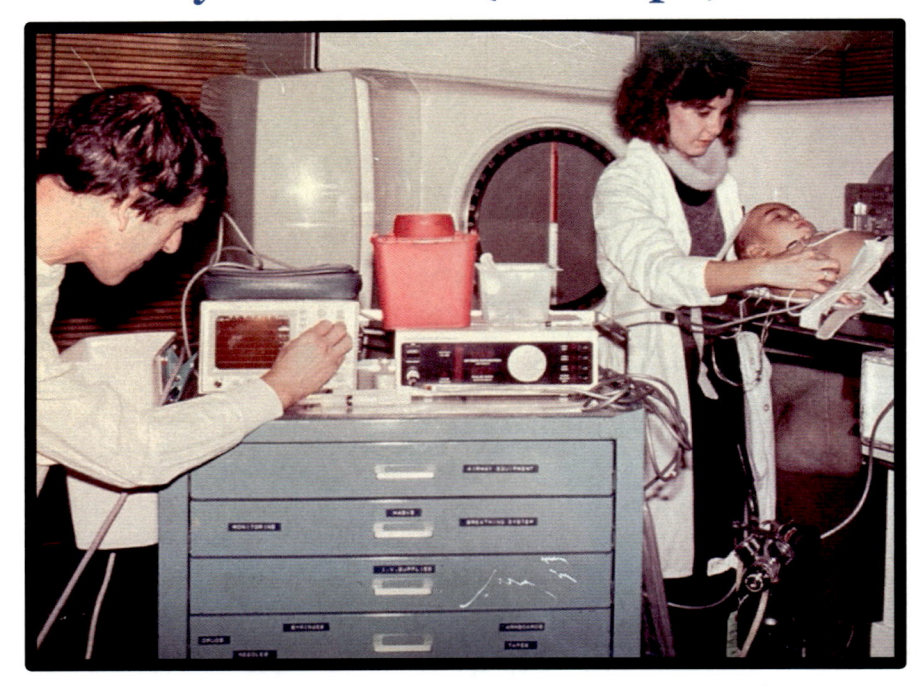

Stanley Samuels and Kristi Peterson performing anesthesia in the radiation suite (1988).

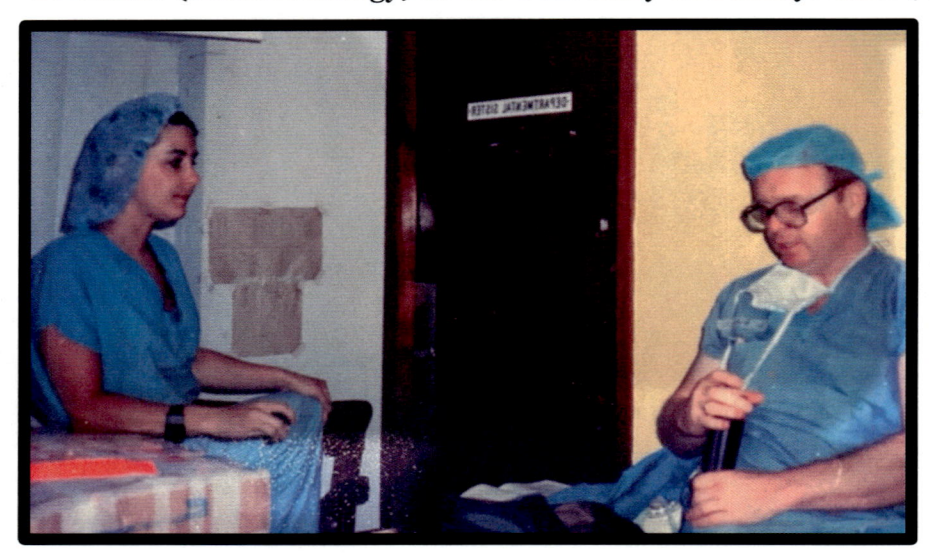

John Redpath and Kristi Peterson on an Interplast mission in Jamaica (1988).

"There were no anesthesia machines, so we used a bag + mask + vaporizer to anesthetize children with cleft lips, palates, and burns injuries."

"Perhaps the fondest memories of my 11 years with Stanford Anesthesia were the opportunities to be in the middle of several trials and innovations in cardiac anesthesia. The first of these was the introduction of aprotinin which was, for a while touted as the "magic bullet" for controlling blood loss after cardiopulmonary bypass. I suppose there are some who still regret its removal from the market!"

"We were interested in achieving early tracheal extubation in pediatric cardiac surgery, which led to our study of the use of regional anesthesia in these patients. It was the laudable willingness of both the anesthesia and cardiac surgical teams to be bold and innovative that led to the remarkable result of extubating 89% of patients in the operating room, with no incidences of sustained neurological problems in 224 consecutive cases. To me, the Department always lived by the counsel that work, like life, begins at the end of one's comfort zone. I salute the Department's long history of contributions to the specialty."

Glenn Douglas Rennels was born in Culver City, CA. He attended Dartmouth (BA, Mathematics, 1977) and earned his medical degree from the Geisel School of Medicine at Dartmouth (MD, 1980). He received a PhD (Medical Information Science, now known as Biomedical Data Science) from Stanford (1986). He did an internship (Internal Medicine) at Berkshire Medical Center (1980-1981), then completed his Anesthesiology residency at Stanford (1986-1989). After training he was simultaneously appointed an Assistant Professor (Computer Science) at the Massachusetts Institute of Technology (MIT) and an Assistant Professor (Anesthesia) at MGH/Harvard Medical School (1989-1990). He left and joined the Permanente Medical group (1990-2013) and was Chief Technology Officer for TPMG (1999-2006). Glenn was awarded the Cecil Cutting Leadership Award (2007). That award recognizes the achievements of physicians who have distinguished themselves as leaders at TPMG. Glenn retired in 2013.

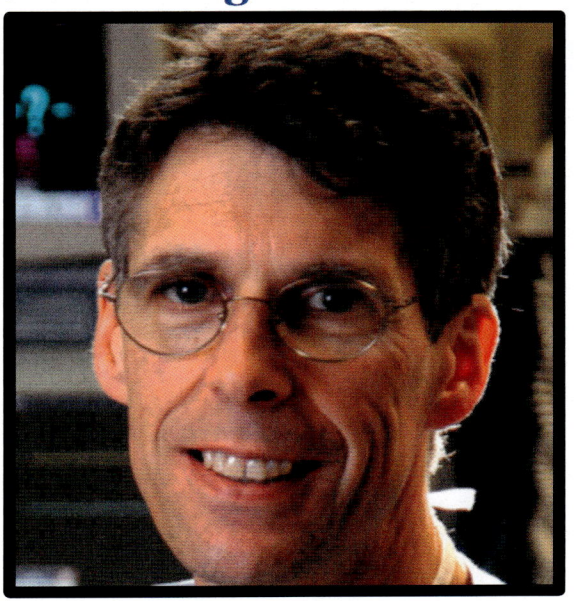

The Cecil Cutting award reads: "Dr. Rennels foresaw the power that the Internet could bring to a medical practice." When many were just learning about information technology for the first time, Glenn Rennels, MD, was already using IT to enhance medical care. Dr. Rennels' considerable expertise helped transform The Permanente Medical Group TPMG into one of the most technologically sophisticated medical groups in the country. His skill and vision in using information technology to improve care to patients became evident soon after he joined TPMG in 1990. After nearly a decade of developing various innovative IT systems, he was tapped to become TPMG's first Chief Technology Officer in 1999. With his leadership, Physician Home Pages, the Personal Physician Selection Online, eConsult, eRx, and eChart were developed and deployed regionwide. Each of his contributions helped facilitate the transition to KP HealthConnect, the electronic medical record system that promises to further enhance

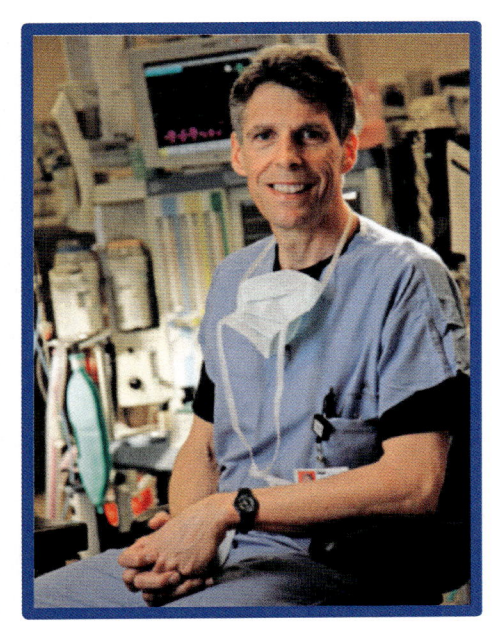

patient care and service throughout Kaiser Permanente. Dr. Rennels also was instrumental in creating the role of Assistant Physician-in-Chief for Technology – a critically important leadership position as Kaiser Permanente continues to implement KP HealthConnect in Northern California. Dr. Rennels recently stepped down from the CTO position in order to resume caring for patients in the Anesthesiology Department at Santa Clara, but he still keeps an eye on emerging technology and is committed to being an influential voice in TPMG.

DARTMOUTH
THE MAGAZINE OF THE GEISEL SCHOOL OF MEDICINE AT DARTMOUTH SPRING '16

ALUMNI ALBUM

In Pursuit of Dual Passions

By Kimberly Swick Slover

Glenn Rennels's colleagues thought it was "a lunatic move" when, in 1990, he gave up an endowed chair at MIT to work in computer technology at The Permanente Medical Group (TPMG). But for Rennels (Med'80), this was the ideal way to unite his dual passions for medicine and artificial intelligence.

After medical school, Rennels went on to earn a PhD in medical information science and complete a residency in anesthesiology at Stanford University, followed by his appointment to MIT's Cabot Chair for Artificial Intelligence in Medicine. But he was drawn to TPMG by the opportunity to practice anesthesiology, while also helping to transform the organization into one of the nation's most technologically sophisticated medical groups.

Rennels and his colleagues designed a popular application that acts as the equivalent of match.com for patients in search of primary care doctors. Later, as TPMG's chief technology officer, he led the development of eConsult, a complex and novel computer system in which he takes obvious pride.

"When a primary care physician refers a patient to a specialist, eConsult facilitates specialty care before the patient leaves the PCP's office," Rennels explains. "Immediately, eConsult asks the primary care doctor problem-specific questions designed by the specialist. Then eConsult specifies x-rays and labs to be completed prior to the specialist appointment, books the appointment, gives instructions for interim care, and prints patient-education handouts pertaining to the problem."

All 5,000 doctors in Rennels's group embraced eConsult because it enables the PCP and specialist to become a close-knit team, accomplishing more together than when they were working separately.

After 23 years at TPMG, Rennels recently stepped down to work independently, with plans to pursue the next innovations in medical technology. He believes his location in Silicon Valley could be a fertile environment for growing his own startup on the next frontier of health care.

"The conveniences provided to patients when they can connect with doctors via video links such as FaceTime are tremendous, especially as the population ages," Rennels says. "For a 75-year-old patient, it's onerous to troop into a doctor's office. It's exciting to think that through the use of video conferencing and wearable sensor technologies, some of those interactions could be done from a patient's home, making the physical distance to the doctor's office less of an obstacle to care."

For Rennels, software design and medicine are "creative and wonderful processes."

"I love them both and have devoted my career to finding touchpoints between the two," he says.

George E. Wakerlin Jr was born in Chicago. He attended the University of Iowa (BS, 1978). In college he was awarded the Nile C. Kinnick Memorial Scholarship (1976) and placed 10th in the NCAA national high-bar competition (1976). He received his medical education at Stanford (MD, 1985) followed by an internship (Flexible) at SCVMC (1985-1986). He completed his residency (1986-1989) followed by a Fellowship (CCM) (1989-1990) at Stanford. He originally worked as an independent anesthesia contractor (1990-1993), then as a staff anesthesiologist at Kaiser – Vallejo (1993-2022). He briefly returned as an independent contractor (2022-2023) and retired in March 2024. He is a life-long tennis enthusiast.

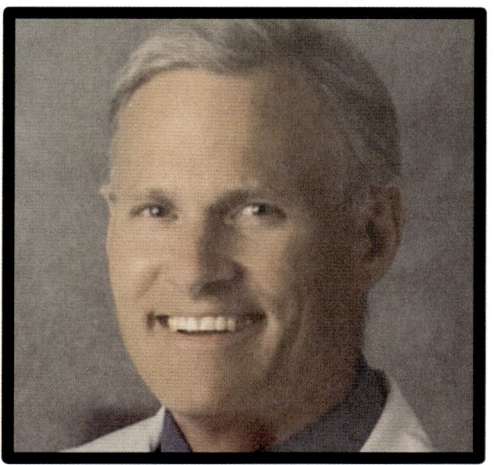

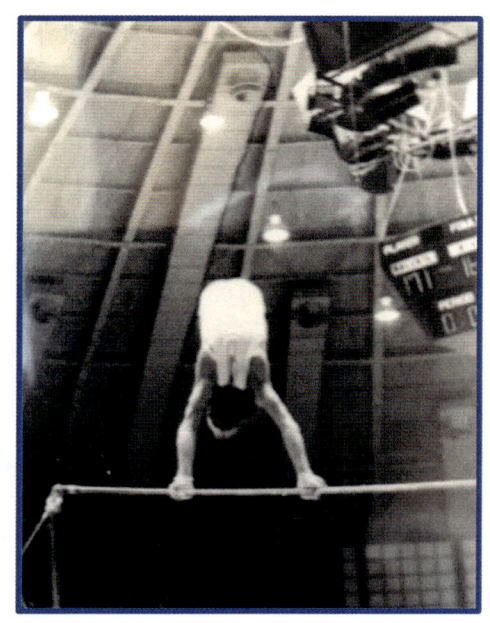

"I had a fascination with ultrasound starting at Stanford, it continued throughout my practice. Its biggest value was when I was an ICU Attending at Kaiser in the OR anesthetizing unstable patients. While on call I got short of breath at age 43. My workup - EKG, CXR - were negative. I was told "it's just Kaiser". I turned the echo on myself and found my own atrial septal defect. It was repaired at UCSF by a pediatric cardiologist in 1998 (clamshell closure). I'm still here!😁"

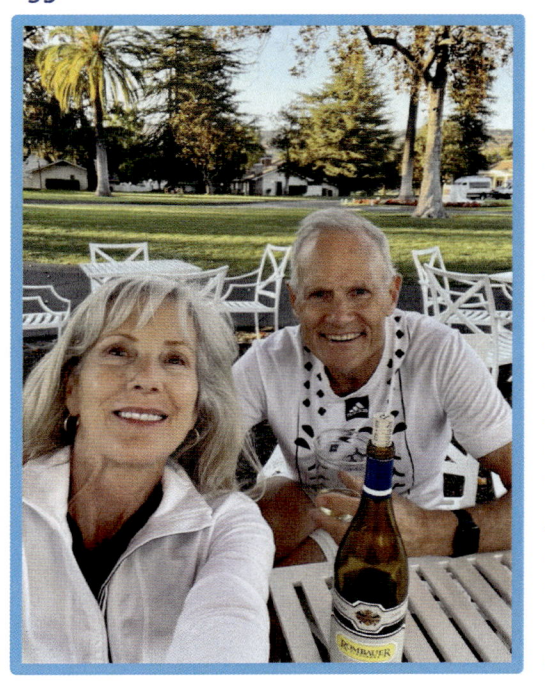

"Fred Mihm/ SF Zoo 1988; Siberian tigress needing hysterectomy for bleeding; 10 mg/kg blowdart x3; before finally falling asleep, then 20+ foot leap from back to front of large cage fully 8 feet upright, grabbing the bars loudest ROAR ever; Fred after 5 seconds of group paralysis said, "I don't think those bars are thick enough". Residents into cage for iv start and more ketamine before the 200-yard transport to the OR; mask induction with forane and an 8-liter bag; then Fred performed manual intubation, deep anesthesia (no muscle relaxants), Fred's arm to elbow inside the tigress; Fred's words to me, "George, your residency depends on your holding the (spring loaded inter-canine) device steady!!!"

Steven L. Shafer attended Princeton University (AB, Biology, 1978) and received his medical degree from Stanford (MD, 1983). He interned (General Medicine, 1983-1984) and then did his Anesthesiology residency at the University of Pennsylvania (1984-1986). He was Chief Resident his final year. He then completed a Fellowship (Clinical Pharmacology) at PA-VAH under the mentorship of Donald Stanski (1986-1988). Steve was appointed to the staff at the VAH (1987) as a Clinical Instructor (Anesthesiology). He was promoted to Assistant Professor (1988-1994), Associate Professor (1994-2000), and then full Professor (2000-2007).

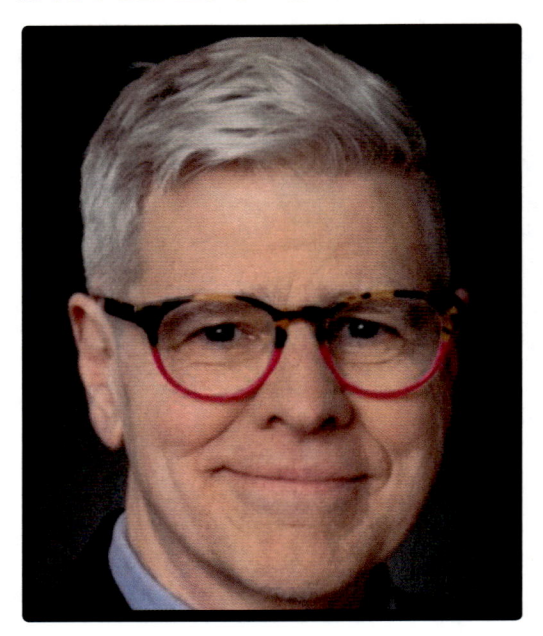

He left for a position as Professor (Anesthesiology) at Columbia University College of Physicians and Surgeons (2007-2012), but returned to Stanford in 2012. At Stanford he did research in the clinical pharmacology of intravenous anesthetics and the development of novel methods of pharmacokinetic and pharmacodynamic analysis. He taught residents clinical anesthesia and worked with many Fellows teaching research methodology. Dr. Shafer was also an Adjunct Associate Professor (Bioengineering and Therapeutic Sciences) at UCSF (2001-2022).

Steve is a pioneer in target controlled intravenous (TCI) anesthesia. He created mathematical models that characterize drug behavior. Early in his career he created and then placed the program *STANPUMP* ('STANford infusion PUMP') in the public domain. STANPUMP is an open-source software platform for anesthetic drug TCI, as well as the pharmacokinetic engine for most, and perhaps all, commercialized TCI systems worldwide. More recently he developed *STANPUMPR*, an R implementation of pharmacokinetic algorithms for many of the commonly used perioperative drugs.

Dr. Shafer was Editor-in-Chief of Anesthesia & Analgesia (2006-2016). He has been an editor for the journals Anesthesiology, Clinical Pharmacology and Therapeutics, the British Journal of Anaesthesia, the Journal of Pediatric Anesthesiology, and is currently the Editor-in-Chief of the ASA Monitor (2020-Present).

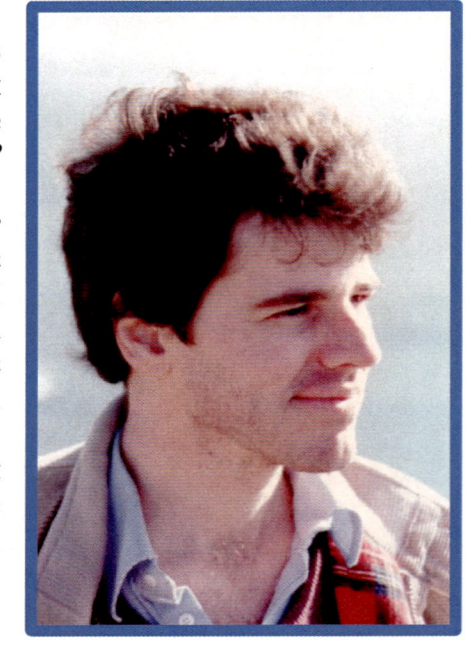

Steve Shafer during his Fellowship at Stanford (1986)

"My work in publication policy and ethics follows my years as editor-in-chief of Anesthesia & Analgesia. From 2006-2016 we uncovered two of the most prolific serial academic fraudsters in history - Joachim Boldt and Yoshitaka Fujii. I finished my term as at A&A with the unenviable record of retracting more papers for research fraud than any previous editor of any journal, ever. This led to a lasting interest in

publication policy and ethics. In collaboration with others, I continue to develop statistical models to detect fraud, and serve on multiple editorial boards to offer guidance on publication policy and ethics."

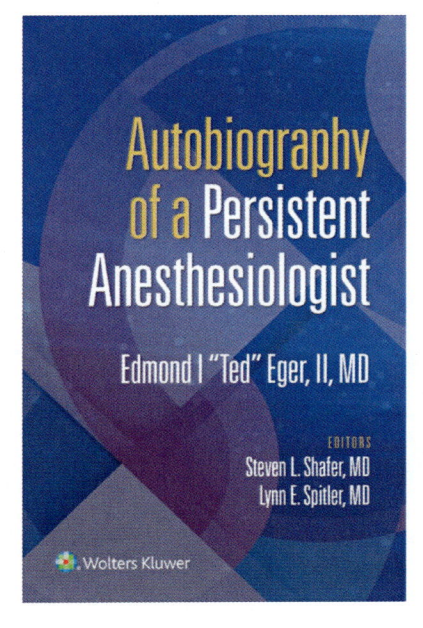

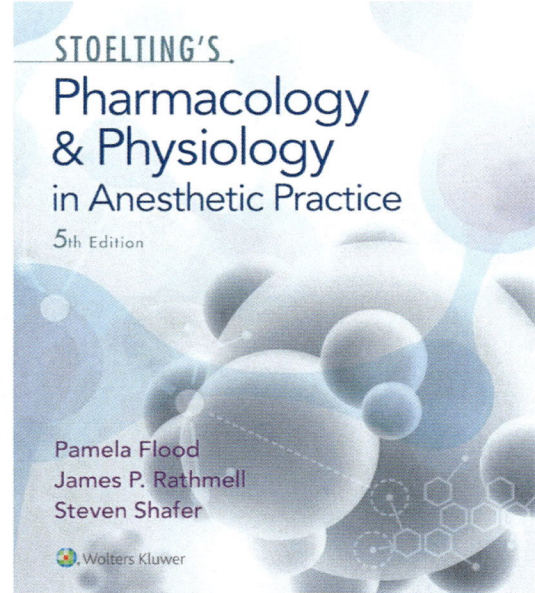

He has been on numerous committees for national organization and was the President of the International Society of Anesthetic Pharmacology, the Vice-President of the World Society of Intravenous Anesthesia, and on the Board of Directors of FAER. He was the Director of the Center for Scientific Integrity, and the Director of the World Association of Medical Editors. He has more than 200 peer reviewed research publications, dozens of chapters in medical textbooks, and he co-edited several books on pharmacology.

Dr. Shafer is the Founder of Soft-Pack, Inc (1976-1981). Softpack developed accounting, inventory control, job costing, and project management software for small manufacturing companies. He is the founder Aesculapius Systems (1982-1988). Aesculapius developed software to assist in the documentation of patient history and physical examinations. It also linked to early databases of disease signs and symptoms. He was also a founder of PharmacoFore (1991-1998). He is also a co-founder of Signature Therapeutics (2003-2014).

Signature Therapeutics, Inc. is a biopharmaceutical company focused on creating best-in-class medicines that address unmet needs in the areas of pain management and anesthesia. The goal of the company is to improve patient care by developing molecules that retain the efficacy of commonly used pain and anesthetic agents while reducing or eliminating unwanted side effects and safety concerns using their proprietary abuse-resistant Bio-MD™ opioid prodrug technology.

Shafer is a co-Founder and former Vice-President for product development for Pharsight Corporation (1991-2001) and helped develop Pharsight's commercial products, including WinNonlin, WinNonmix, and Pharsight's information products.

His professional interests include data modeling and at the start of the COVID-19 pandemic he would send weekly modeling updates on COVID-19's world-wide morbidity and mortality to members of our Department.

He was the recipient of the Department's Faculty Teaching Award (1990) and the Ellis Cohen Achievement Award (2020). He has been invited to lecture at hundreds of national and international meetings. He is only one of two anesthesiologists (the other is Jim Eisenach) who have delivered all three of the named lectures at annual ASA national meetings (FAER/Helrich Lecture (2009), Severinghaus Lecture (2015), and Rovenstine Lecture (2021)). He has been awarded the Bernard H. Eliasberg Medal, Mt. Sinai Medical Center (2006), a Lifetime Achievement Award from the International Society of Anaesthetic Pharmacology (2011), and the Lewis Sheiner Award, International Society of Pharmacometrics, Washington, DC (2015).

Shafer appeared as an expert witness for the prosecution at the Michael Jackson manslaughter trial.

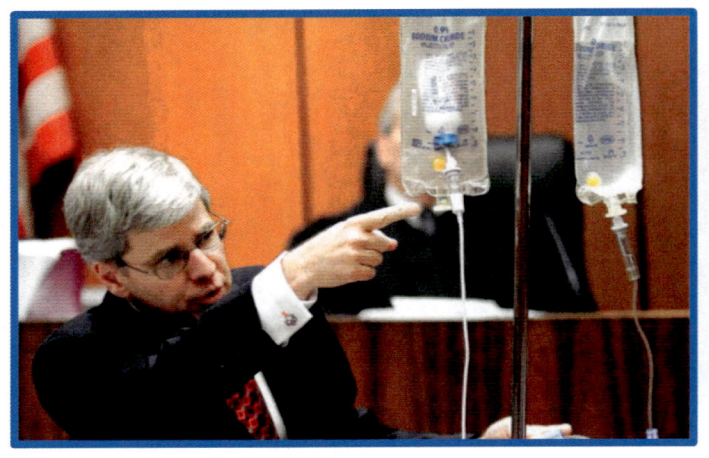

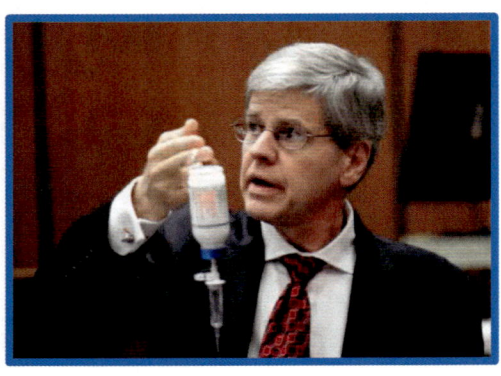

"I developed an interested in the role of clinical pharmacology to criminal law following my testimony on behalf of the State of California in the trial of Conrad Murray for the death Michael Jackson. I continue to provide pro bono testimony in criminal cases involving anesthetic drugs."

Steve retired as Emeritus Professor, Department of Anesthesiology, Perioperative and Pain Medicine in 2023. He and his wife Dr. Pamela Flood, a former Stanford Professor of Anesthesiology live in a bucolic farmhouse in Port Angeles, WA.

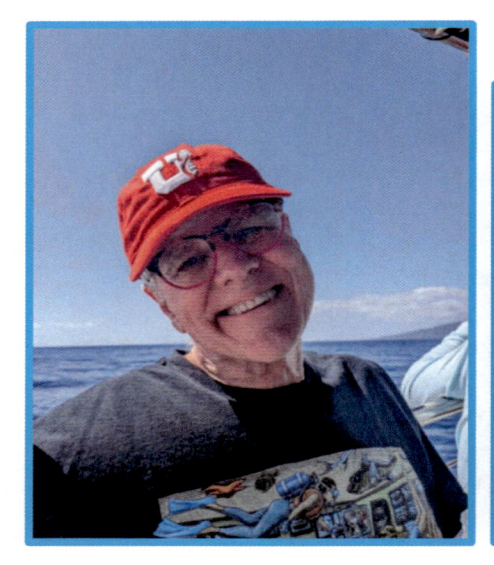

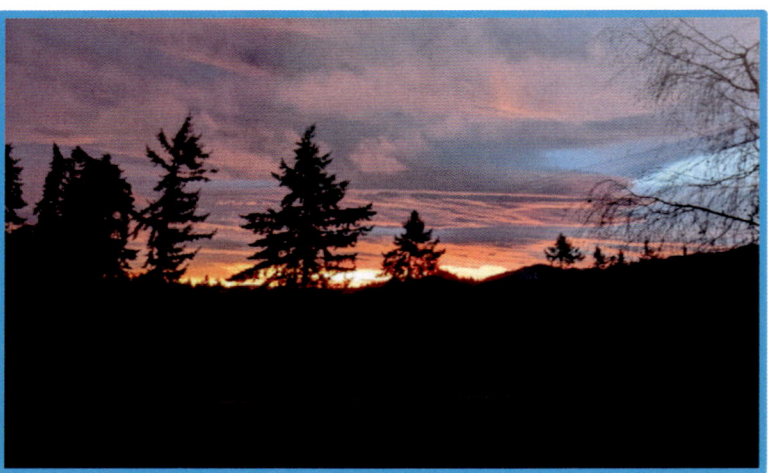

Lawrence Charles Siegel earned a BS (Electric Engineering) at MIT, then received his medical degree from the Harvard-MIT Program in Health Sciences and Technology (MD, 1983). After internship (Internal Medicine) (1983-1984) he completed a two-year Anesthesiology residency at the University of Pennsylvania (1984-1986). He spent an additional CA3 year of Fellowship training at Stanford (1986-1987). In 1988 he was appointed a tenure-line Assistant Professor (Anesthesiology) eventually rising to Associate Professor. In 1996 he left Stanford to become Chief Technical Officer for Heartport, Inc., Redwood City (1996-2001). He has been the Chief Medical Officer (CMO) at several other medical equipment companies.

Two CA1 residents starting in 1986 did not complete their training.

Frederick Jonathan Long attended Harvard (MD, 1985) and did an internship (Surgery) at the Icahn School of Medicine at Mount Sinai Hospital (1985-1986). He completed six months of an Anesthesiology residency at Stanford (7/1/86-12/16/86). He quit the program and did a residency (Psychiatry) at Mount Sinai, NY (1990-1993). He practiced psychiatry in New York City.

Robert Joseph Cosgrove attended the University of Miami School of Medicine (MD, 1985). He did an internship (Transitional) at Healthsouth Metro West Hospital (1985-1986) and was a Stanford Anesthesiology resident (1986-1988). He did ' 'improper behavior'.

CHAPTER 6

RICHARD A. JAFFE

We lost a dear friend and colleague in June 2023. Richard Jaffe's many contributions to patient care and to the sub-specialty of Neuroanesthesia cannot be overstated.

Richard A. Jaffe (deceased) was born in Alameda, CA, on September 22, 1947. He grew up in Hayward. He graduated from UC-Berkeley with a bachelor's degree in Vertebrate Zoology. He then earned a master's degree (Biology, 1971) from California State University-East Bay.[1-2] His degree dealt with a new technique of continuous measurement of testicular blood flow in a conscious rat. In 1976 he received a PhD (Neurophysiology) from UCSF. His PhD was entitled 'Electrophysiologic and pharmacologic properties of mammalian sensory neurons'.[3]

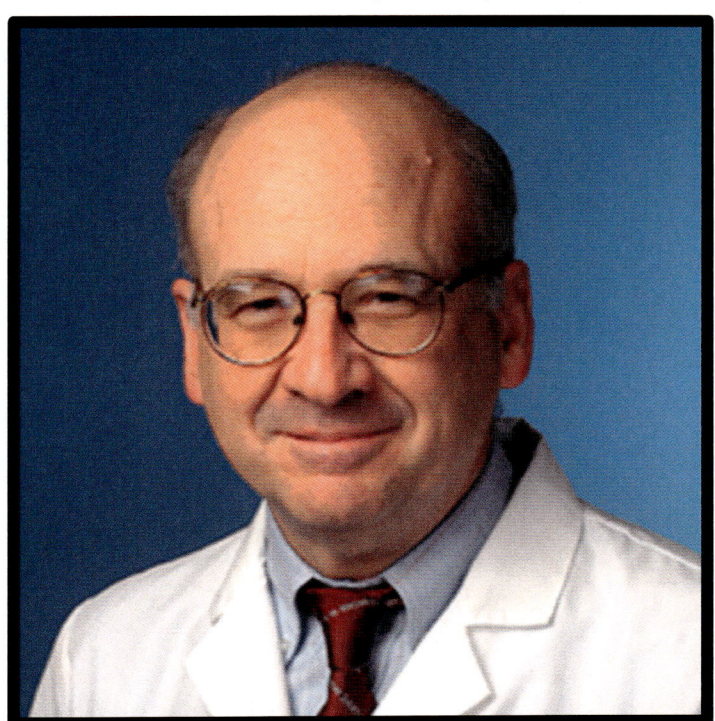

John Brock-Utne: "After earning his master's degree Richard was accepted at UCSF to do a PhD. He needed a car and asked his father to lend him money to buy one. "What do you know about cars?" was his father's reply. Richard said, "It is a horseless carriage with 4 wheels." At that point his father put his hands up and Richard thought that was the end of that. A week later a tow truck drove into the family's driveway with a wrecked car. The wreck was dumped onto the driveway and the tow truck disappeared. His father appeared and said, "I bought you this car for $25. You make it work and I will pay for all the parts that are needed". We all who know Richard how he responded to a challenge. Of course he succeeded."

After his PhD at UCSF, he and his wife Judy left for Washington where he was appointed an Assistant Professor (Physiology) at Washington State University (WSU) and the Director of the Neurophysiology laboratory at the Pacific Northwest National Laboratory. In 1981 he was promoted to Associate Professor at WSU.

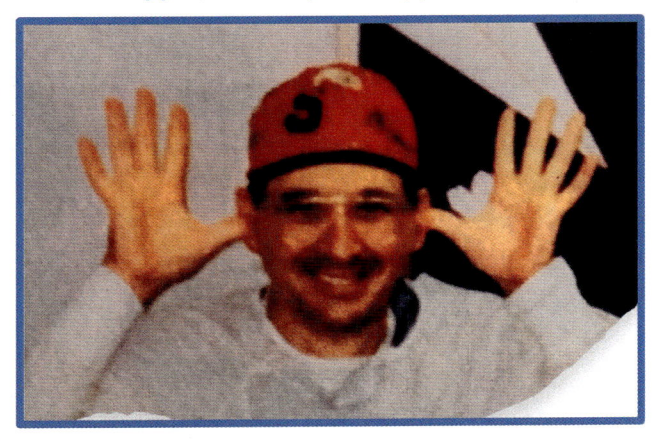

Even as a resident, Richard Jaffe always had a smile.

In 1983 at 36 years of age, he decided to attend medical school. Due to his background, he was able to earn his medical degree from the Miller School of Medicine at the University of Miami in just 2 years (MD, 1985). He interned at Providence St. Vincent Hospital, Portland, OR (1986) and then came to Stanford for his Anesthesiology residency (1986-1988).

Once his training was complete, he was appointed to the faculty as an Assistant Professor (Anesthesiology) in 1989. In 1994 after working on neurosurgical cases with his mentor Phil Larson, Jaffe was made Chief of Neurosurgical Anesthesia at Stanford. Richard Jaffe quickly rose through the academic ranks and was promoted to Associate Professor, and then full Professor in 2000. He was also by courtesy a Professor of Neurosurgery.

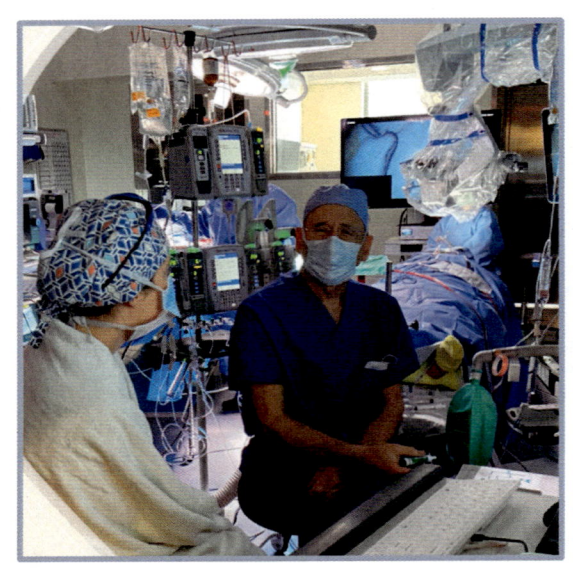

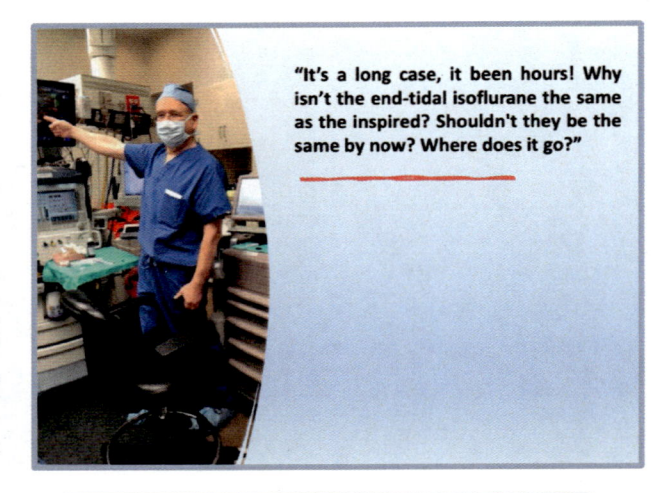

"It's a long case, it been hours! Why isn't the end-tidal isoflurane the same as the inspired? Shouldn't they be the same by now? Where does it go?"

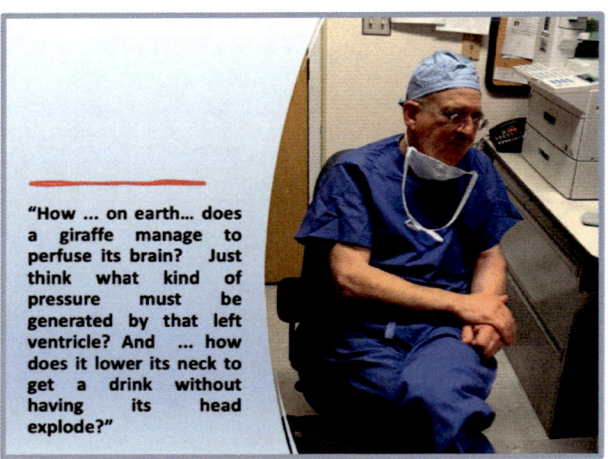

"Ok ... just one more question, and then I'll let you have lunch."

"The President has been flying on Air Force One to visit the Queen of England and suddenly the plane is taken hostage by terrorists! You are armed with only a bottle of isoflurane. How many milliliters of isoflurane would you need to safely anesthetize everyone on the plane and extract the president?"

"How ... on earth... does a giraffe manage to perfuse its brain? Just think what kind of pressure must be generated by that left ventricle? And ... how does it lower its neck to get a drink without having its head explode?"

In addition to working with anesthesia residents during their Neuroanesthesia rotation, Jaffe trained many clinical Fellows. Several of Jaffe's Fellows have continued in our Department and remain the core of its Neurosurgical Anesthesia Division.

Sarah Stone (Former Resident and Neuroanesthesia Fellow) – "He loved his job and coming to work – his work was really important and meaningful to him. He loved to teach more than anything."

Many will remember that Richard always had a slightly mischievous grin just before he would ask an impossible question to an unsuspecting resident or Fellow. The questions were at times so far out that even he might not have known the answer. His goal was to make you think.

Jaffe's specialty was administering anesthesia during extracranial to intracranial bypass procedures for Moyamoya disease working with neurosurgeon Gary Steinberg. He was often the first to test new technology in the ORs. Jaffe published numerous peer reviewed papers in both the areas of Neurophysiology and Anesthesiology. With colleague Stanley Samuels, they edited 'The Anesthesiologist's Manual of Surgical Procedures' first published in 1994. That book is now a classic anesthesia textbook and is in its 6th edition.

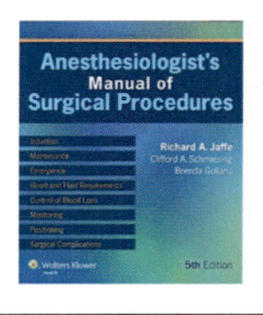

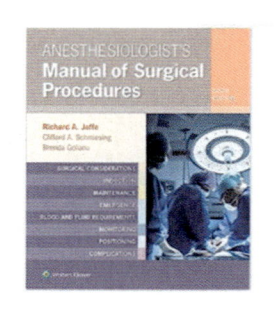

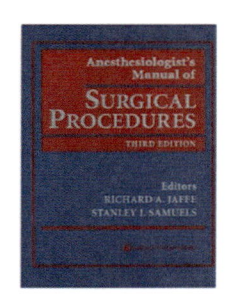

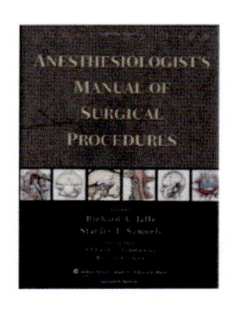

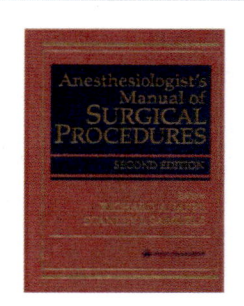

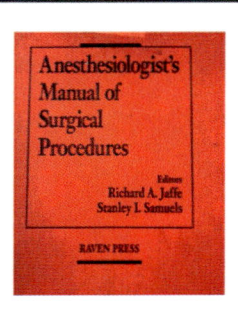

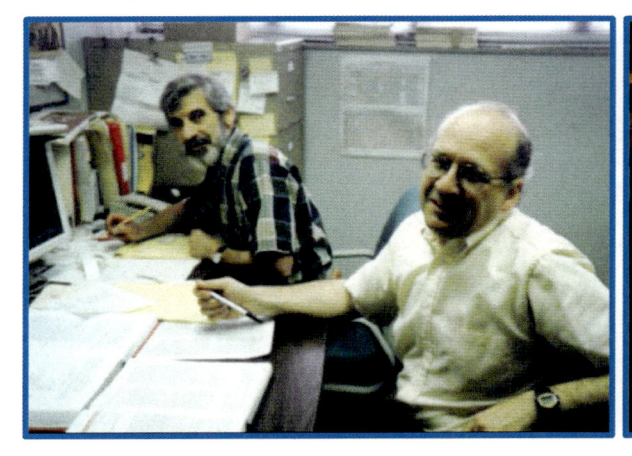

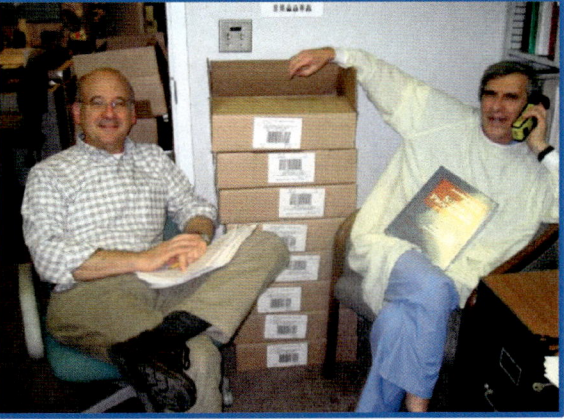

Stanley Samuels and Richard Jaffe published the 1st edition of their book "The Anesthesiologist's Manual of Surgical Procedures" in 1994. It is currently in its 6th edition.

101

Brian Bateman (Current Chair, Department of Anesthesiology, Perioperative and Pain Medicine) – "Jaffe was extremely well known worldwide for his work in neuroanesthesia, particularly for his textbook. It was one of the first books I purchased many years ago. He was particularly beloved as a teacher of the residents and was someone the residents respected tremendously."

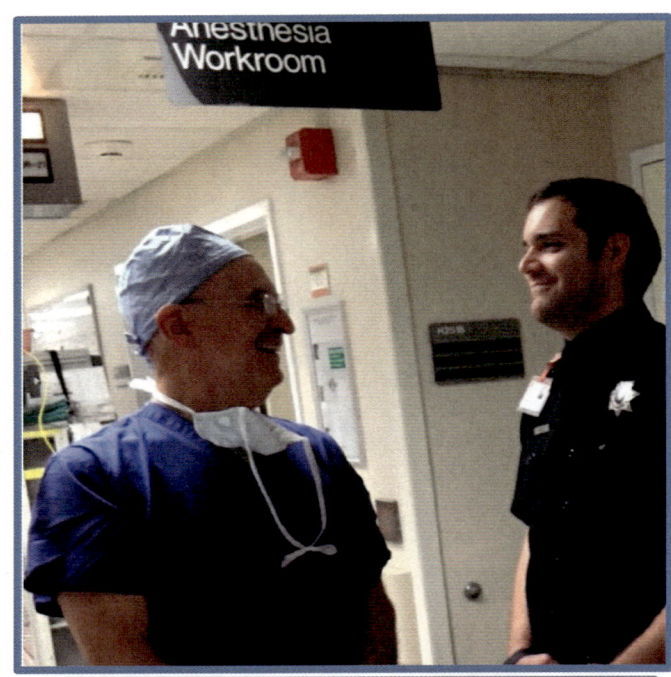

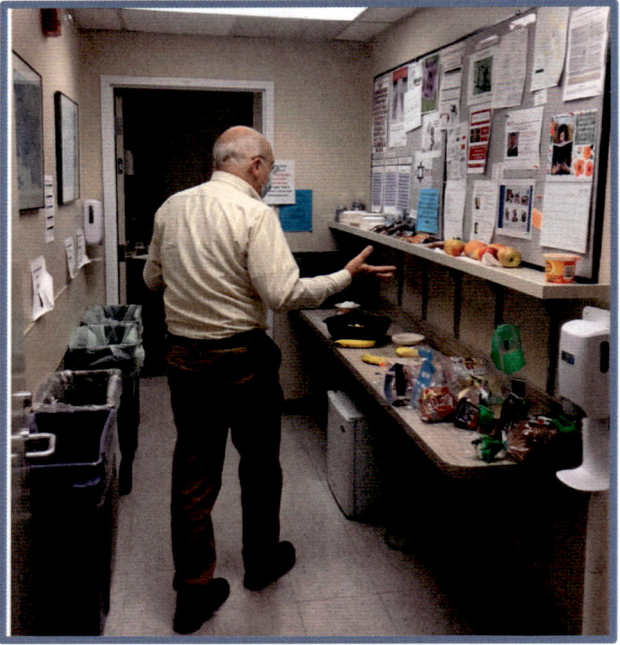

At the hospital Richard was never pompous. He had a wonderful sense of humor and an engaging personality. He was friends with everyone – nurses, physicians, technicians, as well as hospital employees like cleaning staff and orderlies. He knew most by their first name and he would always be prepared to stop and have a chat.

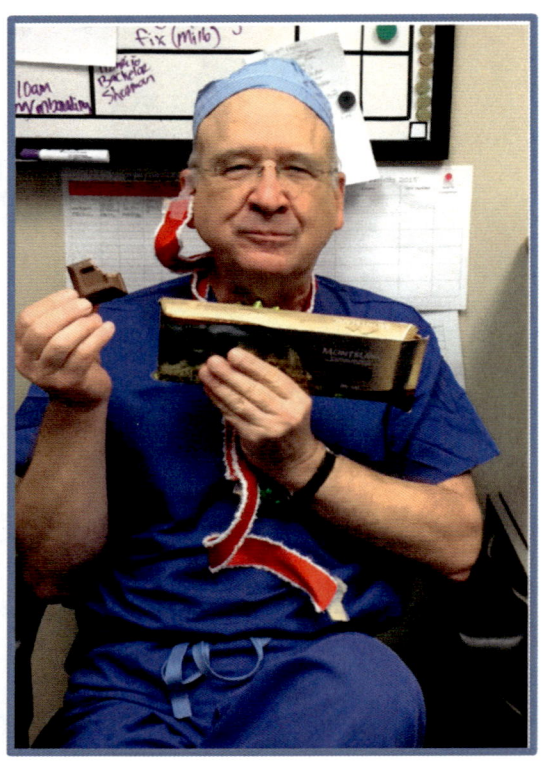

Everyone knew he was obsessed with chocolate, and he frequently received gifts of chocolate and baked goods from people he worked with.

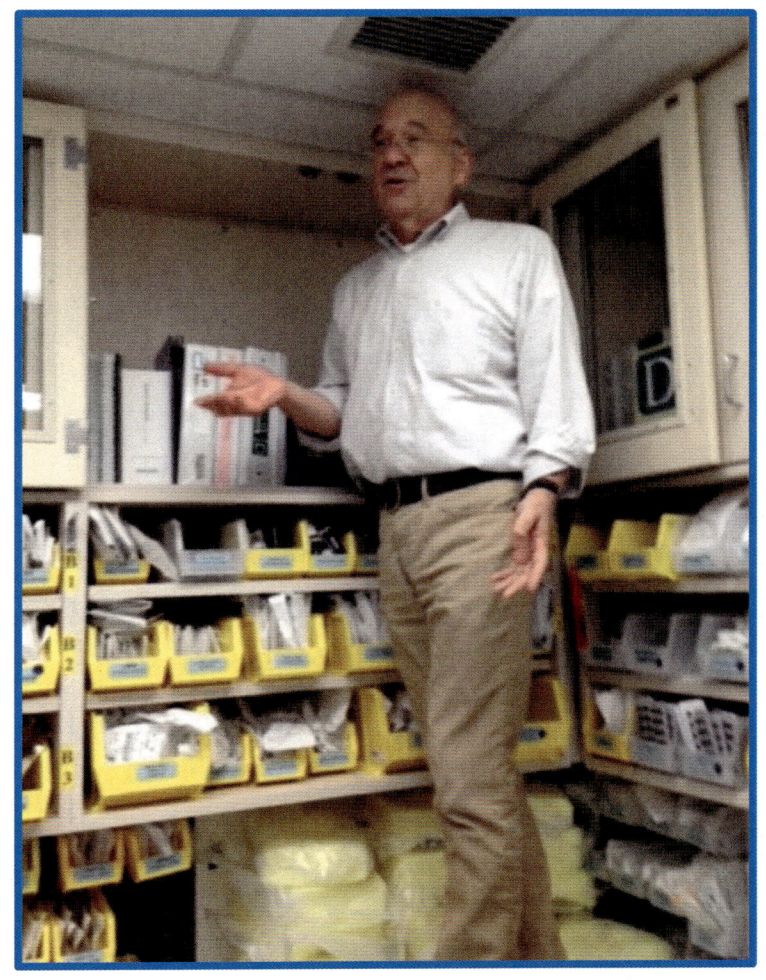

John Brock-Utne (Colleague) – For the anesthesia faculty he was a person people would go to for advice on clinical matters. For our residents he was an icon among their teachers."

Jaffe became ill in 2020 during the Covid pandemic. Even while confined to his home he continued up until his death advising faculty and residents on complex cases by telephone.

Judy (wife) – "He didn't want anyone to see how bad his illness was. He could go from feeling really bad - and then somebody from work would call, and he would just be his regular old hardy self, all full of energy and smarts."

Just weeks before his death Anesthesiology News highlighted Jaffe and co-investigator John Brock-Utne's years-long fight to revise guidance regarding the storage of spiked intravenous bags. (**see: Anesthesiology News, March 7, 2023 - Elimination of the USP 1-Hour Rule: A Spike Through the Heart of the Matter**). The recommendation was to dispose of IV bags after only one hour if at room temperature. Jaffe and Brock-Utne demonstrated that there was no risk of infection even after nine days at room temperature. Based on their work, guidelines were revised to allow 24 hours of safe storage, potentially saving the hospital millions of dollars.

John Brock-Utne: "Richard managed to overturn the falsely US Pharmacopeia (USP) mandate of a 60-minute spiking rule for commercial IV bags. In about 2014 USP informed The Joint Commission (TJC) that all IV bags must discarded after 60 minutes if they have not been attached to a patient. The exception would be if the IV bag had been spiked in a Class 5 "clean room". This room classification is the top of the line of cleanliness requiring over 400 air changes per hour. A space suit is required to enter a Class 5 room. To be clear spiking of IV bags in medicine had been going on for over 100 years without any concerns or any evidence about problems with sterility. Richard was very vocal about this madness. So, with no financial support we showed that IV solutions were completely sterile after 9 days even after they were spiked in a busy anesthesia workroom. Based on these results Stanford decided not to build a Class 5 clean room and basically ignored the USP mandate. However, in 2021 the TJC again, quoting USP, said Stanford must have a Class 5 clean room. It was then that Richard with a stroke of genius wrote to the USP and copied the high command of Center of Medicare and Medicaid Services (CMS). He wrote -"Does the USP have any evidence that using an IV fluid bag that had been spiked for more *than 60 min is unsafe? If so then, the USP is obliged to disclose that evidence with its significant implications for patient safety. Failure to do so could have already led to patient harm with a serious medico-legal liability for USP." Within 3 weeks of his writing, USP withdrew their objection to the 60-minute rule. No reason was given! Had this rule not been challenged by Richard every hospital in this country would have to have to build at least one Class 5 sterile room to spike ALL IV bags. Each of these sterile rooms would cost at least $4-5 million, so you can do the math on how much money Richard Jaffe saved the US health budget."*

Richard collaborated with both the basic scientists and clinical anesthesiologists in the Department on studies.[4-5] John Brock-Utne and Richard Jaffe formed an especially close working relationship, and they co-authored more than 30 published papers together.[6-7]

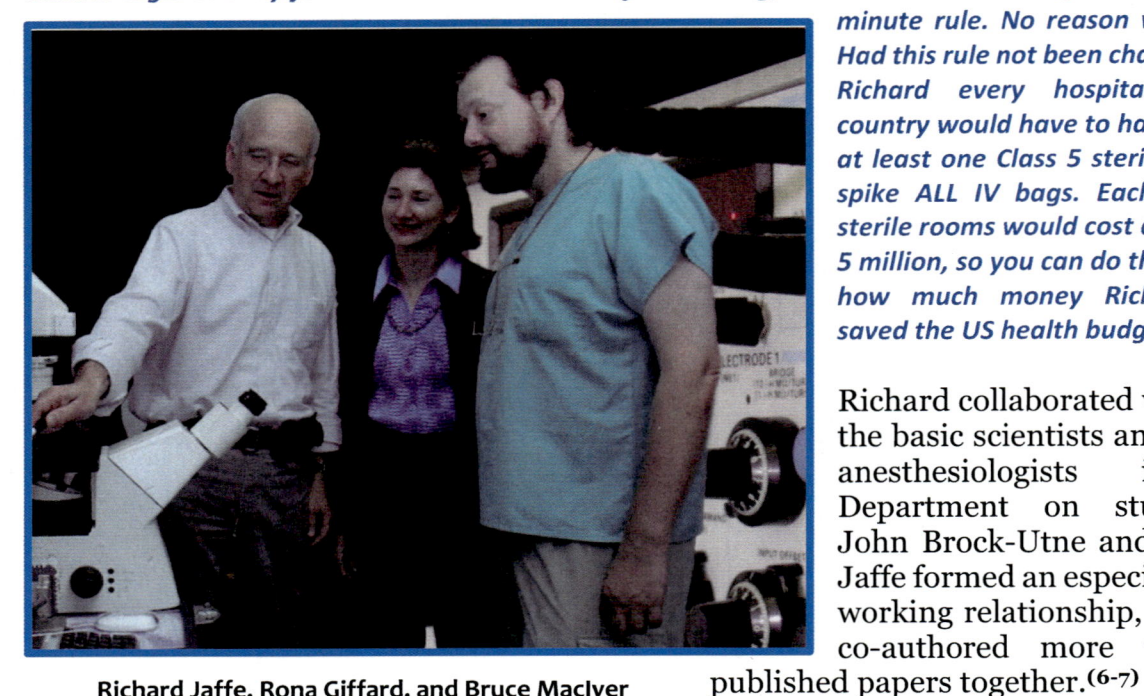

Richard Jaffe, Rona Giffard, and Bruce MacIver

John Brock-Utne recalls – "I first met Richard in January 1989. His intellectual curiosity and his ability to ask the right research questions were what most impressed me at that time. Together, in 1990, we managed to get the first HP ultrasound machine into the Stanford ORs for research purposes, under the direction of the then Chair Barrie Fairley. We published several clinical studies using this new technology and commenced a prolific research relationship. We continued working together for the next 30+ years.

Richard Jaffe's clinical and technical skills both inside and outside the neurosurgery suite were impressive. All our residents will recall he taught subclavian line placement in the era before and after the use of ultrasound made internal jugular line placement the standard for central venous access. He felt an IJ line would interfere with positioning his neurosurgical patients.

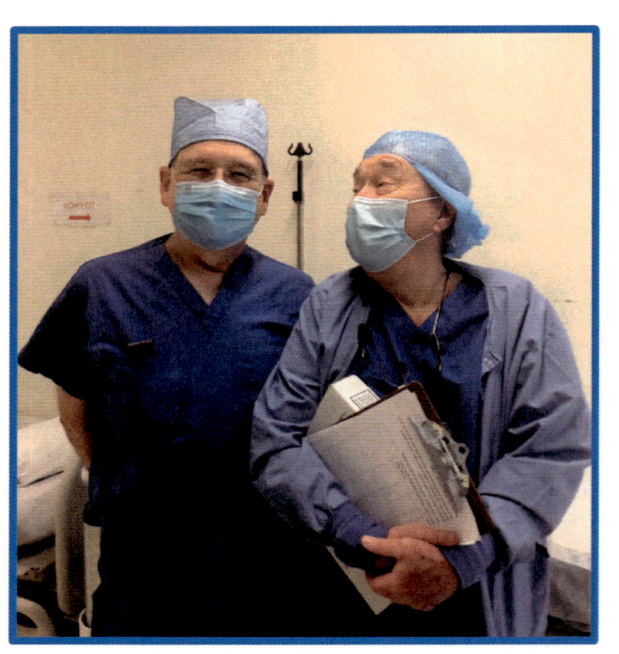

Richard and John Brock-Utne with a hoard of chocolates

104

Brock-Utne – *"One night we were both on call (1st and 2nd) at Stanford. The board was empty, and we thought this was our opportunity to go home. Suddenly there was a "code blue" call from one of interventional radiology rooms. When responded and entered a very dark room. We found a very large patient who was severely cyanotic. Her underlying diagnosis was a Superior Vena Cava Syndrome. Her neck was severely swollen. The Rapid Response Team (RRT) had attempted to secure an airway but were unsuccessful. A quick assessment with the laryngoscope confirmed the RRT findings. A tracheostomy set had been produced and an ENT surgeon had been called. We were told that it would be another 10 minutes before he would arrive. Richard said: "Well we better get on with an emergency tracheostomy". Richard dissected with his fingers and identified the trachea so I could place a 5.0 endotracheal tube. The patient survived and went home. Richard, however, was never tired of telling the story that I had nicked his finger when I cut into the patient's trachea! The entire procedure took 2-3 minutes."*

Richard Jaffe won the H.B. Fairley Teaching Excellence Award in 1994, 2011, and 2012 – the only three-time award winner in the history of the Department.

Richard and wife Judy enjoyed traveling to Europe and Hawaii. They drove to the Oregon coast for three weeks every year walking along the beaches and hiking through the woods. He also enjoyed gardening at his Stanford campus home. He was a collector of 6–8-foot metal dinosaurs that he placed all around his garden. He was an accomplished wood and metalworker and an avid nature photographer. Many people didn't know that Jaffe was also a certified magician and airplane pilot.

After his death his former residents and Fellows published a book entitled "In Memory of Richard Jaffe". It contains photographs and emotional tributes from scores of his trainees, colleagues, and friends.

His contributions to clinical care, education, and research were recognized by hospital and school leadership with a Celebration of Life which was attended by hundreds of people.

Lloyd Minor (Medical School Dean) – "Richard Jaffe's skill as an anesthesiologist was instrumental in the successful treatment of thousands of neurosurgery patients. He was incredibly devoted to his residents and their education. He will be dearly missed."

Ronald Pearl (Former Department Chair)– Richard was always looking to improve clinical care, the department, the hospital, and the medical school. He created a leading neuroanesthesia division that has saved countless lives and trained hundreds of anesthesia residents not only to provide safe neuroanesthesia but to think through problems that occur in the operating room."

YOU ARE INVITED TO A

Celebration

IN HONOR OF

DR. RICHARD JAFFE

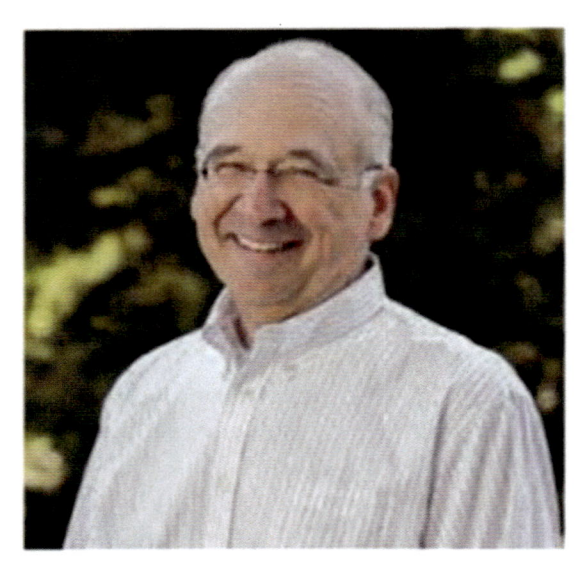

FRIDAY, JULY 14

6:00-8:00PM

Faculty Club
439 Lagunita Dr, Stanford, CA 94305

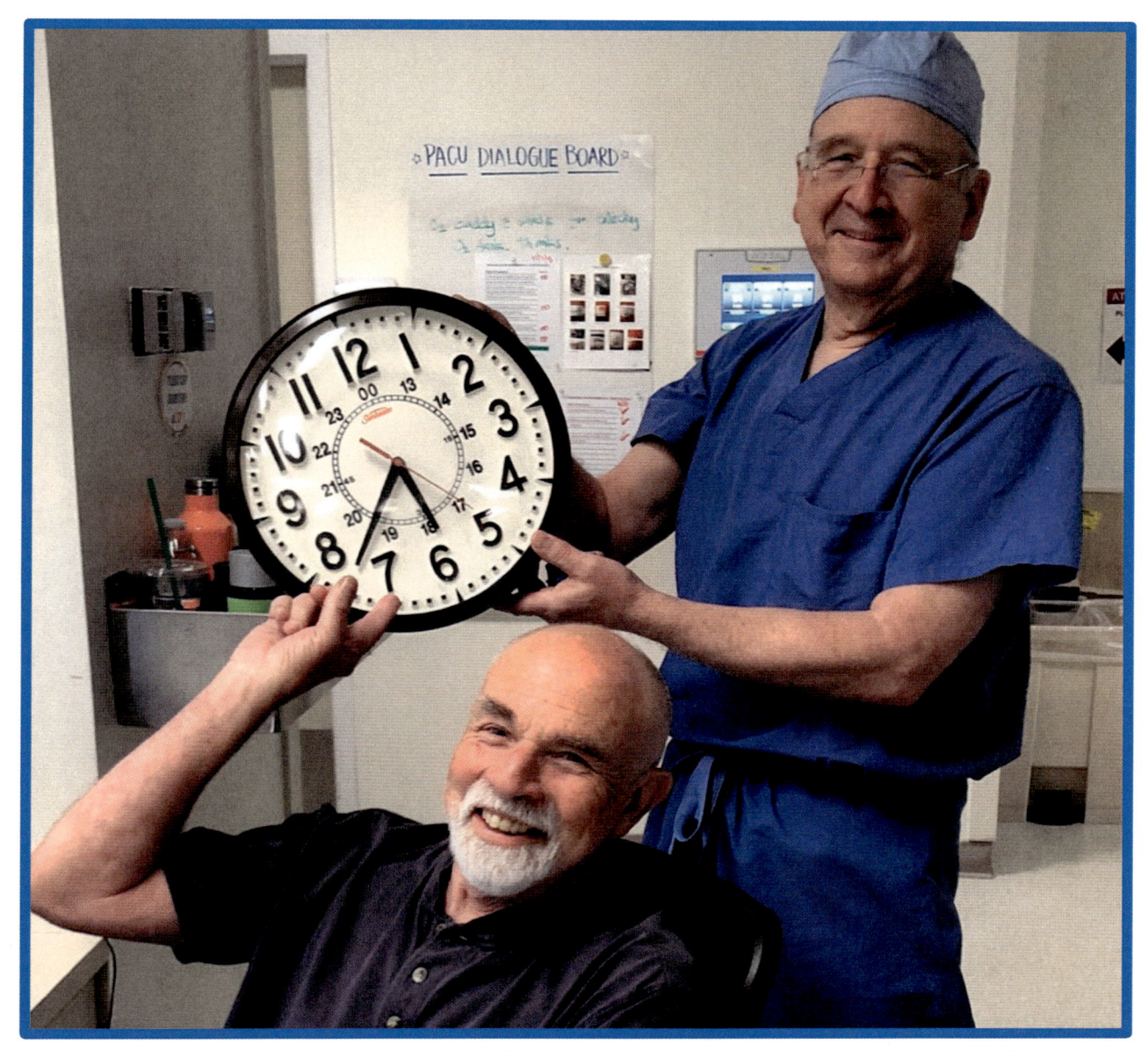

Richard indicates that Jay Brodsky is still at the hospital is after 5 pm when he is <u>not</u> on call.

Jay Brodsky … "Richard was a close colleague and a very dear friend. We enjoyed playing pranks on each other. Each time a new edition of his Manual was published, I would write a ridiculous review that he would then send to his publisher. The latter would always believe the review was real. Richard would often cut and paste photos of me on cartoons. The OR Scheduling Office has a collection of these photos on the wall."

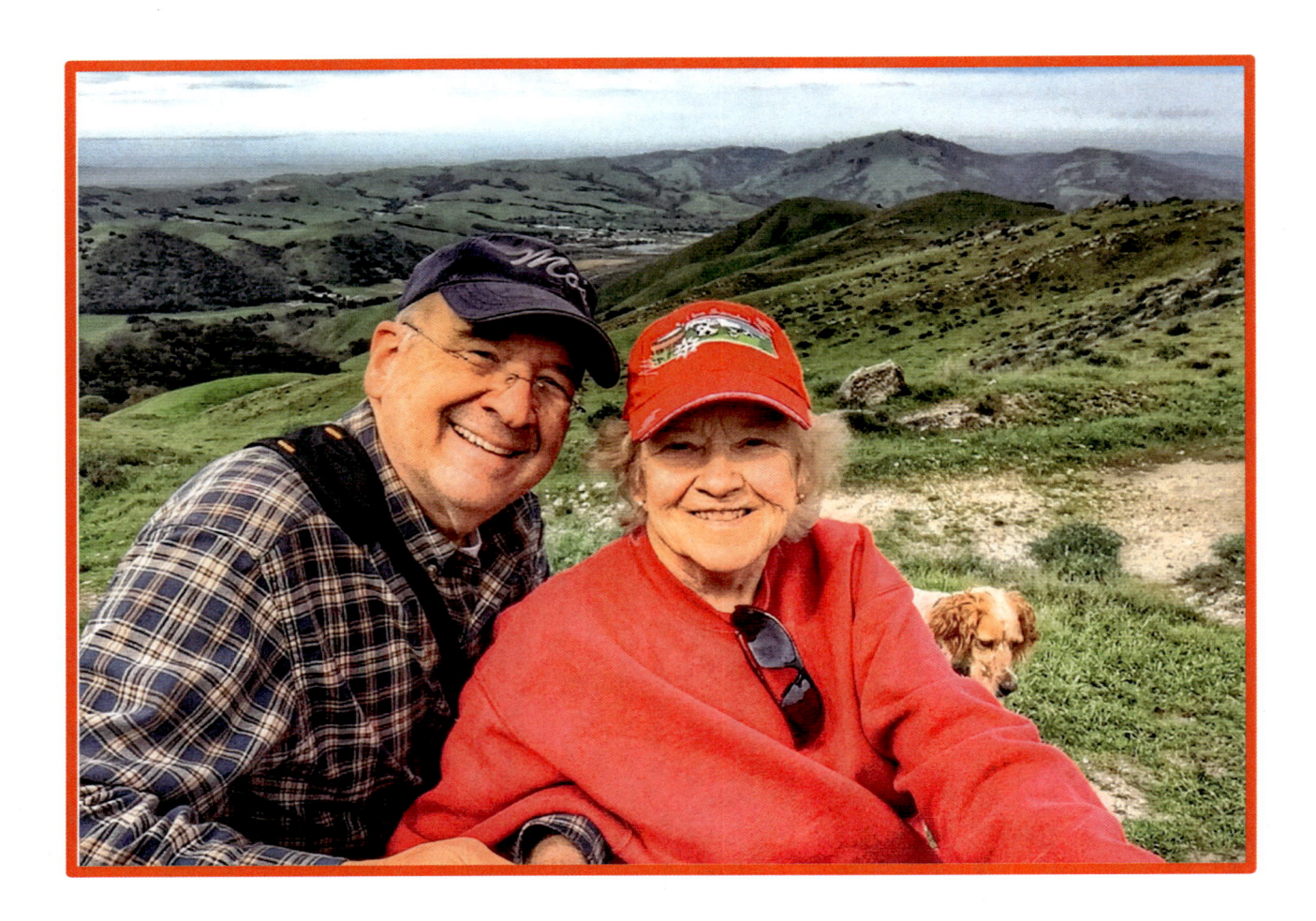

REFERENCES

1. Jaffe RA, Free MJ. A miniature friction flowmeter for use in rat testicular artery and other small vessels. J Appl Physiol (1972) 32:571-573.
2. Jaffe RA, Free MJ. A simple endotracheal intubation technic for inhalation anesthesia of the rat. Lab Anim Sci (1973) 23:266-269.
3. Sampson SR, Nicolaysen G, Jaffe RA. Influence of centrifugal sinus nerve activity on carotid body catecholamines: microphotometric analysis of formaldehyde-induced fluorescence. Brain Res (1975) 85:437-446.
4. Jaffe RA, Pinto FJ, Schnittger I, Siegel LC, Wranne B, Brock-Utne JG. Aspects of mechanical ventilation affecting interatrial shunt flow during general anesthesia. Anesth Analg (1992) 75:484-488.
5. MacIver MB, Bronte-Stewart HM, Henderson JM, Jaffe RA, Brock-Utne JG. Human subthalamic neuron spiking exhibits subtle responses to sedatives. Anesthesiology (2011) 115:254-264.
6. Brock-Utne JG, Sanford J, Jaffe RA. Overregulation Revisited. Anesth Analg (2017) 124:1743.
7. Brock-Utne JG, Smith SC, Banaei N, Chang SC, Alejandro-Harper D, Jaffe RA. Spiking of intravenous bags does not cause time-dependent microbial contamination: a preliminary report. Infect Control Hosp Epidemiol (2018) 39:1129-1130.

CHAPTER 7
1987

On April 19th, 1987, *The Simpsons* cartoon was first shown on The Tracey Ullman Show airing on the newly launched Fox television network. In March, the first Starbucks outside the USA opened in Vancouver, Canada. By 2022 there were 35,711 Starbucks worldwide in 84 countries. President Ronald Reagan delivered his famous speech at the Berlin Wall on June 12th where he implored Soviet Union leader Mikhail Gorbachev to "tear down this wall," urging him to include the reunification of Germany as a part of Gorbachev's 'perestroika' (restructuring). At Mecca on July 31, a demonstration by Iranian pilgrims against the "enemies of Islam" resulted in Saudi police shooting demonstrators causing a stampede that resulted in 402 deaths. The first Intifada in the Israeli-Palestinian conflict began in the Gaza Strip and West Bank on December 8th. Other noteworthy events that year included the FDA's approval of fluoxetine (Prozac) for use as an antidepressant, and the Nobel Prize in Literature being awarded to Russian poet Joseph Brodsky thus becoming the first Brodsky to win that esteemed prize. The 1987 season went down in the record books as one of the finest in Stanford's baseball history as the Cardinal under head coach Mark Marquess set a then-school record with 53 wins and captured the College World Series championship.

Senator Joe Biden made the first of many unsuccessful attempts running for President, while a smiling mayor Bernie Sanders believed that music was a "powerful way to communicate with the downtrodden masses".

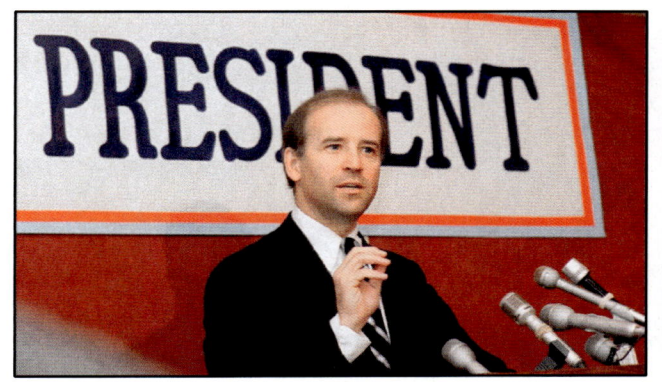

Senator Joseph Biden (D-Delaware) speaks in Boston during a presidential primary campaign trip through New England (1987).

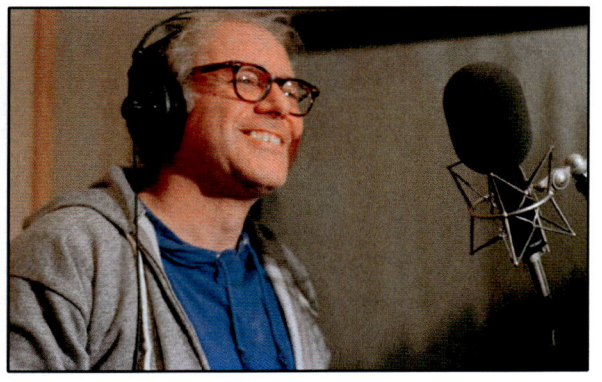

An *extremely rare* photo of a smiling Bernie Sanders, then mayor of Burlington, Vermont. He is pictured singing during a recording session in Nov 1987 taping 5 songs and a discussion of his "philosophy" (1987).

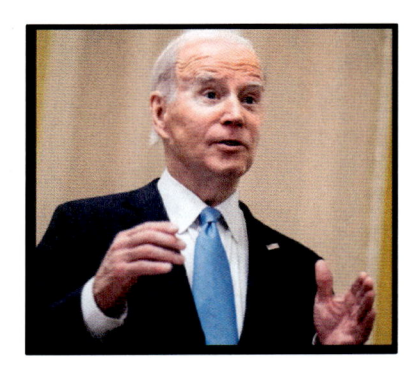

President Joe and Senator Bernie (2023)

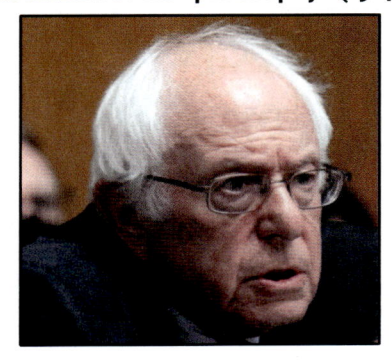

On May 24th, 1987, an unknown number of Stanford anesthesia residents were among the more than 800,000 people who crowded onto the deck of the Golden Gate Bridge to celebrate the 50th anniversary of the bridge's opening.

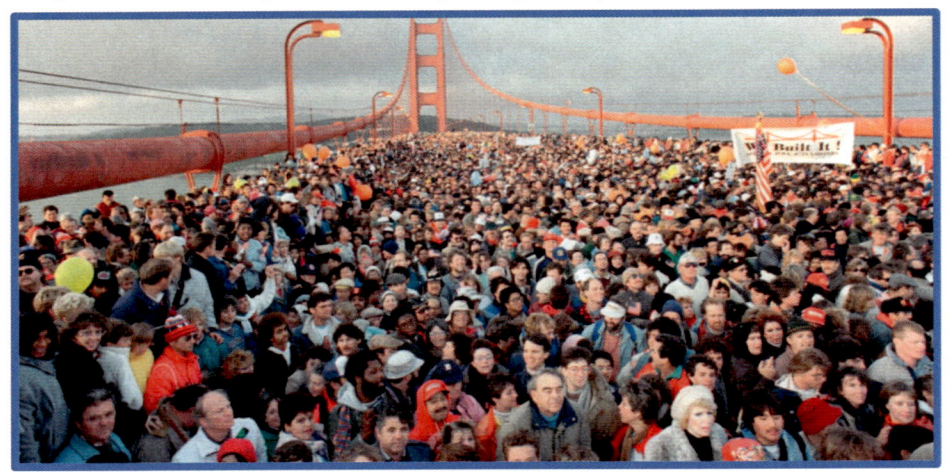

A crowd estimated to be more than 800,000 people on the Golden Gate Bridge

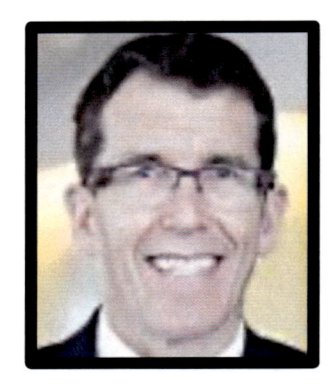

John Hoffman Archer graduated from Stanford (MD, 1986). He interned and completed his Anesthesiology residency (1986-1989) and was Chief Resident his final year. He did a Fellowship (Pediatric Anesthesiology) at Stanford (1989-1990). He worked at Saint Christophers Hospital for Child and Adolescent Health and the Society Hill Anesthesia Consultants, Philadelphia, PA.

Carolyn Anita Bahl received a BA (Biophysics) from the University of Pennsylvania (1976-1980) and then attended Stanford Medical School (MD, 1986).

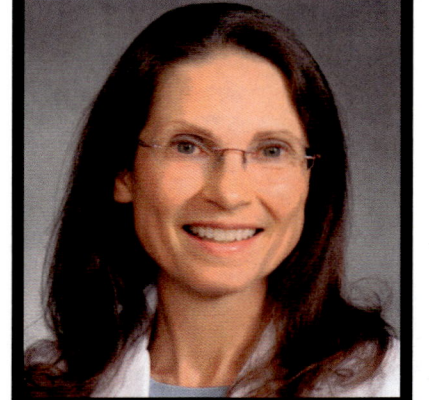

"When I was a medical student at Stanford, my first clinical rotation was two weeks of OR anesthesia. I loved everything about it, from those important pre-op moments with a patient, to fast paced high stakes situations, to hands on care, to seeing physiology in action, to discussing backpacking routes on breaks. I was hooked. I went on to do a rotation in the Pain Clinic where I did my first epidural with Dr. Lorne Eltherington, and when they closed for construction, I was able to finish the rotation in OB where I was able to do my first labor epidural with George Albright, as well as get a personal lecture on the cardio- toxicity of bupivacaine.

Needless to say, the superb experience as a medical student greatly influenced my choice of Anesthesiology as a career."

She interned (Internal Medicine) at Kaiser - Santa Clara (1986-1987) and then did her Anesthesiology residency (1987-1990). She worked at Kaiser – Santa Clara (1990-1992) and South Sacramento Medical Center (1992-2020). She was on the Department's volunteer clinical faculty (1990-1992). Carolyn retired in 2020. Her interests include outdoor sports, health and fitness, gardening and reading.

- *I was very grateful to continue at Stanford for my residency. Two very special programs that I was able to be a part of were the Critical Care Transport Team, transporting critical patients or harvesting organs for transplant, and going on an Interplast trip.*
- *One of my best memories was going with a Stanford anesthesia team to Peru to provide for children having cleft palate and cleft lip repairs. Parents would walk for days and camp outside the hospital for their child to have a chance for repair. Supplies were limited and we had to wash and reuse endotracheal tubes. IVs were disconnected at an extension and used for another patient. One young boy had significant bleeding post op and we had to rush him back to the OR late at night. We ended up packing the nasopharynx with a tampon to stop the bleeding. A family member donated the whole blood needed for a transfusion. I'll never forget the hug from that little boy the day we left.*
- *One of my worst memories was the attending at Santa Clara who would surreptitiously turn off flow to the copper kettle vaporizer on the anesthesia machine to see how long it would take the resident to notice something was amiss.*
- *There were not many female attendings when I was a resident, and it was wonderful to have Drs Audrey Shafer and Sheila Cohen as role models. Audrey was also my faculty mentor and a great support to me during my training.*
- *The anesthesia program increased from 2 to 3 years just after I started. The training was still set up to cover all the bases in the two years, so I had the opportunity to do a six-month concentration in Pediatric Anesthesia, effectively a Fellowship without the research. With that focus, I started my career with TPMG at Kaiser - Santa Clara. I was fortunate to be hired by the department Chair, Dr. Sonja Sorbo (a former Stanford resident and Fellow), who met me for lunch while on maternity leave. When I had my first child, Dr. Sheila Cohen was my anesthesiologist, coming in from home to place my labor epidural, and standing by as I narrowly avoided an emergency C-section.*
- *When life circumstances led me to Sacramento, I transferred to the South Sacramento Kaiser to start up OB anesthesia for a soon to open Labor and Delivery Department. From that point on, OB anesthesia became my "baby". I have a lot of gratitude to Dr. Cohen, not only for a strong foundation in this area, but also for the Stanford OB anesthesia resident's handbook, and more than a few conversations as I worked through the nitty gritty of covering all aspects of providing anesthesia care in what quickly became a very busy Labor and Delivery suite. The pediatric training did not go to waste, as for a time we also managed all the neonatal resuscitations.*
- *Over the years, much changed in the practice of OB anesthesia, and we adapted and evolved to maintain cutting edge care. I was part of the Perinatal Patient Safety Project at our hospital and for the Kaiser Northern California region, and the statewide*

California Maternal Quality Care Collaborative, working on multidisciplinary teams to ensure safety in routine and emergency care through protocol, training, and simulations. We went on to become a Level 2 trauma center and developed plans for trauma care in the pregnant patient.

"I am so grateful to my attendings and mentors for a solid preparation for a challenging career. While I loved all the technical and intellectual aspects of anesthesiology, it was the connection with patients, in what was often a life defining event for them, that has made it most rewarding."

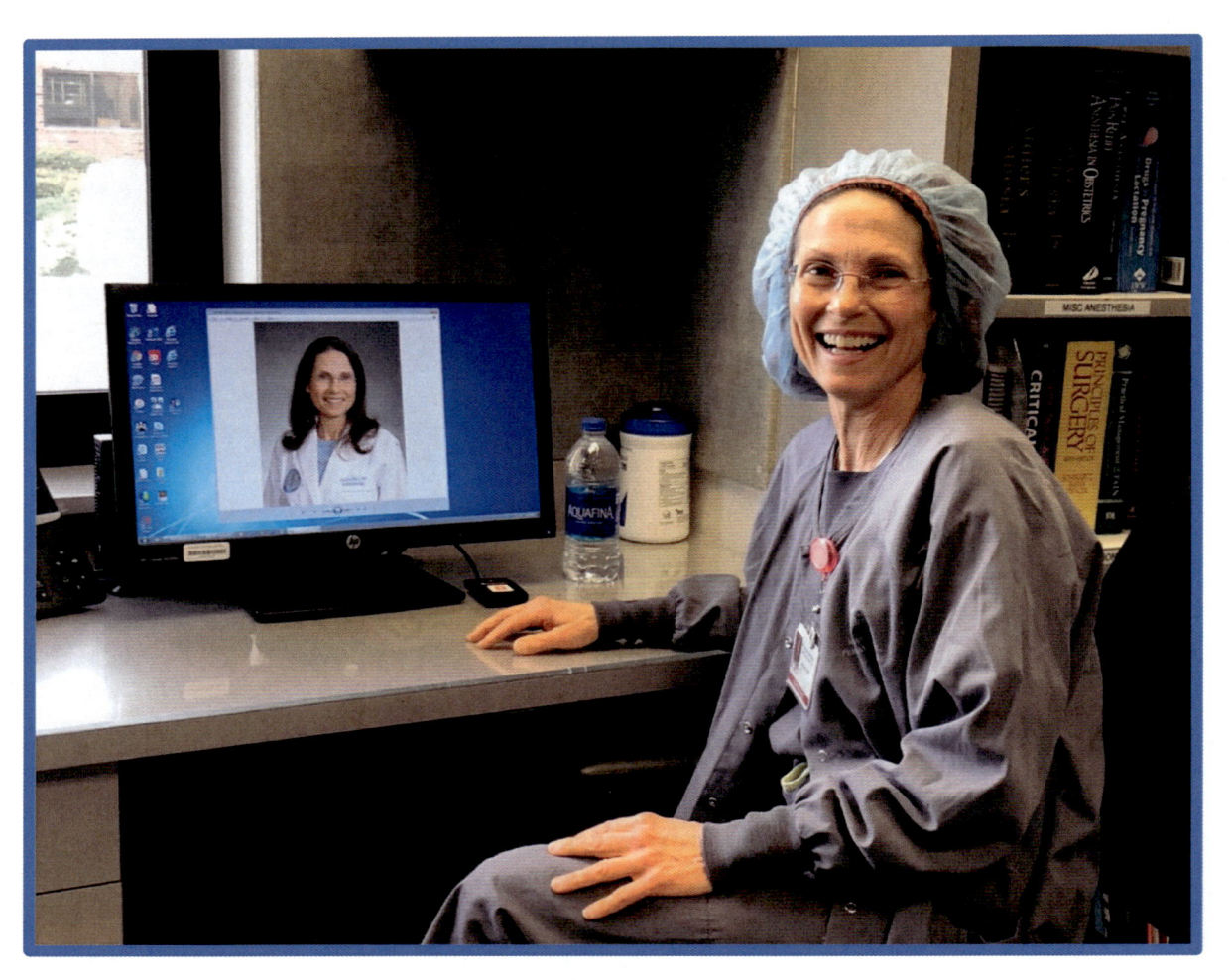

Last day at work

"A poem I wrote the night before my last day of work as I reflected on my career in anesthesia."

ON THE EVE OF RETIREMENT

For thirty years I've done my best
At last it's time to take a rest
From weekend calls and night time pages
From lack of sleep that surely ages
From missing meals and staying late
From policies I had to rate
From memos, meetings, metrics too
And running off to codes called Blue

On February twenty nine
I'll leap into a lifestyle fine
To be outside on days with sun
To hike or bike or take a run
To grow a garden, flowers fair
To pause a bit and breathe fresh air
To watch a bird or smell a rose
To walk the beach and stretch my toes
Then when it rains, I'll find a book
Or into closets take a look

I'd like to help out those in need
And spend more time with family
No doubt some trips to far off places
To see new lands and greet new faces

But what a life I leave behind:
Colleagues who are good and kind
C-R-N-As and anesthesia docs
We are a team and we do rock!

The tech on standby at my side
Handing me the faithful glide
The nurses bright who have my back
And let me know when orders lack

The chance to aid a baby's birth
Or ease the pain of labor's work
The surgeon with an urgent case
Off to the OR we must race
And when I know not what to do
Consultants come and see me through

The patients who will shed a tear
But trust in me despite their fear
I take their lives within my hands
To gently guide through "Lala" land
And bring them back to light of day
To live and love and work and play
A privilege both so raw and real
An honor I shall always feel

In many ways it's hard to leave
So part of me will also grieve
For I have loved my work and friends
And now it's coming to an end

Into the new life now I leap
But cherished friends I'll alway keep
My cherished friends I'll always keep.

Juliana Barr has a BS (Biomedical Engineering) from USC. She received her medical degree from John Hopkins University (MD, 1984). She completed residencies in Internal Medicine at the University of Utah (1984-1987) and Anesthesiology at Stanford (1987-1990). She then spent a year as a CCM Fellow at Stanford (1990-1991). After completing a post-doctoral research Fellowship (Clinical Pharmacology) at the PA-VAH, she joined the faculty as a staff anesthesiologist and intensivist at PA-VAH (1992).

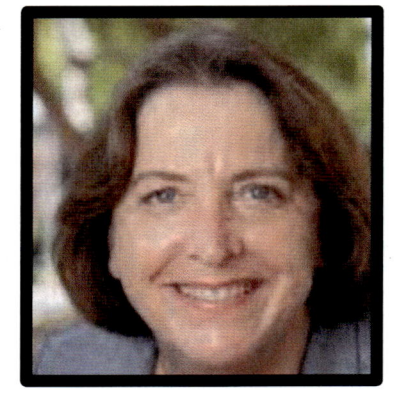

Dr. Barr co-founded the Stanford Critical Care Medical Student Core Clerkship and was Director (2005-2015) and Associate Director (2015-2019) of the clerkship. She previously served as Chair of the Society of Critical Care Medicine's (SCCM) Ethics Committee and Patient and Family Support Committee, and she co-authored the SCCM's *'Patient and Family Support Clinical Practice Guidelines'* (2007). She was also the lead author of the SCCM's *'Clinical Practice Guidelines for the Management of Pain, Agitation, and Delirium in Adults Patients in the Intensive Care Unit'* (2013). She is a founding member of the 'SCCM ICU Liberation Campaign' to promote widespread adoption of these guidelines. She co-authored a landmark study which demonstrated significant improvements in ICU patient outcomes following implementation of these guidelines. Dr. Barr has previously participated in several national collaboratives to improve ICU patient care and outcomes, including the IHI's *'100k Lives and the 5 Million Lives Campaigns'*.

At Stanford she co-founded the first intensivist-led ICU Team at the PA-VAH (1993) and she created the VA ICU Nurse Practitioner Program (2011). She has served as the Medical Director of the PA-VAH Respiratory Therapy Department for over 25 years, and as Medical Director of the VAH ICU NP Program since its inception. She has also been a member of the Stanford Faculty Senate, the medical school Admissions Committee, and the Human Subjects Committee. She is currently a member of the ASA's Committee on Performance and Outcome Metrics. She is currently a Professor Emerita (Active) of Anesthesiology, Perioperative and Pain Medicine at Stanford.

Walter David Bernard graduated from the University of Missouri - Kansas City School of Medicine (MD, 1986) and interned (Internal Medicine) at University of Wisconsin Hospitals and Clinics (1986-1987). He was a Stanford Anesthesiology resident (1987-1990). Dr. Bernard worked in Springfield, OR region affiliated with Northwest Anesthesia.

Patricia Elizabeth Curtis attended David Geffen School of Medicine at UCLA (MD, 1986), interned (Internal Medicine) at CPMC (1986-1987), and did her residency at Stanford (1987-1990). She worked for PAMF at El Camino Hospital, Mt. View, CA.

Ernest Hayward Jr was born at Fort Bragg, NC. As an undergraduate he attended Marquette University, Milwaukee, WI (BA magna cum laude and Phi Beta Kappa, Liberal Arts, 1981). He was in the Stanford University Medical Scholars Program (1983) and graduated from the Stanford School of Medicine (MD, 1986). He interned (Internal Medicine) at Cedars-Sinai Medical Center (CSMC) (1986-1987) and was an Anesthesiology resident at Stanford (1987-1990). Dr. Hayward worked as a staff anesthesiologist at Mission Hospital, Mission Viejo, CA (1990-1993). He then worked at Kaiser – Harbor City as Chief of Anesthesiology (1993-1997). Since 1997 he has been with California Anesthesia Associates (1997-Present). He was Chief of Anesthesiology at Memorial Care Saddleback Medical Center, Laguna Hills, CA (2007-2010). At Saddleback he was also Chief of the Medical Staff (2012-2013) and Medical Director of Surgical Services (2013-2016). He was Lead

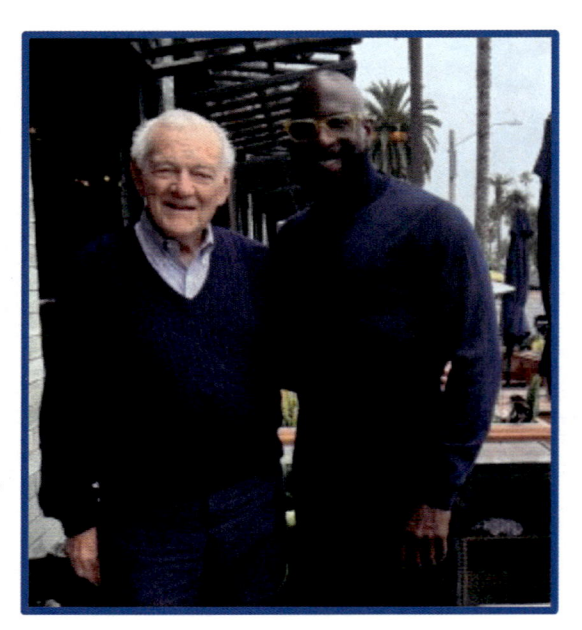

Recent photo of Phil Larson with Ernest Hayward

Anesthesiologist for MemorialCare for five hospital campuses (2013-2016). In that role he helped design, test and implement the electronic anesthesia module.

He has been a long-time sponsor of Tias Arms, a non-profit supporting the daily life experiences of South African orphans with HIV and AIDS. He enjoys travel, singing in several choral groups, playing piano, and indulging in physical fitness challenges including marathons and cycling.

"I have two wonderful sons. Andrew is a graduate of Embry-Riddle Aeronautical University Class of 2012. He is a Blackhawk helicopter operations specialist and serves in the Army National Guard Reserve. Vincent is a graduate of Emory University School of Medicine, Class of 2023. He is specializing in Internal Medicine. My sons' successes are my happiest achievements."

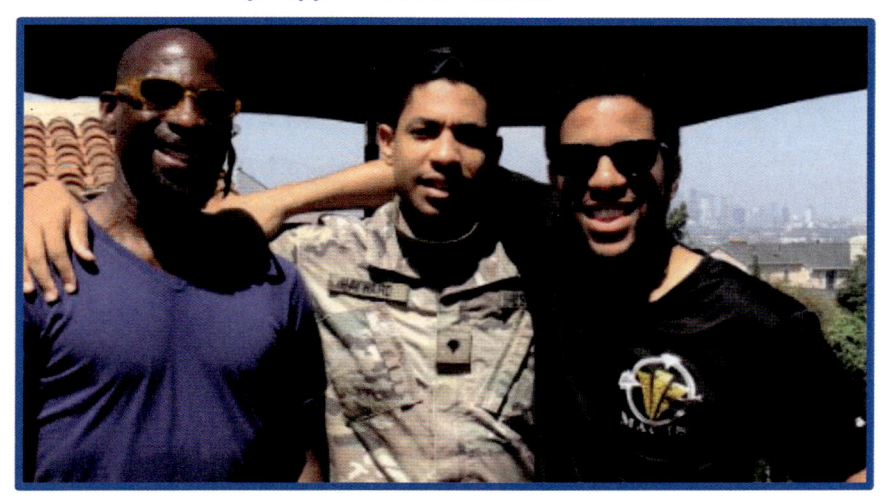

(L-R) Ernest Hayward Jr with sons Andrew and Vincent

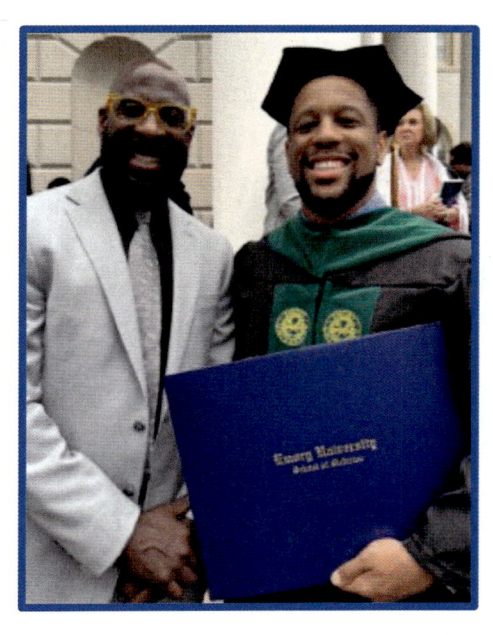

Doctors Ernest and Vincent Hayward at Vincent's graduation from medical school

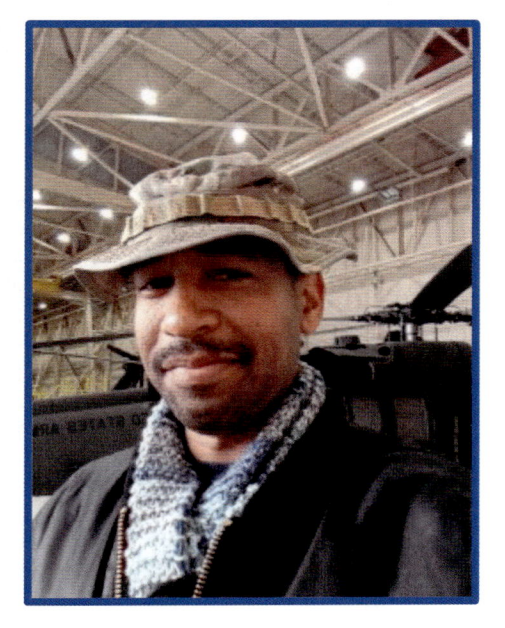

Andrew is a Blackhawk helicopter operations specialist and serves in the Army National Guard Reserve.

"Dr. Mervyn Maze mentored me through research and showed me the art of presenting our work. Drs. Janet Wyner and Sheila Cohen elevated the bar for clinical excellence and safety. Dr. Myer Rosenthal stressed precision in our assessments and concise communication in our management strategies. Dr. Phil Larsen's knowledge of airway management prepared me to approach even the most difficult patients confidently."

Curtis Orland McMillan

was born in Washington, DC. He attended Harvard College (AB, 1980) followed by a Rotary Fellowship (Health Economics) at the Sorbonne, Paris (1980-1981). He then graduated from Stanford (MD, 1981-1986) and interned (Internal Medicine) at McGill University, Montreal (1986-1987). Following his Anesthesiology residency at Stanford (1987-1989) he did a Fellowship (Pediatric Anesthesiology) at Boston Children's Hospital (1989-1990) and another at the Hospital for Sick Children/Toronto General Hospital (Pediatric and Adult Cardiac Anesthesia) (1990-1991). Later in his career he did another Fellowship (Regional Anesthesia) at Cork University Hospital, Ireland (2015-2016).

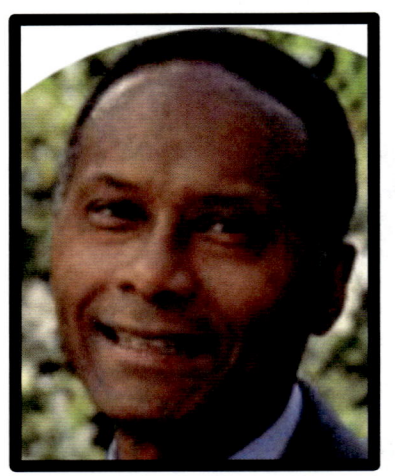

He initially did freelance anesthesia at various SF Bay Area hospitals (1991-1997). He then worked at Sutter, Santa Rosa (1997-2000). He has been at CPMC - St. Luke's Campus, San Francisco since 2000 (2000-Present).

His interests include snowboarding, cycling, tennis and photography. He is a volunteer with ReSurge (formerly Interplast) and has been on medical missions to South America and Asia.

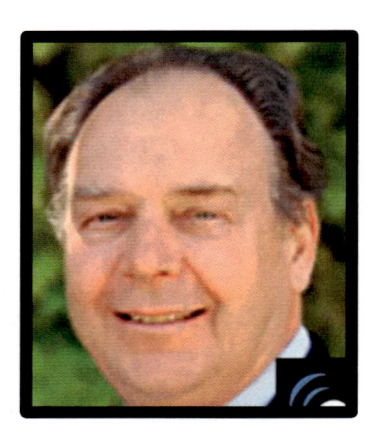

Friedrich "Fritz" Ekkehart Moritz

is another Stanford Medical School graduate (MD 1986) who chose Anesthesiology. He interned at LA County-Harbor - UCLA Medical Center (1986-1987) and then did his residency (Anesthesiology) at Stanford (1987-1990). He worked at SCVMC as Chief of Anesthesiology and later at Sutter Maternity and Surgery Center, Santa Cruz.

Marilyn Jeannie Roper

is a graduate of UCLA (MD, 1976) and completed an Anesthesiology residency at Stanford (1987-1990). The only information we have from the Internet is that a Dr. Roper practiced in Charlottesville, VA.

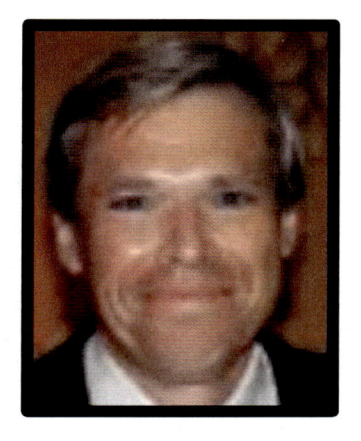

Charles Henry Tadlock was in the Medical Scientist Training Program National Institute of Health (NIH) (1980-1989). During that period, he graduated from Stanford Medical School (MD, 1986). After interning (Internal Medicine) at St Mary's Hospital and Medical Center (1986-1987) he completed his Anesthesiology residency at Stanford (1987-1990). He worked in Nevada and California. Charles founded an ambulatory surgical management company, Epiphany Surgical Solutions (2007). He practiced pain management and was the Nevada representative to the American Academy of Pain Medicine. Charles also collaborated doing research with the Department of Cellular and Developmental Biology at the University of Arizona Tucson, AZ (2017-Present). He lists his interests as jet pilot, high performance driving, scuba diving and running.

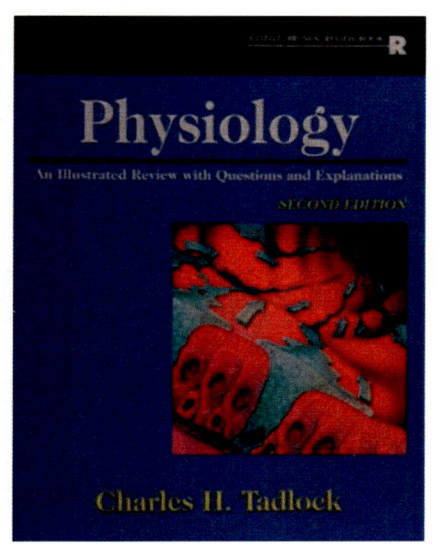

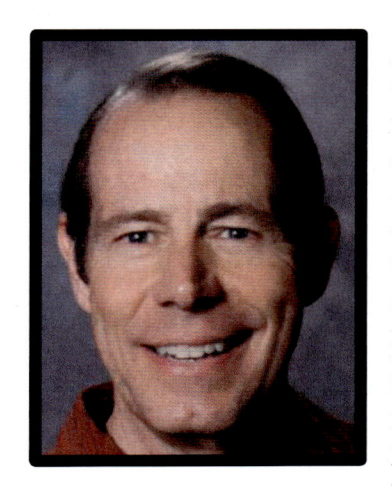

Bradley Jonathan Thomas attended Amherst College (BA, French Literature, 1976) and did postgraduate work at UCD (MS, Biochemistry, 1980). He began his medical education at the Royal College of Surgeons, Dublin, Ireland (1981-1983) and graduated from UCLA's David Geffen School of Medicine (MD, 1985). He interned (Internal Medicine) at CPMC (1985-1986) and did his Anesthesiology residency at Stanford (1987-1990). He initially did anesthesia locums work in the SF Bay Area (1990-1994) but then worked at Tahoe Forrest Hospital (1995 -2021). He was on the Board of Directors at the hospital (2009-2012) and was President of the Board (2011). Brad is now retired. He enjoys skiing (alpine, Nordic, and backcountry), biking, hiking, camping, and gardening. His other interests are in music – he plays the guitar the harmonica and sings and is currently in two rock bands.

"I made a movie parody of Apocalypse Now involving a harrowing quest to reach a "gone rogue" anesthesia attending physician in the far off O.B. department. I played the Martin Sheen character."

John Brock-Utne, "Bradley was at Candlestick Park for the World Series game when the earthquake struck. He was sitting high in the rafters. He assured me he was the very first person out of the ballpark."

Kristi Ann Watson attended SUNY - Stony Brook (MD, 1986), did an internship (Transitional) at UCSD (1986-1987), and a Stanford Anesthesiology residency (1987-1990). She worked in Arizona for Old Pueblo Anesthesia and then joined Oro Valley Anesthesia.

Three residents completed only a CA3 year of training at Stanford in 1987.

Donald William Milne was born in Toronto. He was an undergraduate at the University of Toronto and received his medical degree from the Michael G. DeGroote School of Medicine, McMaster University (1984). He interned and completed his first two years of Anesthesia residency at McMaster University (1984-1987 and did a CA3 year at Stanford (1987-1988). He initially practiced in Ontario, Canada. He was then Chief of Anesthesia at Waynesboro Hospital in Pennsylvania for 10 years. He then worked in Florida then returned to the SF Bay area working at Highland Hospital, Oakland, and Kaiser - Santa Rosa.

"One of my fondest memories of his time at Stanford was anesthetizing an orangutan at the San Francisco zoo."

Forbes Innovation Consumer Tech:

This Doctor Says The Apple Watch Saved His Life. *A doctor in California says his Apple Watch helped him identify a heart condition that led to a life-saving bypass operation. The doctor is Dr. Donald W Milne, an anesthesiologist who works at the Antelope Valley Hospital in Lancaster, CA. He wrote to Apple CEO Tim Cook to explain the story of how an Apple Watch effectively saved his life. Milne was working out on an elliptical trainer and noticed unusual shortness of breath, and then saw an ST depression in the Watch's echocardiogram app's reading. This is an abnormal heart pattern an echocardiogram sensor can catch, but a normal LED-based optical heart rate monitor can't. "I have the first generation of the Apple Watch to be able to do heart monitoring. I know that the primary intended use is to monitor for atrial fibrillation. As a 66-year-old anesthesiologist I use my watch for many occasions," said Milne. "I had no history of any heart disease prior to this incident." Apple added an electrical heart rate sensor to the Watch in its Series 4 hardware, released in 2018. "An appointment with my primary care physician obtained a resting ECG in her office that was normal. However, upon showing the tracing with the ischemia she agreed and referred me to a cardiologist at John Muir Concord Hospital," says Milne. "He agreed as well with the assessment and upon having an angiogram the finding of critical diffuse coronary artery disease was found, and I am now scheduled for a 5-vessel bypass and aortic valve replacement on July 13, 2020." You might not have the same level of ECG reading insight as Dr. Milne, but it proves there's more to the Apple Watch's hardware than just monitoring your heart rate during a run or gym exercise.*

Carl Edward Noe attended the University of Texas Health Science Center at San Antonio (MD, 1984). He did an Internship (Rotating) at Texas Tech University Health Sciences Center, Lubbock, TX (1984-1985) followed by two years of Anesthesiology residency at Texas Tech (1985-1987). He transferred to Stanford for his CA3 year doing Cardiothoracic Anesthesia (1987-1988), followed by a Fellowship (CCM) at Stanford (1988-1989). He returned to Texas Tech University and did an additional Fellowship (Pain Management, 1989).

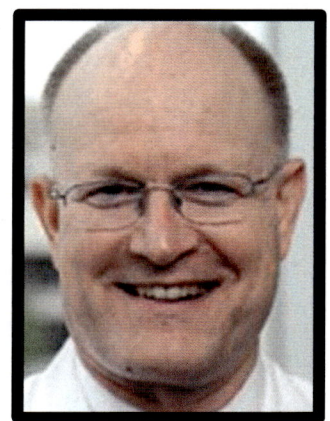

Dr. Noe is a Professor in the Department of Pain Management and Anesthesiology at UT Southwestern Medical Center and serves as Medical Director of the Eugene McDermott Center for Pain Management. He is a founding member of the Texas Pain Society, and is a member of other professional organizations, including the American Pain Society, Texas Medical Association, and Texas Society of Anesthesiologists.

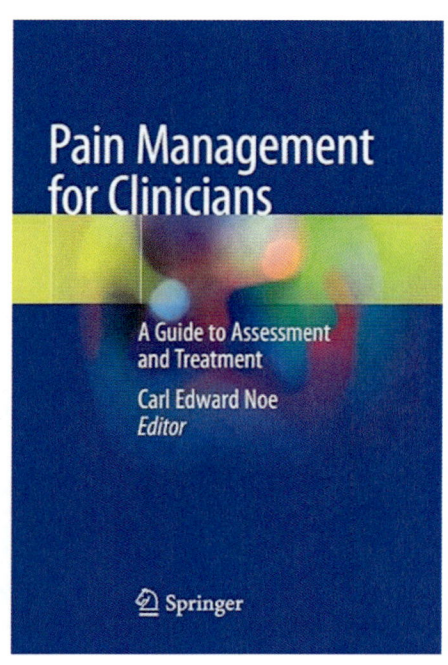

Stephen Travis Peake is a graduate of University of Oklahoma College of Medicine (MD, 1981). He completed a CA3 year (Cardiothoracic Anesthesia) at Stanford (1988-1989) as part of his residency at the US Naval Hospital, San Diego. Dr. Peake works in Chattanooga, TN. He has held several executive positions with insurance companies.

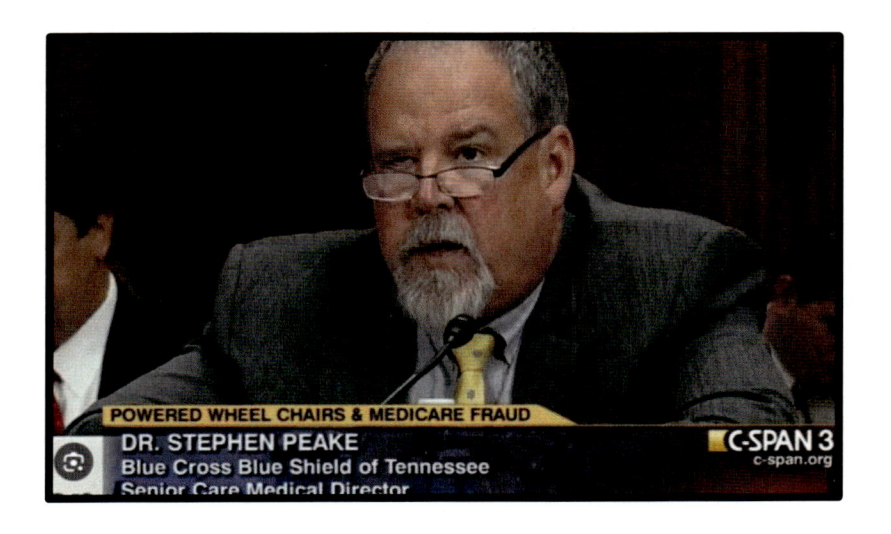

Leo I. Stemp was born in Brooklyn. He was an undergraduate at Brooklyn College, CUNY (BS, Chemistry, 1978) and a medical student Harvard (MD, 1983). He interned and did an Internal Medicine residency at the Mount Sinai School of Medicine, NYC (1983-1986). That was followed by a Fellowship (CCM and Trauma) at the Shock Trauma Center, University of Maryland (1986-1987). He started his Anesthesiology residency at Stanford but left (7/1/87-12/31/89) during his CA3 year to complete training at Emory University (Adult and Pediatric Cardiothoracic Anesthesia, 1990-1991) and Pediatric Cardiothoracic Anesthesia at Boston's Hospital for Sick Children (1991). He was a cardiothoracic anesthesiologist at the Cleveland Clinic (1991-1993). Leo was co-founder and an intensivist with Western Mass Critical Care, PC (2001-2019) and a critical care physician and anesthesiologist at Holyoke Medical Center, Holyoke, MA (2019-Present).

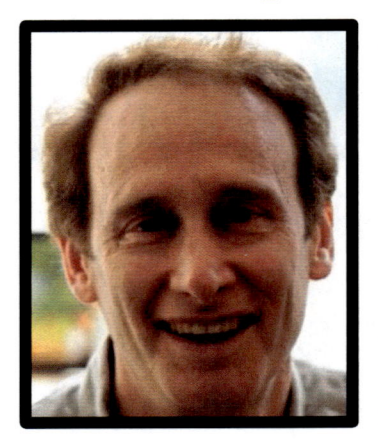

"My fondest memories from Stanford were working with Chuck Whitcher and with Phil Larson. And while I would imagine it's a common experience among clinicians after 30-40 years of practice that most of what they do today has little resemblance to what they did in training, I'm cognizant of the influence of Dr. Whitcher and Dr. Larson to this day.

The lasting influence that Phil had on both my practice in Critical Care and in Anesthesiology extends from steadiness under fire, to fiberoptic intubations and prone tracheal extubations. I remember in particular Phil telling me about a case he served as an expert witness on, a patient with a bowel obstruction who had a massive aspiration because an NG tube wasn't put down to decompress his stomach prior to induction. Some years ago, I was called to electively intubate a patient who was having an upper GI bleed, prior to an EGD. We couldn't put down an NG tube because it might cause bleeding. It was obvious that an awake fiberoptic intubation was the only safe way to go. Despite not having done one in 10 or maybe 20 years, it went fast and smooth, suitably impressing the ICU staff who'd never seen one before.

This is what I wrote in memoriam about Chuck Whitcher in 2014: "Chuck Whitcher's repute at Stanford was as an ENT anesthesiologist, but to be honest, I have no recollection from my rotation with him whether or not we did anything anesthesia-wise that was unique to ENT surgery in particular during that short month. Rather, my recollection is that Chuck Whitcher was THE master of vapor anesthesia. Not before, nor since, have I encountered an anesthesiologist who knew vapor dynamics like he did, who practiced with the meticulousness he did, or who could teach vapor anesthesia like he did. I remember the six-channel recorder, and how Dr. Whitcher used it to teach us vapor dynamics. To this day, I do closed circuit on every case I do, even hearts, the exact way he taught me. Nothing else I learned through two residencies and three fellowships has had such an impact on and longevity in my practice career. A decade after I left Stanford, I was doing most of the ENT anesthesia at a county hospital, doing weekly 12-14-hour radical neck cases with continuous cervical epidurals with morphine and bupivacaine, with spontaneous ventilation with low dose closed circuit vapor anesthesia for the entire case duration, and loving it. Those cases were the professional highlight of my week. Truth be told, if it wasn't for Chuck Whitcher, I would have been with the 99% of anesthesiologists who have no clue how to expertly manage anesthesia gases, and probably would have stopped practicing anesthesia long ago from shear boredom. To this day, I think about him almost every one of the dozens to hundreds of times I turn a vaporizer dial during a case. I hope he's looking down and smiling that at least in one

hole-in-the-wall corner of the earth, a guy he taught is doing it right, that patients are benefiting because of it, and that I'm extraordinarily grateful to have been his student".
   I can't say how grateful I am to both Chuck and Phil for the lasting impact they've had on my practice."

The resident class starting in 1987 was unusual in that two residents began their anesthesia training and then resigned from the program, and another was dropped from the program because of substance abuse problems.

Jean Gordon attended Princeton University and then earned a PhD (Mathematics) from Dartmouth College. After four years as a college Professor (Mathematics) at Williams College she moved to California to merge her mathematical expertise with the field of medicine. She graduated from Stanford (MD, 1986), interned (Internal Medicine) at CPMC, and started a Stanford Anesthesiology residency (1987). During her CA1 year (7/1/87-3/23/88) she took a leave of absence and never returned. She subsequently did a residency (Dermatology) at Stanford (1992-1995) and has worked as a dermatologist in Mt. View, CA, affiliated with El Camino Hospital.

Lynne M. Scannell was an undergraduate at UCD (BS, Zoology/Animal Biology, 1980) and graduated from Washington University School of Medicine (MD, 1984). She completed a residency (Pediatrics) at Stanford (1984-1987). She began an Anesthesiology residency but resigned after 7 months. (7/1/87-1/31/88). She has worked at several hospitals in California as a pediatrician.

Diana Mansfield Runyan is University of Texas graduate (MD, 1982). After an internship (Transitional) at Scripps Mercy Hospital, San Diego (1982-1983) she began a residency (Anesthesiology) at UCSF and came to Stanford as a CA2 Anesthesiology resident in 1987. She did not complete our program due to substance abuse problems. She subsequently completed a residency (Occupational Medicine) and worked as an occupational medicine specialist in Santa Clara, CA.

CHAPTER 8
1988

In 1988 one of the world's first computer viruses, the '*Internet Worm*' (also called the '*Morris Worm*) was written by Cornell University student Robert Morris. It resulted in the first felony conviction in the US under the 1986 Computer Fraud and Abuse Act. The first prime time wrestling match in 30 years saw Andre the Giant beat Hulk Hogan. Pam Am 103, a transatlantic flight travelling to Detroit from Frankfurt, via London and New York was destroyed while flying over the town of Lockerbie in Scotland. A bomb planted by a Libyan operative exploded killing everyone on board plus 11 people on the ground. In other terrorist news Osama bin Laden and Ayman al-Zawahiri met that August in Peshawar, Pakistan, and created Al-Qaeda. In 1988 the USSR withdrew its 115,000 troops from Afghanistan, more than 8 years after Soviet forces entered the country. Unfortunately, future history proved that the United States did not benefit from the Russian experience in Afghanistan.

On February 10th a 3-judge panel of the 9th Circuit Court of Appeals in San Francisco struck down the Army's ban on homosexuals, declaring they should receive the same protection against discrimination as racial minorities. In December the first World Aids Day was held to remember those who had suffered from the illness. James Hansen, a NASA climatologist, made awareness of the '*Greenhouse Effect*' to the American public after telling Congress that worldwide temperature increases were a sign of human alteration of the atmosphere. In May Surgeon General C. Everett Koop released a report declaring that nicotine was as addictive as heroin and cocaine. The first US test tube quintuplets were born in Royal Oak, MI. That year

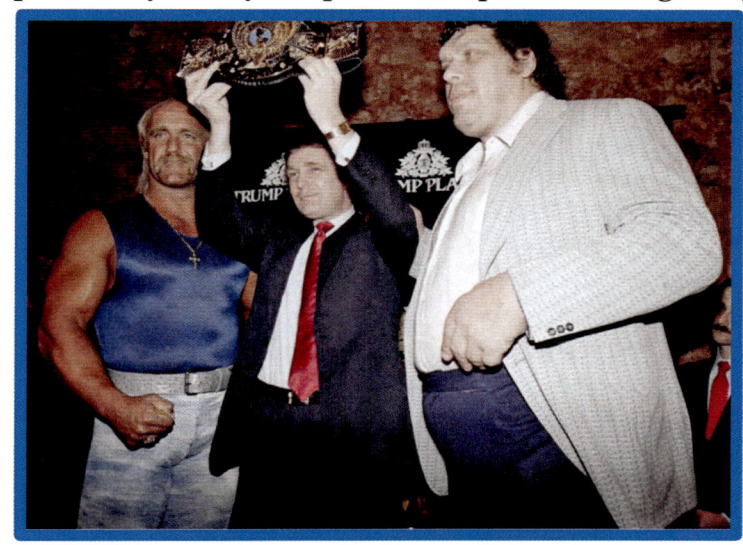

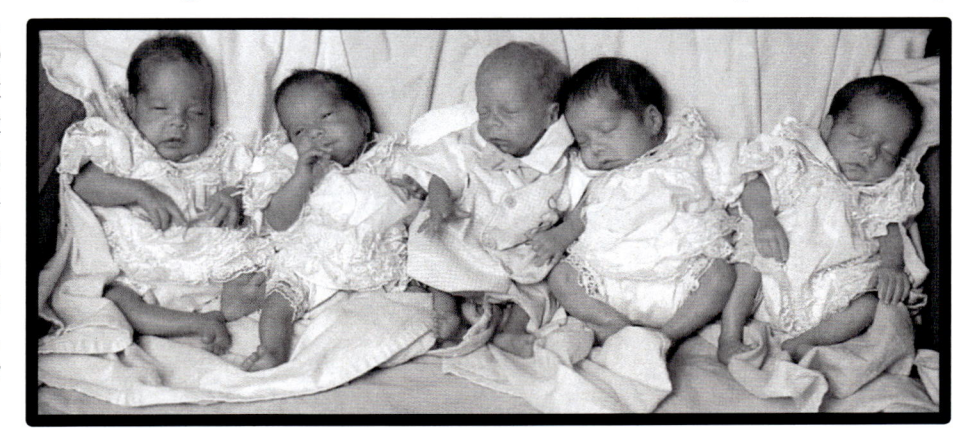

March 15th, 1988, real-estate developer and future President Donald Trump holds the World Federation Wrestling Championship belt flanked by Hulk Hogan and Andre the Giant.

123

Magnetic Resonance Imaging (MRI) became available for the first time at Stanford Hospital.

Wayne Raleigh Anderson

graduated from UCSD (BA summa cum laude, Biochemistry and Cell Biology, 1983) and from medical school at UCSD (MD, 1987). He did an internship (Internal Medicine) at UCLA Medical Center (1987-1988) and then his Stanford Anesthesiology residency (1988-1991). At Stanford he did a Fellowship (Molecular Mechanisms of Immunological Mediated Diseases, 1988-1992). He also has an MBA (Accounting and Finance) from the George L. Graziadio School of Business and Management, Pepperdine University (1995-1997). He worked at Mammoth Hospital, Hillcrest Medical Clinic, and Ventura County Hospital before briefly returning to Stanford in 2020 as a Clinical Instructor (Anesthesiology). He is President of Smart Medical Devices, Inc., Las Vegas, a medical R&D company that developed the SMARTdrill, a more sensitive device than handheld drills used in orthopedic surgery.

John Brock-Utne – "One morning I was working with Wayne. He seemed not to be his usual jolly self. He was moving slowly and had difficulty bending over. After inquiring he admitted that he had fallen of his mountain bike late Sunday. A large road rash covered his whole right leg, abdomen, and upper torso. I sent him to the ER and told him to get seen and go home. Only after I was stern, did he agree. They built them tough in those days." **The rest of the story ...** *Anderson, "The story above happened on the Wednesday before Thanksgiving. Dr. Brock-Utne sent me to the ER at the beginning of my day shift - I was diagnosed with a cellulitis and possible osteomyelitis from a bicycle accident I had on Woodside Road about 10 days earlier. I left the ER AMA with IM antibiotics instead of IV antibiotics so I could cover my call shift and not stick somebody with it on Thanksgiving - problem was after I left the ER, by the time I got to OB Dr. Howard had started to put an epidural in a patient for a C-section. He was so mad at me and would not talk to me. He threatened that I would have to repeat that OB month. Luckily, Dr. Brock-Utne and Larry Siegel stuck up for my and introduced the ER records into the conversation, so I did not have to repeat that month."*

Raymond Richard Gaeta

did his undergraduate work at Stanford (BS, Biological Science, 1980) and is a Stanford School of Medicine graduate (MD, 1985). He completed an internship (Internal Medicine) at Stanford (1985-1986) and then did residencys in Internal Medicine (1986-1988) and Anesthesiology (1988-1991) both at Stanford. He won the Department's Outstanding Resident Award (1991). He completed Fellowiships in CCM (1991) and Pain Management (1991-1992). He was appointed an Assistant Professor (Anesthesiology) (1992-1996) and promoted to Associate Professor (1996-2011). He was a Division Chief of the Stanford Pain Management Service (1996-2008) and President of the Stanford Hospital Medical Staff (2001-2003). He was also Chair of the School of Medicine Faculty Senate (2003-2005).

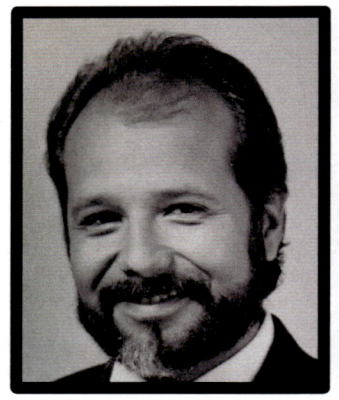

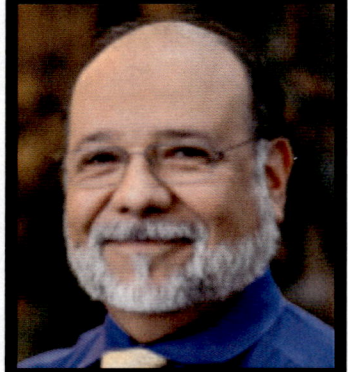

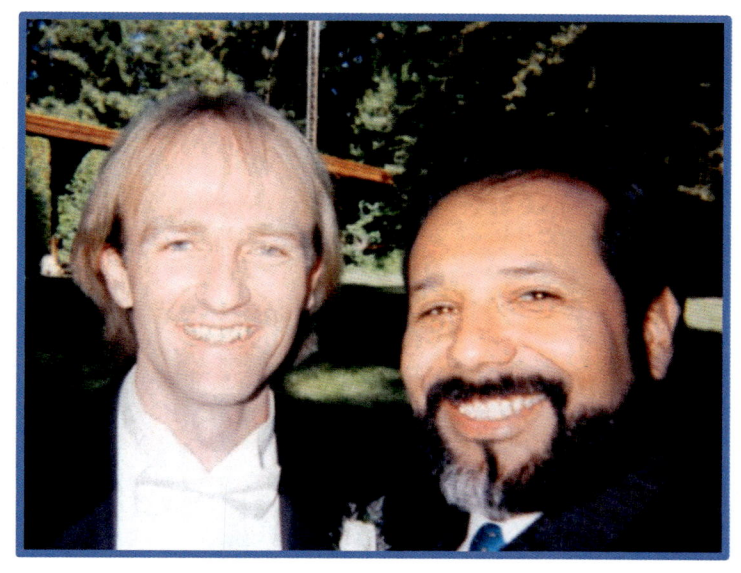

Ray was President of the American Association of Pain Program Directors (2009-2001) and on the ABA Pain Medicine Board Examination Committee (1997). After leaving Stanford he was Regional Medical Director of Bill Brose's HELP Program (2011-2018), and President of American Telepain Consultants (2018-2019). He currently works at the PAMF as Department Chair (2019-Present).

"The colleagues that I met during my time Stanford remain a wonderful memory. I remember fondly the transport service and the many flights for donor harvest and patient transport."

Gerald "Jerry" A. Holguin

was born in Los Angeles. He was an undergraduate at UCLA (BA cum laude, Biology, 1976-1981) and a UCSF medical student (MD, 1985). He did his internship and residency (Internal Medicine) at SCVMC (1988) followed by an Anesthesiology residency (1988-1991). He worked at Northwest Kaiser - Portland, OR, (1991-1999) and was Department Chairman his final 6 years there (1993-1999). He then completed a Fellowship (Pain Management) at OHSU (1999-2000). He moved to Minneapolis, MN, and worked as a staff anesthesiologist for Northwest Anesthesia (2000-2016), then with American Anesthesiology of Minnesota, Minneapolis - St. Paul Area, working part-time from 2016 to 2020. He returned to OHSU as a Clinical Instructor (2020-2021). His interests were regional and obstetrical anesthesia and management of chronic pain. He retired in September 2021.

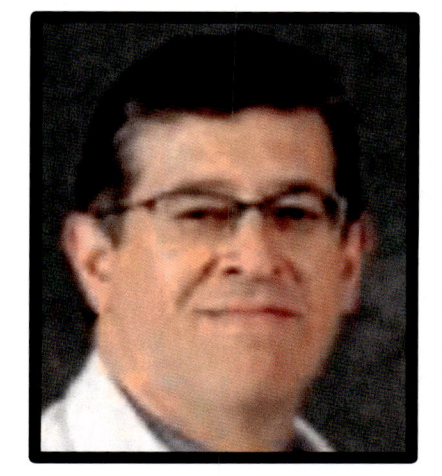

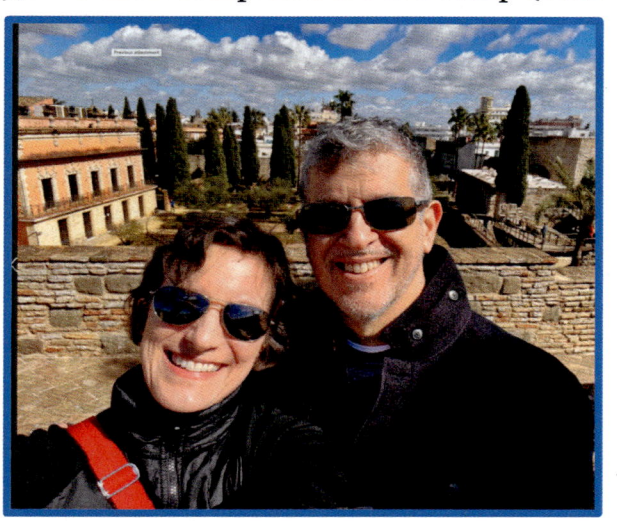

Recent trip with wife Carol in Jerez, Spain

His interests and activities include conversational Spanish classes, classic guitar lessons, cycling and hiking. He also has a "fancy" for Burgundian pinots. He is a volunteer for the Refugee Care Initiative in Portland.

"I have so many warm memories of my residency years that I just can't list them all. So many great teachers/attendings who were patient, intelligent and humorous. That, of course, includes Jay and John (and no, I'm not sucking up; I really mean it). But also, folks like Mike Rosenthal, David Gaba, and Rich Jaffe. So many great lessons and clinical pearls you provided me which I carried and utilized throughout my career. Thank you for helping shape me into the competent anesthesiologist I became and for instilling in me the desire to continuously learn and improve. You all made a big difference in our lives and careers."

"I think one of the most humorous antidotes I can remember is the epidural my wife, Carol, received in July 1991 from the OB fellow (whose name I can't remember and who had already been practicing anesthesia at SCVMC for a few years) and under the "supervision" of Barrie Fairley. I assured my wife that she was getting care from an experienced anesthesiologist and the Chairman of my department. First, the fellow/experienced SCVMC attending had significant difficulty placing the epidural in my thin wife. Then when it was finally placed, they dosed it with the infusate de jour (fentanyl 25 mcg only) which didn't work at all. They then "rescued" it with local which led to a numb right leg and a "natural" childbirth."

"A memorable experience was a number of anesthesia textbooks falling off the shelves all around me in the ICU call room during the Loma Prieta earthquake of 1989."

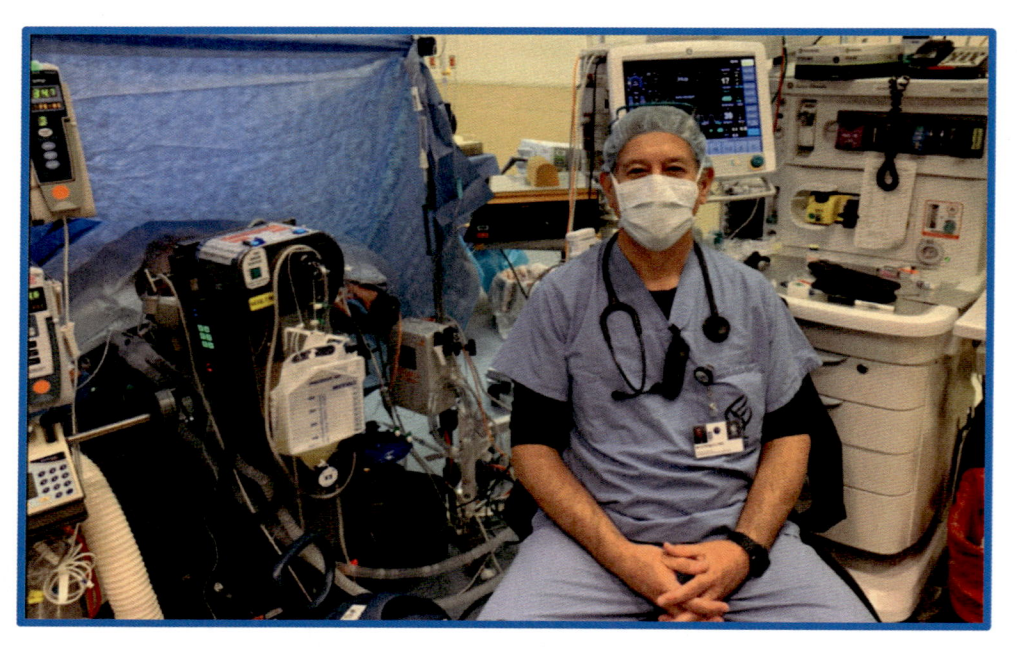

Jerry Holguin final day working as an anesthesiologist

Steven Keith Howard was born in 1961. He attended UC - Santa Barbara (BA, Pharmacology, 1983) and Chicago Medical School (MD, 1987). He interned at CSMC and came to Stanford as an Anesthesiology resident (1988-1991). After residency he did a Fellowship (Simulation and Patient Safety) with David Gaba at the PA-VAH (1992). He joined the faculty at the PA-VAH and remained on the staff for his entire career (1991-2023). He retired in 2023 as Professor Emeritus, Department of Anesthesiology, Perioperative and Pain Medicine.

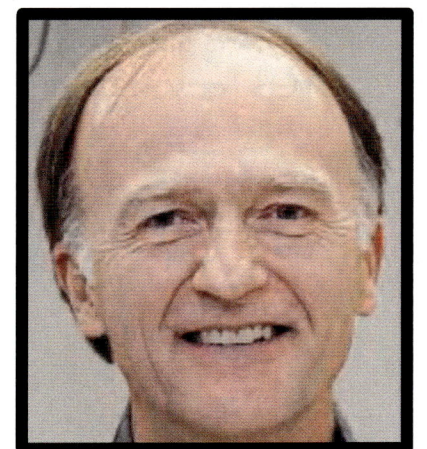

"I creatively went straight through college, medical school, and residency without doing any "work." So not much work history before Stanford. During residency, I became friends with Dave Gaba who lured me into doing a Fellowship with him (the Dead concert at Frost sealed the deal). His work in simulation and crisis management was exciting and I thought I would spend the first part of my career helping with that. During Fellowship I was offered a staff position at the PA-VAH (as Don Stanski was "looking into" the Chair's position at Stanford). I recall Jeff Baden telling me that I could take the position, work the same amount of clinical days and make more money, but I would not get the Fellowship award at the end of the year – I took the money!"

"There was really no "after Stanford" but I did retire on June 30, 2023. Currently, I still work as a fee basis anesthesiologist at the PA-VAH and teach our residents simulation."

Steve worked closely with David Gaba and is one of the early pioneers in Crisis Management. Steve and David are co-authors on the definitive text on this subject.

He was a member of numerous national committees including the ASA Educational Track Subcommittee on Professional Issues (2008-2016), the ASA Committee on Occupational Health (2014-2021), the Scientific Evaluation Committee of the Anesthesia Patient Safety Foundation (APSF) (2008-Present), and the ASA Abstract Review Committee on Patient Safety and Practice Management (2012-2016). He was Chair of the Scientific Evaluation Committee (APSF, 2013-2020). He was also on the Professional Advisory Committee of the Malignant Hyperthermia Association of the United States (2009-Present) and on the editorial board of the journal Simulation in Healthcare (2011- Present).

"We had a publication appear in the New England Journal of Medicine and a huge fatigue study that was published in Anesthesiology. We were pretty excited about both. I have always wondered how many people actually read those articles (including my close relatives)! Academic medicine is an interesting beast it turns out, but the academic currency is the all-important publication!

"I enjoy fly fishing in Alaska with my father and then with my extended family after they saw our catch each year. Travel with family – Italy, London, and Kauai are my favorites. Live music, Giants baseball, and my constant love of running. Hanging with my wife Jenifer (my best friend) and our daughter Rachel is the way I will always choose to spend free time."

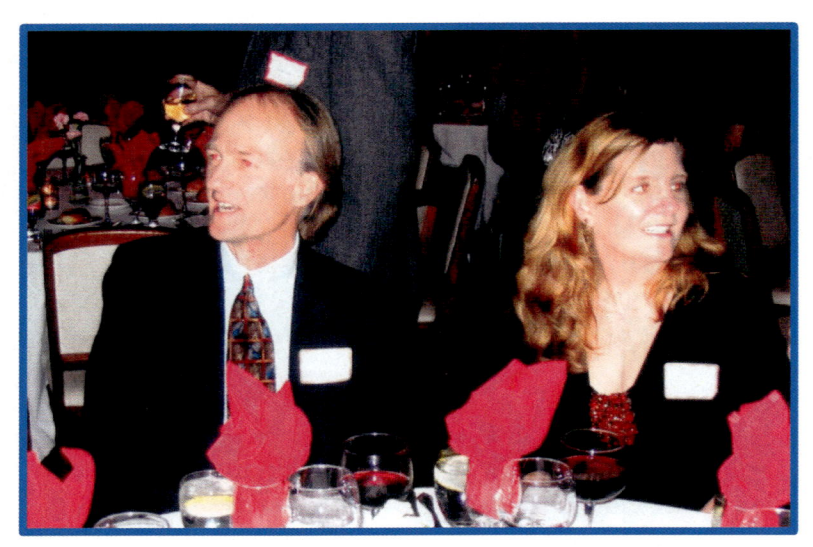

Steve and Jenifer at an Anesthesia department event.

"For whoever would listen, I am on record as stating that I was "over" taking call for a few years before I retired. It was always the possibility of the train wreck coming through the door even though that rarely happened. How many professional athletes stay around too long? In our job, staying around too long can be lethal. I chose to do it the Buster Posey way and bow out before the fall! All the crap surrounding COVID made this decision even easier."

"Since retirement, I can do whatever I want! It is quite refreshing not having to put in call and vacation requests. Retirement allows me to do what I have always liked which is to really get back into running. No, I DO NOT do marathons. I am a middle-distance runner and prefer racing on the track – 800, 1500, 3000, 5000 meters, with an occasional mile thrown in. I will do local road races up to 10K depending on the season. I was recruited to join a nationally ranked track club (SoCal Track Club) and we recently won the men's national indoor championship in Chicago!"

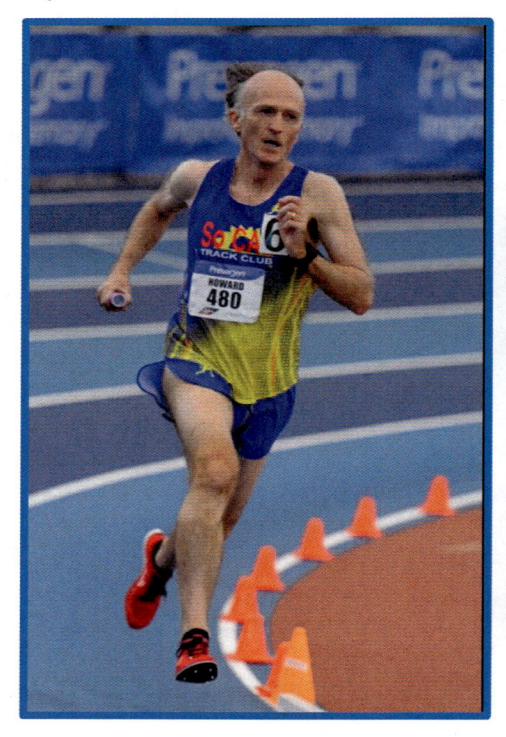

Steve Howard the National Masters indoor track and field meet in Chicago, March 2024

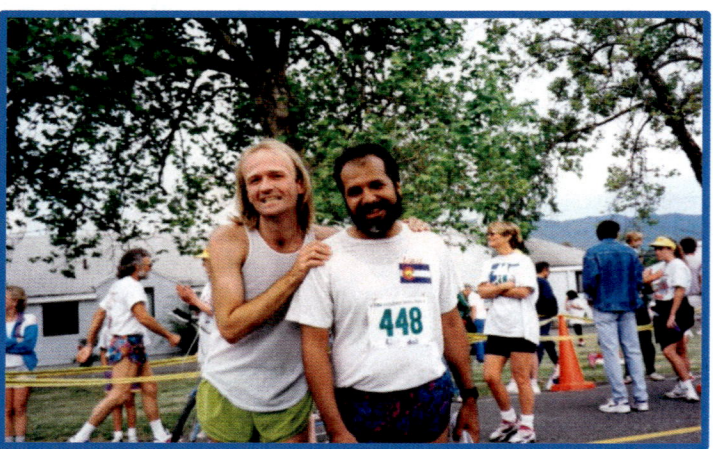

Steve and Ray Gaeta at a track meet during their residency

128

Memories:
The rules of anesthesia were maybe the most important things I learned as a CA1. Dave Gaba was the keeper of the list of rules and passed this on to me at an impressionable stage. There is copy of this somewhere and trust me, they are important. Here are a few that I can remember:
- *Always change a losing game, never change a winning game (Big Bill Tilden).*
- *Keep it greasy, it'll go down easy (Frank Zappa).*
- *You can't anesthetize a rumor (Kent Garman).*
- *The most important piece of equipment is a stool.*
- *Don't use sux outside of the OR unless you are damn good.*
- *You got the 'DMA' which is the 'daily miracle of anesthesia' (the return of spontaneous ventilation from a previously paralyzed patient) which was usually followed closely by the 'MOT' which is the 'moment of truth' (when to extubate the trachea).*

"Mike Rosenthal on service in the ICU when every third night I would get slammed. Seeing him standing in the doorway during morning rounds grinning (you know the look) and shaking his head while we actively treated the latest sick patient. Then coming in and getting his hands dirty with us."

"Withdrawing support on three patients on one of my post-call days. One was a kid who was younger than I was who died from AIDS. That was horrible at best."

"Working with Ron Pearl doing a redo MVR. Prior to going on his break to eat his donut, we went over what to do if the cardiac surgeons cut through the "wrong thing." Sure enough, the wrong thing was cut through and we proceeded to crash onto CPB. Talk about training in the moment!"

"I have so many memories of the residents that I have had a part in training. I cannot name them all because I know I would inadvertently leave somebody out. We have had great young anesthesiologists pass through our program! One story though – one of my research assistants went on to go to Harvard Medical School and he became friends with a guy named Chris Miller. When Chris was interviewing, he contacted me and wanted to come by the PA-VAH and shadow me in the OR. He came into an open AAA that I was doing with Jen Basarab-Tung. Chris ends up at Stanford and was a spectacular resident and Fellow and we became good friends. His last rotation was at the PA-VAH, and we were together for his last call – sure enough, after going home at the end of the day, Chris calls me to tell me that there was an urgent AAA that needed to go. What a great way to bookend his time as a resident – it was even in the same room!"

"Teaching in simulation has taken me to many interesting places and is also where I have met some of my closest academic friends. My best working days are teaching with people like Dave Gaba, Ruth Fanning, Kyle Harrison, Sara Goldhaber-Fiebert, Naola Austin, and the rest of our clan. Our group has taught Anesthesia Crisis Resource Management to anesthesiologists from around the world and this type of training has become commonplace in many academic centers. For those who do not know – it started at the PA-VAH/Stanford. There are also some great spinoffs from this work – OB Sim, Neo Sim, and the Stanford Emergency Manual to name a few."

"My first exposure to Jay Brodsky as a CA1 was at an Organon-sponsored Giants game out in the parking lot at a tailgate – "Hi Dr. Brodsky, my name is Steve Howard, I am a new CA1." To which he responded, "I don't work with CA1s!" No words! Jay later in my residency asked Stanley Samuels and me to provide the anesthetic for his mother (no pressure). There was a reason to look carefully at her larynx on DL, so

I looked and when Stanley went to look "we" gave her a lip laceration. I thought I would never hear the end of it. As I recall, she did great after her surgery but as some of you may know, Jay has a way of reminding you of things ..."

Ted Robert Kreitzman (deceased) graduated from Rutgers College (BA, German, 1983) then Rutgers Robert Wood Johnson Medical School (MD, 1987).

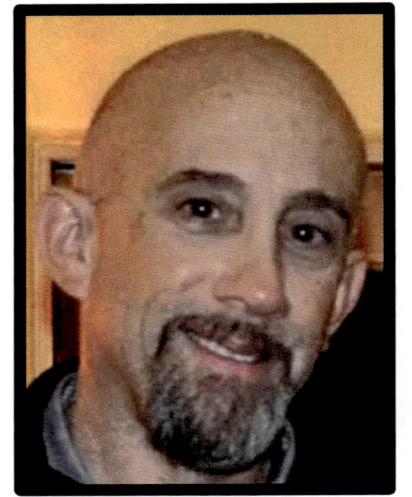

His obituary relates that he decided to become a physician when his high school guidance counselor told him "It's not like you are going to become a doctor." Instead of discouraging him, it spurred him to pursue a career in medicine.

He completed an internship (Internal Medicine) at Rutgers (1987-1988) followed by his Anesthesiology training at Stanford (1988-1991). He is listed as on the faculty at Stanford (1992-1993). Dr. Kreitzman worked with Metro Anesthesia Consultants, Phoenix, AZ, at Banner-University Medical Center and St. Joseph's Hospital and Medical Center. He served many leadership roles with Metro as treasurer, scheduler, and president. He was the owner of Anzu Technologies, Pune Area, India (2011-2023) a cutting-edge software development company specializing in mobile platform publishing and social networking. Ted was a classically trained pianist and enjoyed jazz. He had a variety of hobbies, including sailing, cycling, scuba diving, skiing, fitness, nutrition, and motorcycles.

Sadly, Ted Kreitzman died at age 62 on August 25, 2023, after a long struggle with glioblastoma.

Emily Ratner, "Fond memories of Ted Kreitzman when we shared an office and he leaving a disgusting, old piece of cake on my desk, because ...? Oh, and during the resident ski trip (I was a beginning skier at the time), Ted took me to a black diamond run, looked at me and said "good luck" then went down the hill. I am so saddened by his recent passing."

Jerry Holguin, "A sweet memory is of fellow resident Ted Kreitzman volunteering to videotape my wedding in 1990 in lieu of an expensive Palo Alto videographer. He was a real mensch."

Linda Rose Mignano received her medical degree from UCSF (MD, 1987) and did an internship (Internal Medicine) at Kaiser - San Francisco (1987-1988). Her residency training was at Stanford (1988-1991). She worked at Seton Medical Center, Daly City, CA.

"This is about my one regret at Stanford. Sandra Chapman was Chief Resident when she came to me looking for something humorous for the annual faculty roast put on by the 3rd year residents. I told her something that struck me as funny, and she presented it with an academy award worthy performance that received the only standing ovation; everybody stood up. She nailed it. That emboldened me the next year. So, when it again came time to prepare for the faculty roast, I thought about the

disappointment some of the residents had when our annual medical mission with Interplast to South America was cancelled and no one could go. My idea for the roast was to present a series of slides on our South America trip that year, saying how much the residents got out of our medical mission trip down south to the jungle, while showing a slide of the entrance to the Santa Clara facility, and continuing on that theme with pictures of the poor equipment, the primitive conditions, the native population, and anything else I could spoof. I never was able to get there, to take all the photos, and I regret that because I think it would have been fun and a good comic relief for the residents. So that's the one that got away."

"Early in my practice, I had a scheduled C-section on a healthy young woman who reported having some mild asthma, and I had just placed an epidural block and positioned her as usual, when she became tachycardic, her pressure fell, she complained of not being able to breathe, and told me it was her usual asthma symptoms. She had the normal lead 2 monitoring and it just showed tachycardia. It would seem that the block was setting up, she needed fluids, a pressor, and bronchodilator for her asthma, perhaps brought on by stress. She was crashing fast though, and thanks to Sheila Cohen and Stanford University for making sure I left there knowing a thing or two about both OB and hearts, I instinctively realized this onset was too fast for the block to be at fault; counterintuitively, I realized she didn't need a pressor, or a bronchodilator. She needed beta blockade, and I gave her esmolol, which corrected everything in seconds. The case went fine, and afterwards I asked her if her asthma medicine helped her attacks. She said no, not really. And with no objective evidence, I spoke to the Obstetrician, gave him my opinion, and recommended he refer her to a cardiologist for suspected conduction system disorder. I also told him she might be curable with physiological oblation. A couple of months later, he thanked me; she underwent testing, was sent to Stanford for oblation, and was cured of "asthma". Woohoo and cudos to the Stanford Anesthesia Department!"

"I did a lot of ballet as an adult and had outstanding training. Like many, I changed to ballroom when olde. There was a woman at the studio where I danced whose ballet career had been under George Balanchine in the New York City Ballet Company. She never said anything to me but told my friend that if I had started young, I would have "been way up there" in ballet. I would never trade my career in anesthesia for being "way up there". Thank you all for your great work."

Emily Florence Ratner

was born in San Antonio, TX. She attended Newcomb College/Tulane University (BS, Biology, 1983). She graduated from Baylor College of Medicine (MD, 1987). Following internship (Transitional) at SCVMC (1987-1988) she completed an Anesthesiology residency at Stanford (1988-1991). She was Chief Resident from 1990-1991.

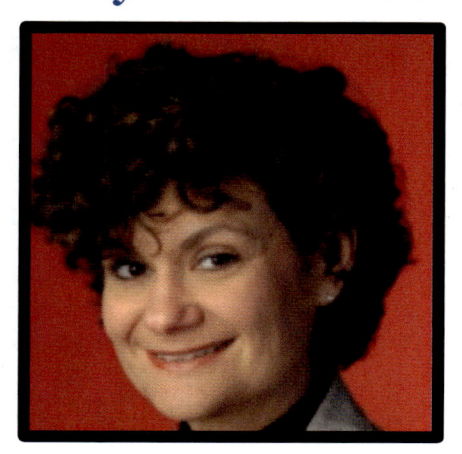

She was appointed Assistant Professor (Anesthesiology) (1992-2001), promoted to Associate Professor (2001-2008), and then Clinical Professor (2008-2014). Emily was a member of the Department's OB Anesthesia group. She was named Interdisciplinary Professor of the Year by the Stanford Department of Gynecology and Obstetrics (1999).

Dr. Ratner trained at the Helms Medical Institute (2004) and was certified by the American Board of Medical Acupuncture (2004). She was a founding co-director of the Division of Medical Acupuncture in the Stanford Department of Anesthesiology. She held that position from 2004-2014. She completed a Fellowship (Integrative Medicine) at the University of Arizona College of Medicine - Tucson (2008-2009) and was then founding co-director of PRIME (Peer Support and Resiliency In Medicine) program in the Stanford Department of Anesthesiology.

In 2015 she left Stanford and was appointed the Director of Integrative Medicine Initiatives at the MedStar Institute for Innovation, MedStar Health, Washington D.C. (2015-Present).

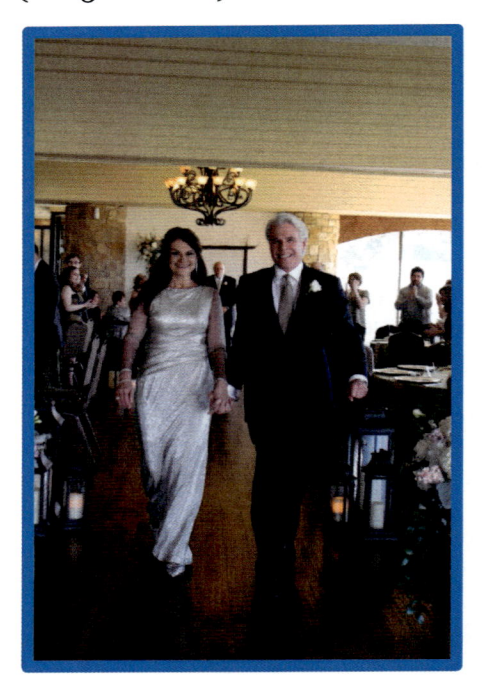

MedStar Health is a not-for-profit health system dedicated to caring for people in Maryland and the Washington, D.C., region, while advancing the practice of medicine through education, innovation, and research. MedStar's 30,000 associates, 6,000 affiliated physicians, 10 hospitals, ambulatory care and urgent care centers, and the MedStar Health Research Institute are recognized regionally and nationally for excellence in medical care. As the medical education and clinical partner of Georgetown University, MedStar trains more than 1,100 medical residents annually.

Emily Ratner is now retired. She enjoys hiking, cooking, gardening, traveling, and basically enjoying life with her now retired husband (Mike Lumpkin). She volunteers with Maryland Medical Rescue Corps, and at an animal rescue organization, at food banks, and at a vaccination center during the pandemic.

Dr. Ratner is a Staff Emeritus Retiree in the Stanford Department of Anesthesiology, Perioperative and Pain Medicine.

"Interesting Anecdotes/Memories Of Time At Stanford - So many!!!"
- *Learning from my teachers and colleagues. Sheila Cohen – "If an anesthetic plan a resident suggests to you doesn't sound right, trust your gut and don't do it!*
- *John Archer - "When riding a bicycle in Palo Alto, act as if none of the cars can see you." This was before I was hit by a car on my bike just in front of Stanford's ER. Thank you John Brock-Utne for walking me back into the hospital! And Ron Pearl's and Frank Sarnquist's leadership."*
- *Being at the VA Hospital during the 1989 earthquake; watching the OR table which was "locked" to the floor move in the opposite direction as the anesthesia machine which was still connected to the patient. Thinking, "How can Kevin Fish appear so calm right now?". Years later, he disclosed to me he was too scared to speak!*

- *Playing frisbee on the front lawn of the VA Hospital with Fritz Moritz after the 1989 earthquake, as we had to be on site, yet there was nothing to do."*
- *In the old, old Stanford hospital building, having to push a gurney uphill to transport patients to the PACU from the OR.*
- *Eating graham crackers and saltines in the PACU in the middle of the night on call when no other food was available.*
- *Sharing an office with Tracey Vogel and having a great time doing so! Having "No Dad's night dinners" with Kristi Peterson, Pat Curtis, and our very young kids.*
- *Having my office being used by female residents who needed a place to pump breast milk; seeing beverages lined up all along the back wall of my office. So glad this isn't needed anymore.*
- *Stanley Samuels and Steve Howard playing a practical joke on me. After I had a patient who no one could not intubate (the ENT docs could not do so either even via bronchoscopy), the patient returned to the OR and was successfully anesthetized. Stanley and Steve left me a note saying they performed a rapid sequence induction and intubated the patient under direct visualization without difficulty on one try … while in fact, they performed an awake fiberoptic intubation! Thanks, guys!*
- *Gordon Haddow's calmness in the face of cardiac chaos and Rich Jaffe's calmness and great sense of humor.*
- *At a big anesthesia party, watching 'The Village People' do karaoke, which included Ron Pearl in costume. Can never, ever forget that one!*

Richard Snyder was born in Springfield, MA. He did his undergraduate work at Bowdoin College (AB, 1982) and graduated from Stanford (MD, 1987). He interned at Kaiser - Santa Clara (Internal Medicine) (1987-1988) and was a resident at Stanford (1988-1990). He did a Fellowship (Regional Anesthesia) at Virginia Mason Franciscan Health, Seattle (1990-1991). He is an anesthesiologist in Seattle, WA, and has been affiliated with Kaiser Permanente Capitol Hill Campus, Swedish Medical Center-First Hill, and Virginia Mason Medical Center all in the Seattle area.

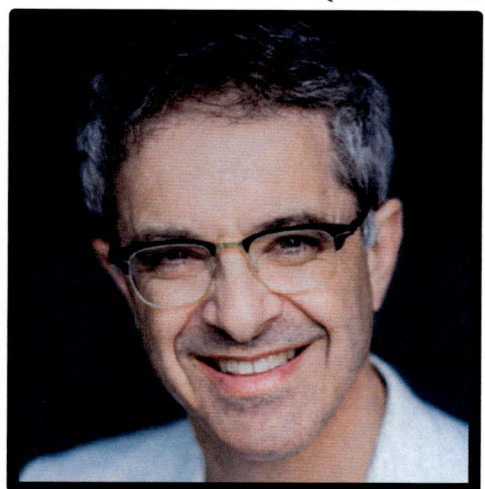

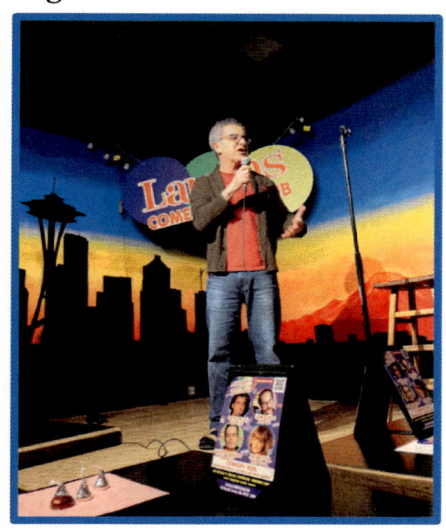

Snyder is also an actor, producer, writer, and comedian. He came to acting at age 50 when he performed a one man show '*In Search of Richard Snyder...*' It was 90 minutes of monologs starting with childhood in the 1960's and ending with meditations on gayness, Jewishness, and the point of it all. He wrote, produced, and acted in the film short '*On the Nature of Hotness*' an exploration into physical attraction over the course of human existence, a multi-media comedy piece which screened in film festivals and won "Best Comedy in Short Film" at the New York City International Film Festival. His second film short *'Neshamah'* in which an estranged brother and sister are forced to confront their ailing father's wish for assisted suicide also won multiple awards and screened at festivals through the country. He has studied Improv at Unexpected Productions, Jet City and Upright Citizens Brigade and has organized and taught workshops at UCLA, Stanford, and international medical meetings on using improv and acting to improve communication in medical settings. He writes a blog *'On Being...'* which chronicles the challenges and funny moments of life. He owns *Otter Be In Pictures, LLC,* a film production company.

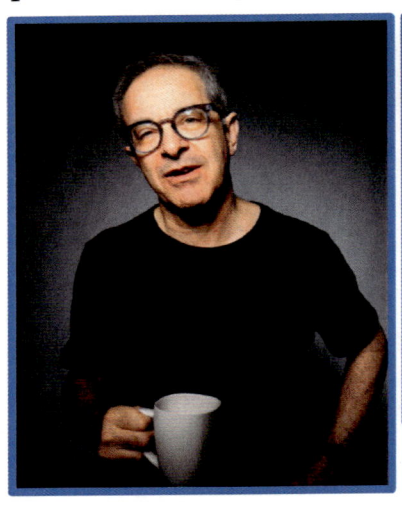

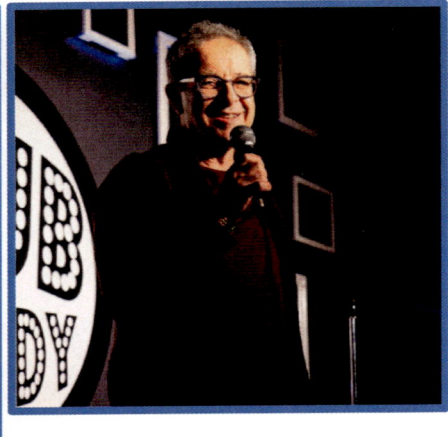

In his spare time, he loves travel to sacred sites such as Israel and Bali, hanging out with his adult children, skiing, comedy, and choral singing.

"I perform standup comedy throughout the Seattle area and once a week create short comedic videos for social media in which I try doing young people trends but fail every time. You can find out all things about Rich at https://richsnydercomedy.com."

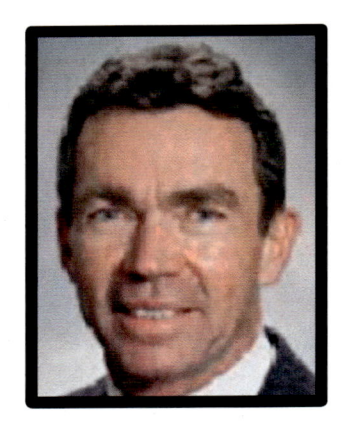

Christopher James Vasil attended Stanford as an undergraduate (AB, 1974) and then medical school at UCSF (MD, 1980). He completed internship and a residency (Internal Medicine) at Stanford (1980-1983). He had a private practice in Internal Medicine (1983-1988), but then did an Anesthesiology residency (1988-1990) and was appointed an Assistant Professor (Anesthesiology) (1991-1993). He worked in anesthesia practice with the GAS Group, Los Gatos (1993-2015) and is currently with PAMF (2015-Present).

Vanessa Thien Vu was an undergraduate at Barnard College, and then attended SUNY - Stony Brook (MD, 1987). She interned (Internal Medicine) at Rutgers Health/Cooperman Barnabas Medical Center (1987-1988). She was a Stanford Anesthesiology resident (1988-1991). She has practiced at Mercy Medical Center, Roseburg, OR, entire career (1991-Present). She was Physician of the Year (2017) and is currently Clinical Administrator/Medical Director of Surgical Services at Mercy Medical Center. She lists timber farming as her outside interest.

"I was doing a neuroanesthesia case for Dr. Frances Conley with the patient in a sitting position. During a requested controlled hypotension, I had to ask to put the patient flat because I had attached the nitroprusside drip, not directly into one of the ports, but at the next IV injection access about 10 cm away. The blood pressure kept dropping when I closed the infusion because of the extra nitroprusside in the line. To Dr. Conley's credit, she remained composed and did not even utter a word. The lesson to always attach a vasoactive drip directly to the CVP port was never forgotten. I did many more cases with Dr. Conley, but she never brought that incident up."

David Paul Whalen graduated form UC-Berkeley and then the Medical College of Wisconsin (MD, 1987). Her interned and did his residency at Stanford (1987-1991). Since 1991 he worked in the Sacramento Anesthesia Medical Group.

Thomas White Cutter graduated from the University of Illinois College of Medicine (MD, 1987) and did an internship (Transitional) at Loyola Medicine MacNeal Hospital (1987-1998). He began Anesthesiology at Stanford but after his CA1 year (7/1/88-6/30/89) he transferred to the University of Chicago (1989-1991). He is affiliated with the University of Chicago Medical Center Chicago, IL, as a Clinical Associate of Anesthesia and Critical Care.

Allen George Gruber a UCSF graduate (MD, 1983), interned (Internal Medicine) at Kaiser - San Francisco (1983-1984), and began an Anesthesiology residency at the University of Washington (1984-1986). He continued his anesthesia training at UCSF (1986-1987) before completing the last 6 months of his CA3 year (1/1/88-6/30/88) at Stanford. He worked int Santa Rosea as a pain specialist until his license to practice in California was revoked (2021).

Adrian George Tedeschi received a medical degree from the Autonomous Universidad de Guadalajara Faculty of Medicine, Mexico (1980). He did an internship (Transitional) at Kern Medical Center (1981-1982). He completed CA1 andCA2 years of residency (Anesthesiology) at University of North Carolina (1986-1988) and his CA3 year at Stanford (1988-1989).

Shale Foster Imeson attended UC-Berkeley and then UCI (MD, 1985). He interned at UCSF/Fresno (Internal Medicine) (1985-1986) and began his Anesthesiology residency at Virginia Mason, Seattle (1986). Imeson completed 6 months of his CA3 year (7/5/88-12/31/88) at Stanford. He has practiced anesthesia and pain management with the Stockton Anesthesia Medical Group since 1989. He served as Chair the Department of Anesthesia at Lodi Memorial Hospital and at St. Joseph's Medical Center, Stockton, where he also served as Chief of Staff (2000-2001). He was President of the San Joaquin Medical Society (2003). He was President of Morpheus Anesthesia, a group of 15 Lodi, CA anesthesiologists (2016) that joined California Emergency Physicians (CEP) America.

CHAPTER 9
1989

George H. W. Bush was sworn in as our 41st President on January 20th, 1989. In March, Tim Berners-Lee submitted a memorandum entitled *'Information Management: A Proposal'* for a system that would eventually become the World Wide Web. A company in Brookline, MA, named *The World*, became the first commercial Internet service provider (ISP) in the USA. It offered direct dial-up telephone connections to the Internet for a monthly fee. The first Global Positioning System (GPS) satellites were placed in orbit that year, and the world's first high-definition television was tested in Japan.

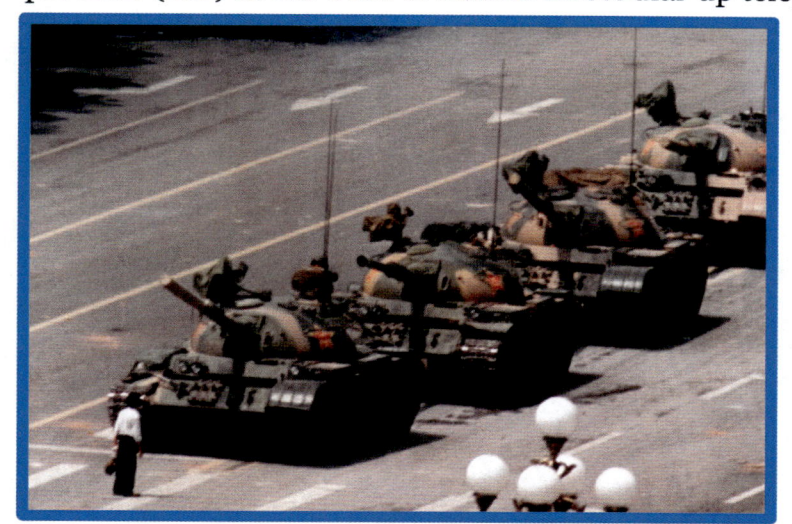

In March the Exxon Valdez spilled 240,000 barrels of oil in Alaska's Prince William Sound. Another ecological disaster occurred on May 15th when the last golden toad was seen in Costa Rica and the species was classified as extinct.

Internationally, in February Iran's Supreme Leader Ayatollah Ruhollah Khomeini issued a fatwa calling for the death of British author Salman Rushdie for his crime of writing *'The Satanic Verses'*. Iran placed a $3 million bounty on Rushdie. The Tiananmen Square protests began in China in May with millions of people demanding greater democracy. Then on June 4th a violent military crackdown took place in Beijing. The following day, an unknown Chinese protester dubbed *'Tank Man'* stood in front of a column of military tanks temporarily halting them. To this day no one knows the fate of the Tank Man, although a rumor persists that is now is a presenter on TikTok. In July, a Tel-Aviv-Jerusalem bus was bombed becoming the first Palestinian suicide attack inside Israel. While in Lebanon, Hezbollah hung U.S. Marine Lt. Col. William Higgins in retaliation for Israel kidnapping Hezbollah leader Abdel Karim Obeid. That same day, the U.N. passed Security Council Resolution #638 condemning the "taking of hostages by either side in a conflict". The resolution apparently was forgotten during the current Israeli-Palestinian crisis of 2023-2024. Not to be outdone, on December 20th the US invaded Panama in *Operation Just Cause* to overthrow dictator Manuel Noriega.

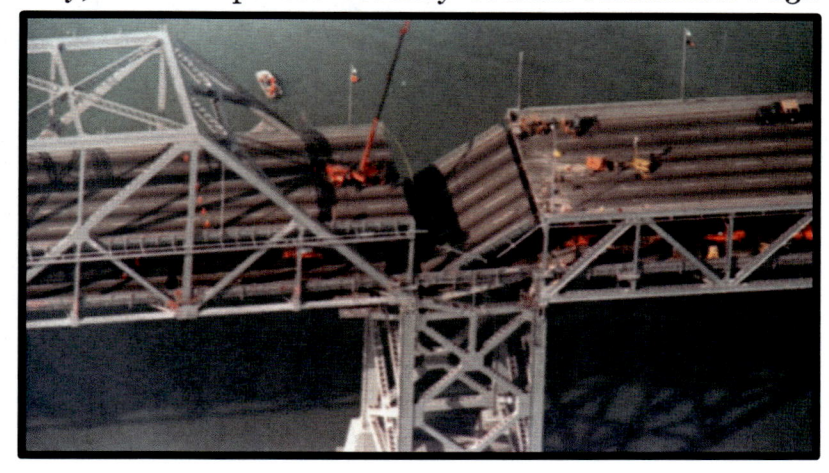

Closer to home, the October 17th, 1989, the Richter Scale 6.9 Loma Prieta Earthquake caused severe damage in the Bay area. Stanford University Medical Center survived the earthquake relatively unscathed, although the PA-VAH suffered approximately $30,000,000 in damages. Game #3 of the 1989 World Series between the Oakland Athletics and the San Francisco Giants, which was scheduled to begin later that evening, was postponed for 10 days.

The addition to Stanford Hospital opened in 1989. Stanford's strategic planners predicted that the 20 new modern operating rooms would be sufficient to meet Stanford's needs for the next 50 years until 2039!

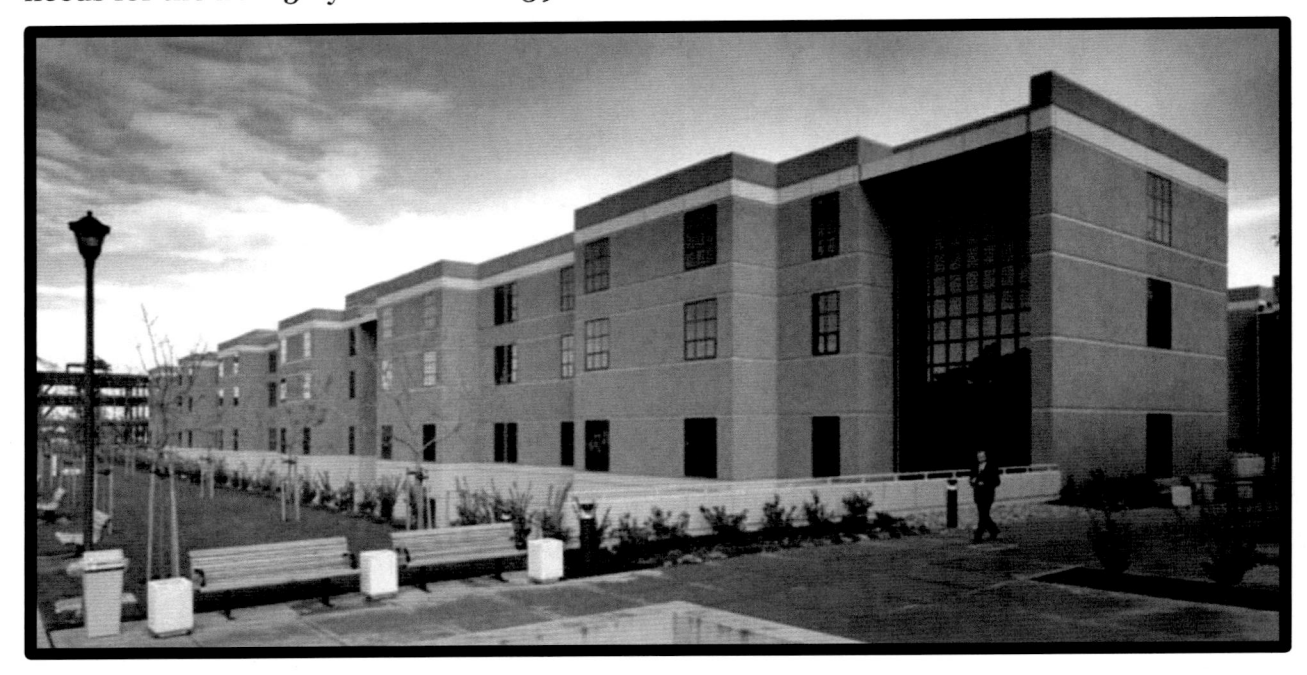

The addition to expand Stanford University Hospital opened in 1989. It was the first modernization project since the hospital opened in 1959.

James Crampton Finn III graduated from Stanford (MD, 1985) and completed a residency (Internal Medicine) there (1988-1989). He then did an Anesthesiology residency (1989-1992) followed by a Fellowship (CCM). He has practiced at Sutter Medical Center of Santa Rosa, Santa Rosa, Petaluma Valley Hospital, Petaluma, CA, Memorial Hospital, Santa Rosa, CA, and Sequoia Hospital, Redwood City, CA.

David Minoru Fujii attended Yale (MD, 1987) and then began a residency (Surgery) in the University of Pennsylvania Health System (1987-1989). He switched career plans and completed a residency in Anesthesiology at Stanford (1989-1992) and a Fellowship (Pediatric Anesthesiology) at Children's Hospital of Philadelphia (1992). Dr. Fuji works in Phoenix, AZ.

John George Kelley was born in Oakland, CA. As an undergraduate, he first attended Chabot College (1975-1976), then UCD (1976-1978) and graduated from the University of San Francisco (USF) (BS, Biology, 1980) and (MS, Biology/Endocrinology, 1980-1982). He was a Staff Research Associate at UCSF at the Francis I. Proctor Foundation for Research in Ophthalmology (1982-1984) and Staff Research Assistant at Stanford University Department of Oncology (1983-1984). He went to medical school at Tulane University School of Medicine (MD, 1988), did an internship (Transitional) at Naval Medical Center, Oakland, CA (1988-1989) and his Anesthesiology residency at Stanford (1989-1992). After training he was a Staff Anesthesiologist at Naval Medical Center, Oakland (1992-1996) and an Assistant Clinical Professor (Anesthesia) at UCSF (1993-1996). He was voted by the residents "Outstanding Clinical Instructor" for two years (1993-1995).

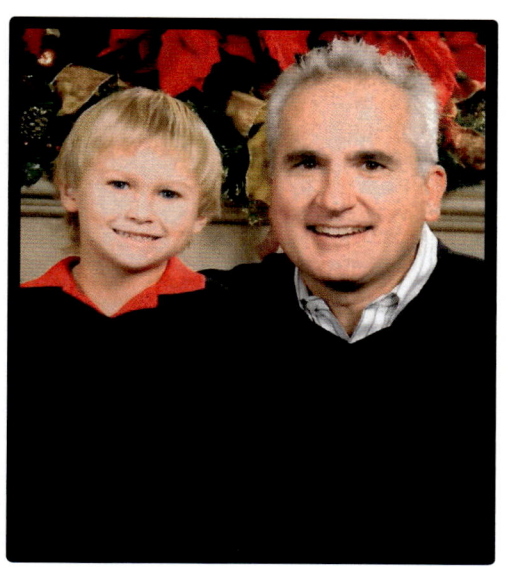

John with John Jr (2008)

"I remember when David Gaba told me that I was the first medical student to ever go through his simulator, almost 40 years ago now."

John was a Lt. Commander in the Medical Corp, US Naval Reserve (1984-1996) and was awarded an Expeditionary Medal, Operation Uphold Democracy, Haiti, in 1994. While in the military he flew FA-18 Hornet fighter jets.

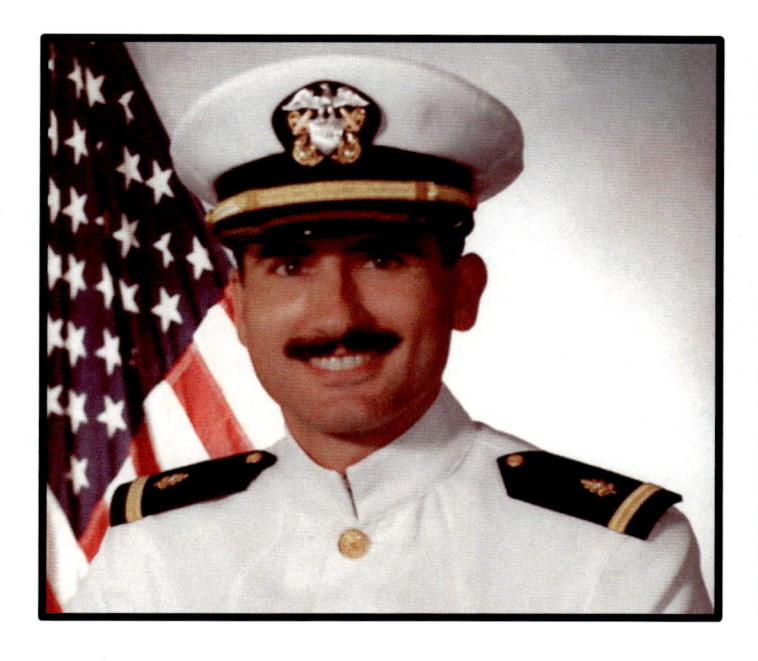

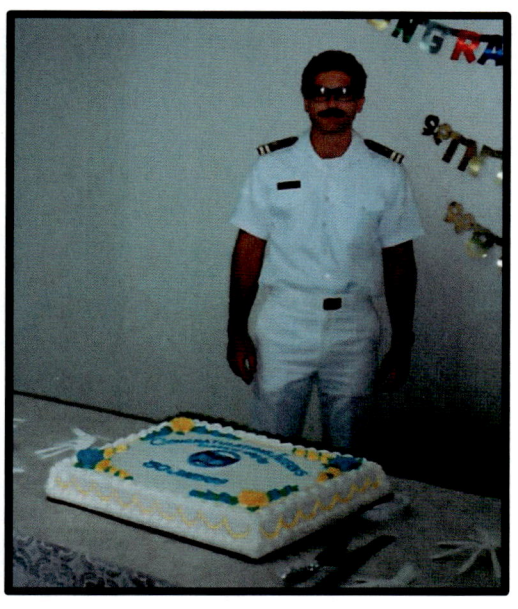

He worked at Community Hospital of Los Gatos (1996-2009), at Good Samaritan Hospital, SJ (1996-Present), and El Camino Hospital, Los Gatos (2009-Present) as an anesthesiologist, pain management and addiction medicine specialist. At Los Gatos he was Chair of the Department of Anesthesia and a member of several hospital committees.

"I thought of the many things I've done in the military. I was stationed at Naval Medical Center Oakland and was also attached to the two aircraft carriers stationed in Alameda, the Abraham Lincoln CVN 72 and Carl Vinson CVN 70. I was also stationed in Rota Spain, which was awesome.

Some of my memories ... When I went to Officer Indoctrination School for months, I was tested daily with rigorous physical fitness goals and academic achievement in the classroom. It was the accumulation of test scores from each day over those months that I was able to achieve Distinguished Physical Fitness Graduate (only six out of 387 received that award), Distinguished Academic Graduate (only five out of 387) received that award and Distinguished Military Graduate. Only two officers out of 387 received all three and I was one of them. The reason I mentioned that is because of my level of physical fitness and academic achievement I was placed on a special MMART military medical alert readiness team where I could get deployed any day to 20-25 of the hotspots in the world at that time.

One example is I was to meet at the Alameda Naval Air Station with my seabag and told that I would be going on a special mission, but that it was highly classified, so I had no clue of where I was going and for how long. I was put on a C-130, rode on wooden seats in the fuselage with ear protection because it was so loud for hours, not knowing where I was going. When we finally landed, I was told that I was at an Air Force Base in Florida. From there we took off in a helicopter, which was even louder still not knowing where we were going. We finally landed right next to the prison on Guantánamo Bay Cuba. We then got onto another helicopter still not being told where we were going. After another lengthy chopper flight which rattles your body continuously plus it is extremely loud, my comrades and I looked out the window and saw an amphibious assault ship the USS Wasp. It supported multiple attack Apache helicopters, Blackhawks, and Harriers, which could take off and land vertically on the deck. I was told that I was the trauma doctor, and to get the operating rooms ready

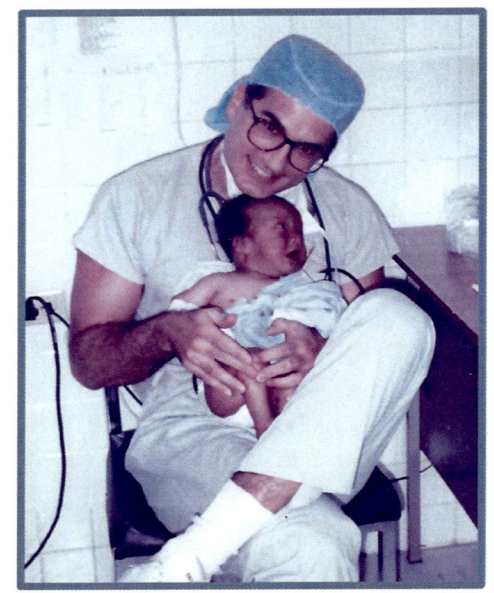

Loja, Ecuador (Interplast) 1992

for mass casualties. I was told that 2500 Marines were on board, and that once I got the ORs ready to go to the bottom of the hall of the ship where the crates of weapons were so that I could join up with the Special Forces from all the various branches. Because of my achievements in both the physical and academic arena, I had the honor of serving with the Navy Seals who respected my level fitness and we're also very proud to show off all the various sophisticated weapons including, but not limited to high caliber machine guns, shoulder held missiles, plastic explosives, etc. We were opening huge wooden crates that had been shipped from the Gulf War. The unit that I was in was typically the one that did the first initial assault, destroying specific targets, such as airport communication centers. etc. I was told that we were waiting for specific orders coming from the President of the United States, Bill Clinton. We were just off the coast of Haiti waiting to invade.

One of the achievements that I'm very proud of is that I went through a year and a half of training, both physically, and in the classroom to get qualified to fly the F-18D Hornet, the same plane that the Blue Angels have flown for years. That was one of the most exciting things I got to do in my life. I used to go to the airshows with my dad every year, and I remember telling my father that I was going to fly the Blue Angel jet when I got older. I made it happen and was the only physician out of our large unit allowed to do so."

Ultra-Rapid Opiate Detoxification (UROD)

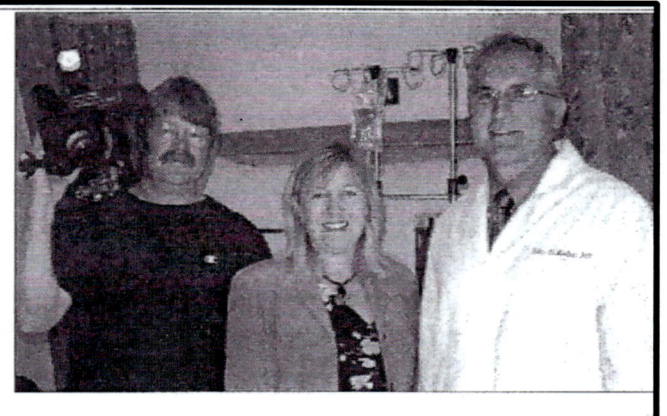

On Tuesday, September 21st, the UROD procedure (performed by Dr. John Kelley, Anesthesiologist at CHLG) was featured on the 5:00 p.m. NBC (KNTV) news. Pictured are Mark, camera man, Marianne Favro, NBC Anchor & Health Reporter & Dr. John Kelley. To learn more about UROD, visit the CHLG website www.communityhospitalLG.

"I was working at Community Hospital of Los Gatos and developed an Ultra-Rapid Opioid Detoxification (UROD) technique to get patients off of their prescription opioids. The patients had the UROD procedure under general anesthesia in the ICU and then went into a comprehensive treatment program with multiple professionals including buprenorphine for opioid maintenance which is a process used routinely now twenty years later. At the time, there were only two anesthesiologists in the South Bay that were certified, myself being one of them, to use the drug for maintenance. My program was featured on the local news."

"I developed an intraoperative epidural implantation technique that I used for decades while doing complex spinal instrumentation surgeries for post-op pain management. These surgeries would last 6-14 hours long but the epidural infusion made it possible for these patients to get up the next morning and participate in PT and OT comfortably. I started this technique in the mid 1990's and continued through 2019. This picture is from 1999."

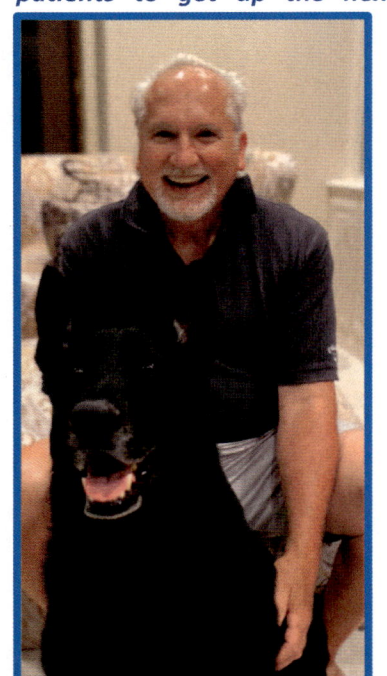

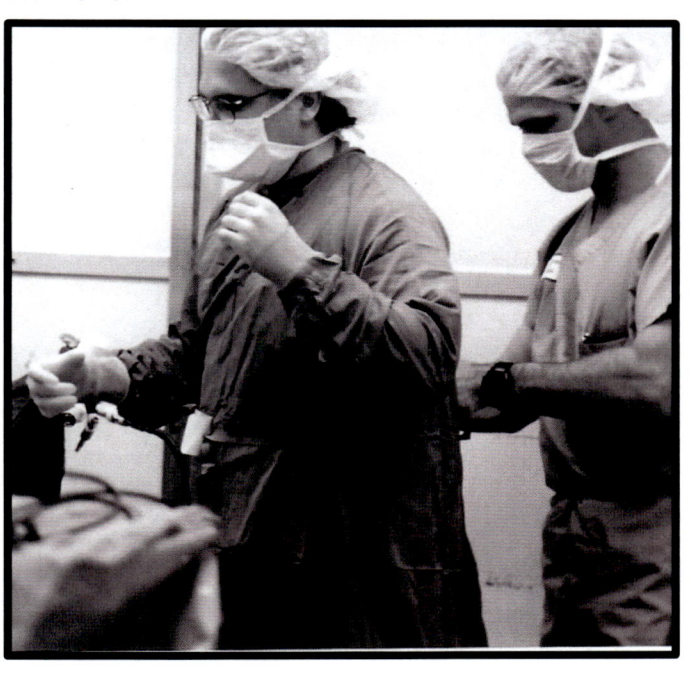

John with his faithful companion Ike

Peter Single Kosek is a 1988 graduate of the David Geffen School of Medicine at UCLA (MD, 1988) and interned (Internal Medicine) at CPMC (1988-1989). He completed his Anesthesiology residency at Stanford (1989-1992). He was briefly on the faculty on the cardiac anesthesia team. He started at OHSU as a member of the adult and pediatric cardiac anesthesia faculty and was interterm Director of Pain Management there. He then focused on pain management full time, left OHSU and founded Pain Consultants of Oregon, Eugene, OR (1998). He joined Oregon Neurosurgery group after closing Pain Consultants in 2017.

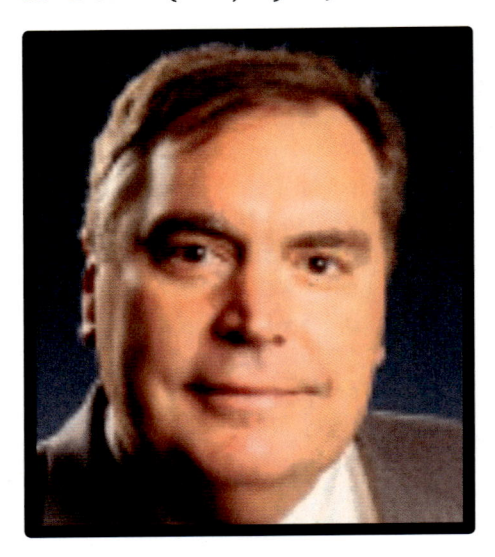

He currently works as a Pain Medicine specialist in Springfield, OR, and practices at Peace Health Sacred Heart Medical Center, River Bend, OR. He holds a courtesy appointment as Professor at OHSU. He is also a principal investigator through the Association of Clinical Research Professionals and has been involved in more than 25 pain-related clinical trials.

Peter has served on numerous boards and advisory committees and was appointed by the governor to the Oregon Pain Management Commission, serving a seven-year term. A former president of the Lane County Medical Society, he was previously a member of the Board of Trustees of the Oregon Medical Association. He has been President of the Oregon Chapter of the American Society of Interventional Pain Physicians, and is now the Chair of the organization.

"I am an avid, if less-than-particularly skilled, a fisherman, beekeeper and gardener. I enjoy being outdoors. In my free time, I can be found searching for ripe tomatoes and salad greens in our greenhouse. Although I haven't convinced my four children to join me, they do eat the vegetables I grow."

Blair Stephen Lee received his medical degree from UCLA (MD, 1988) and interned (Transitional) at Harbor/UCLA (1988-1989). He was a Stanford resident (1989-1992). He works as an anesthesiologist ay Kaiser - Bellevue, WA, at Swedish Medical Center.

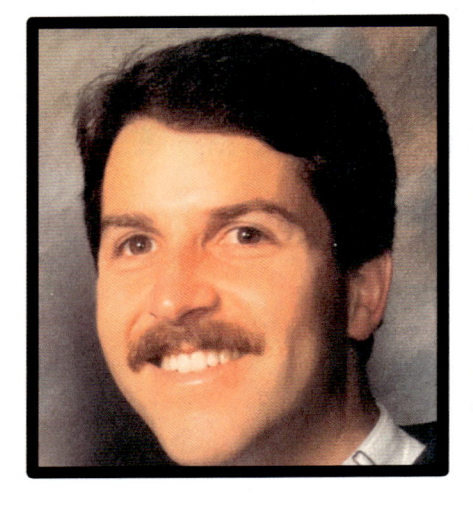

Dennis Michael Lindeborg was born in San Francisco. He attended UCSD (BA, Chemistry, 1984) During college he worked as an oil rig roustabout in Taft, CA (1980-1982) and as a Budweiser truck driver/deliveryman (1984). He graduated UCSF (MD, 1988), and then did an internship (Internal Medicine) at Kaiser - San Francisco (1988-1989), followed by his Anesthesiology residency (1989-1992). He was a Fellow (CCM) at Stanford (1992). He has spent his entire career with the Southern California Permanente Medical Group (1993-Present). He was Anesthesia Chief of Service (1996-2008) and Physician Director of Perioperative Services for Kaiser - Southern Region (1999-2006). His interests include skiing, triathlons, marathons, snowboarding, and golf.

"On my first trip as a Stanford Transport Physician, the helicopter pilot spent the whole elevator ride up to the helipad warning me about motion sickness. Apparently, on the last trip, the pediatric team threw up all over the craft during the flight. As we took off on the warm summer night and my trepidation was peaking, the pilot turned around towards me and said over the intercom, "since it is just you and me, you need to help me avoid any wires I might accidentally hit". I could then feel my pulse quicken as the safety of the Stanford helipad disappeared into the abyss and darkness enveloped the craft. I had no idea how I was supposed to spot an unexpected wire in our flight path to Monterey. When we arrived at the hospital in Monterey it was extremely windy, which caused the pilot to abort multiple landing attempts. She then turned to me and said, "hold on, this is going to be rough". She powered toward the ground and proceeded to practically crash land. I stumbled off the helicopter and wondered to myself what Ron Pearl had gotten me into. Fortunately, I survived the trip and subsequently completed many trips to different locations around the Western US, including Alaska. I really appreciated the enriching experience it provided me and I'm sure many past, present, and future alumni would agree that this was an exceptional opportunity offered by Stanford."

Mei-Ven Chang Lo worked in the Department of Physiology, University of Rochester Medical Center, Rochester, NY, prior to attending medical school at Stanford (MD, 1988). She completed an internship (Transitional) at SCVMC (1988-1989) and her residency (1989-1992). She worked at O'Connor Hospital and Regional Medical Center and is now retired.

Joel Anthony Peelen was a medical graduate of the Medical College of Wisconsin (MD, 1988). He was an intern (Transitional) at SCVMC (1988-1989) and a resident (1989-1992). Joel was Chief Resident (1991-1992). He worked in Templeton, CA (1992-2020) before retiring from clinical practice. He is an avid bikepacker.

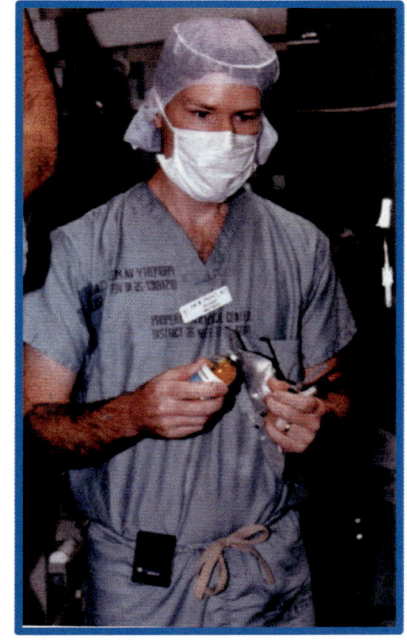

John Buford Pollard received his medical degree from the Duke University School of Medicine (MD, 1988). He was a resident (1989-1982) and Chief Resident (1991-1992). He worked at PA-VAH and is now retired.

Jon Wallace Propst was born in 1957. His undergraduate training was at UCSD (BA, Bioengineering, 1979) and then graduate school at USC (PhD, Bioengineering, 1979-1986). He attended medical school at University of Miami Leonard M. Miller School of Medicine (MD, 1988). He interned (Internal Medicine) at the UCLA-Wadsworth VAH (1988-1989) and did his residency (Anesthesiology) at Stanford (1989-1992). Following residency he completed a Fellowship (Adult Cardiothoracic Anesthesiology) at Stanford (1992). He began private practice at Marian Regional Medical Center, Santa Maria, CA (1992-Present). He plans to retire at the end of 2025. He enjoys travel, golf, gardening and reading.

"I was on call at SCVMC on October 17, 1989, when the Loma Prieta Earthquake occurred a little after 5:00 pm. Fortunately, the hospital did not suffer extensive damage, but we had to check all the operating rooms to make sure everything was in good order. I was able to contact my family to make sure they were doing okay. We had a few cases that night that were mostly orthopedic injuries which were relatively minor."

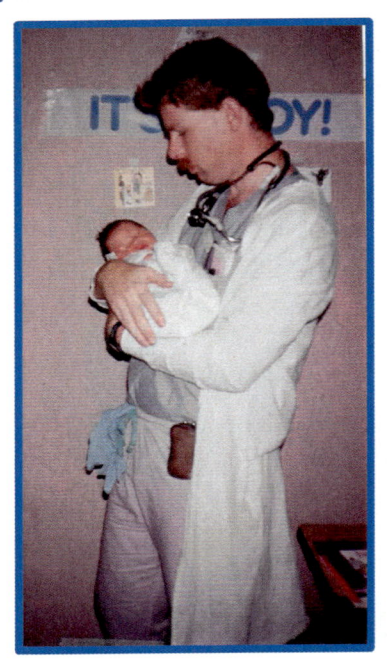

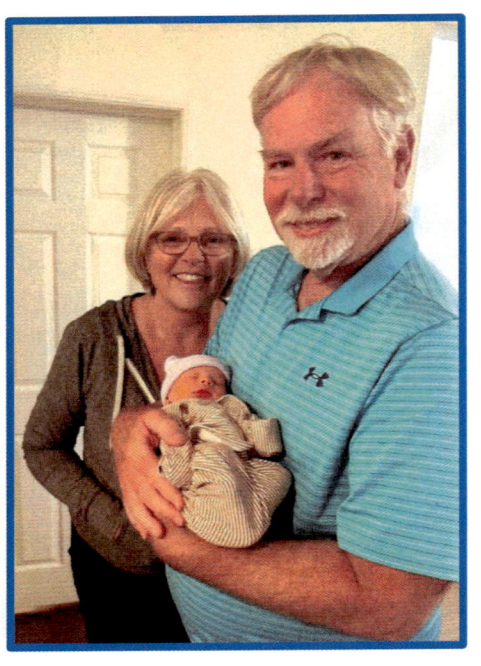

E. Price Stover (deceased) was born in Tallahassee, FL. He graduated Phi Beta Kappa from Stanford University (1982), and then spent two years doing research in endocrinology at Stanford Medical School. He continued his work for the next four years through the Medical Scholars Program while studying for his medical degree (MD, 1988). He completed his Anesthesiology residency (1989-1992) but required rehabilitation for substance abuse during training. He was a Fellow (Cardiovascular Anesthesia) at Stanford (1993). He appointed to the faculty as an Assistant Professor in the MCL as a member of the Cardiovascular Anesthesia Division and was one of the founding members of the liver transplant team. He continued to do research on blood transfusion and coagulation. In 2000 he briefly left the Department for private practice but returned in early 2002. He was a superb teacher appreciated for his sense of humor and fairness. Sadly, he died from a drug overdose at Stanford Hospital while on call during the night of May 24, 2002.

John Brock-Utne, "Many of us attended his wonderful wedding in Burlingame. Price was an outstanding tennis player and tried to attend all major tennis tournaments during his short life. He was an excellent anesthesiologist, who we all respected. So sad."

This residency class was composed of a significant number of trainees that spent only a portion of their three-year residency at Stanford for a variety of reasons. Several began training elsewhere and completed their residency at Stanford, several left before completing their Stanford residency for other programs, and others left the program for medical reasons.

Kirtikumar "Kirti" Gopalji Desai graduated from the Medical College of Wisconsin (MD, 1986). He did an internship (Surgery) and a CA1 year of Anesthesiology residency at Swedish Medical Center/First Hill (1986-1988) then transferred to Stanford for his CA2 and CA3 years (7/1/89-6/30/91). He works at Sutter Maternity & Surgery Center of Santa Cruz.

Wai-Keung Loh was a graduate of the University of Illinois College of Medicine (MD, 1987). His internship (Transitional) was at Loyola Medicine MacNeal Hospital (1987-1988). He completed his CA1 year of Anesthesiology at the University of Illinois College of Medicine, Chicago (1988-1989). He came to Stanford for his CA2 and CA3 years (7/1/89-6/30/91). Dr. Loh was affiliated with Saint Joseph Hospital & Medical Center.

John Raymond Lubben attended Washington University St. Louis School of Medicine (MD, 1986). He interned (Surgery) at Spectrum Health/Michigan State University (1986-1987). He completed his CA1 and CA2 years of Anesthesiology training at Washington University (1987-1989) and his CA3 year at Stanford (7/1/89-6/30/90). Dr. Lubben is an anesthesiologist in Monterey, CA, and is affiliated with Community Hospital of the Monterey Peninsula.

Michael A. Mellenthin Jr

was in Los Angeles. He attended Stanford for his undergraduate education (BS, Biologic Sciences, 1981). He then received his medical degree from UCLA (MD, 1985). He interned (Internal Medicine) at Huntington Hospital (1985-1986) and completed 2.5 years of his Anesthesiology residency training at UCLA (1986-1988). He came to Stanford for the final 6 months of his CA3 year (1/1/89-6/30/89).

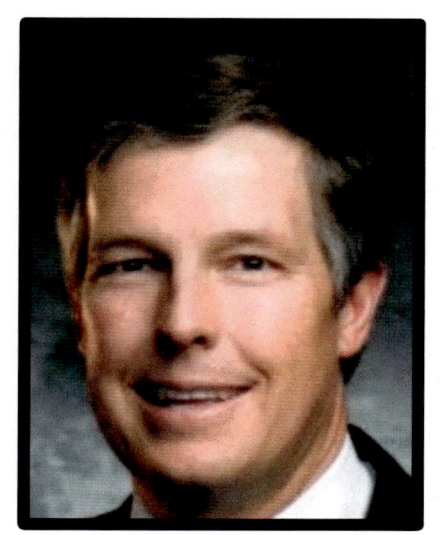

Following residency, he was President of Coast Anesthesia Medical Group (1989-1998), a private group that provided anesthesia services to O'Connor Hospital, San Jose. He was Chair of the Department of Anesthesiology at O'Connor Hospital (1993-1998). Dr. Mellenthin was also an Adjunct Clinical Instructor on our volunteer faculty (1994-2010).

Michael attended the Stanford University Graduate School of Business as a Sloan Fellow (1998-1999). He was Director of Business Development for Neoforma, Santa Clara, CA (1999-2000). (Neoforma provided business-to-business e-commerce services for medical equipment and supplies. He was lead strategist for evaluating partnership and merger/acquisition opportunities within the physician office and alternate care markets.)

He was co-founder and Vice-President of Finance and Risk Adjustment for Benu, San Mateo, (2000-2007). (Benu provides mid-size employers choice of health plan for employees. He managed all internal financial and administrative functions.) During that time, he also worked in the AAMG of Palo Alto (2003-2008).

In 2008 he became Medical Director of Community Anesthesia Providers, Fresno, CA (2008-2014). This group provided anesthesia services for Clovis Community Medical Center and Fresno Heart Hospital, as well as obstetrical anesthesia at Community Regional Medical Center. He returned to the Bay area as an anesthesiologist with Stanford Health Care – ValleyCare Medical Center, Pleasanton (2015-2021).

He has worked providing pediatric dental anesthesia since 2011 at a variety of dental surgery centers and offices. He was CMO for OMNI Anesthesia, Fresno (2011-2013). He was Medical Director of the Fresno Dental Surgery Center providing extensive dental restorative services to underprivileged children of the Central Valley. He was Medical Director of Central California Dental Surgicenter, Atwater, CA (2013-2014). For a short period, he was Chief of Anesthesia at Emanuel Medical, Turlock, CA (2014). He has worked in Oakland and is currently constructing a dental office in the San Jose area.

Dr. Meellenthin is a board member of Tiba Foundation (2021-Present). Tiba Foundation supports locally led initiatives that build robust community health, knowledge, and capacity, to improve access and quality of life in rural Kenya. In that role he travels annually to Matibabu Medical Center, Ukwala, Kenya. He also is involved with Hospital de la Familia and travels annually to Guatemala. He is currently the Chair of their Medical Committee. Other medical missions include trips to Cambodia, Myanmar, and Bhutan.

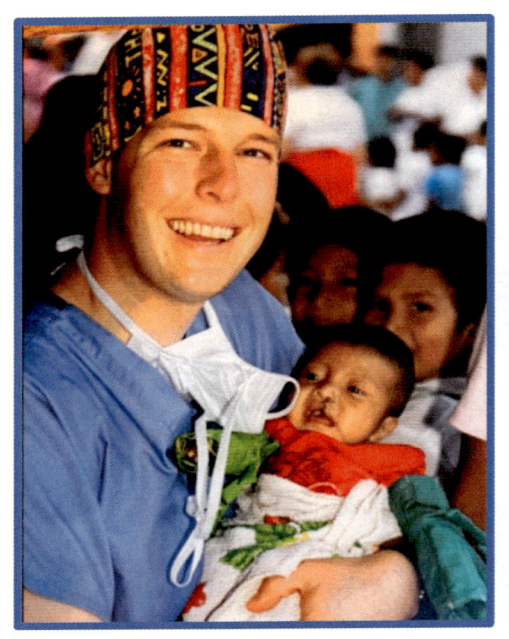

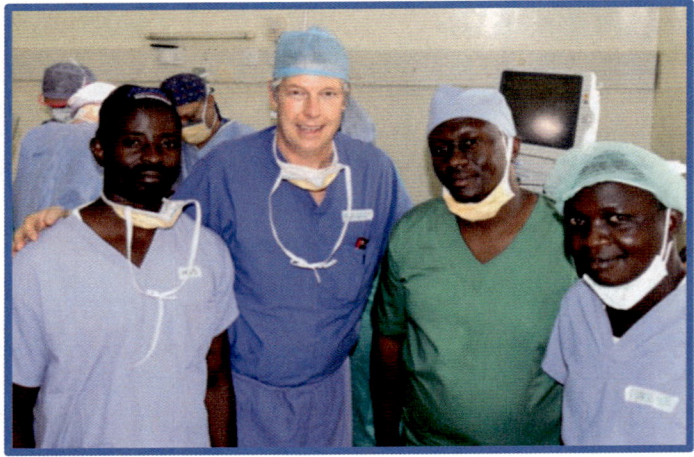

"I was a Stanford Anesthesia resident for only six months, but everyone treats me like I was there the whole three years."

"I remember moving into the 'new' 300 Pasteur OR's in the middle of the six months I was there."

Daniel Raphael Azar was born in Israel and immigrated to the USA at age 3. He grew up in the New York City area, the son of prominent academic anesthesiologist Isaac Azar. Dan attended the University of Pennsylvania (BA, double-major Biology and Biological Basis of Behavior, 1984). He graduated from Icahn School of Medicine at Mount Sinai (MD, 1988). He completed his internship (Internal Medicine) at Kaiser - San Francisco (1988-1989) and then did two years of his Anesthesiology residency (7/1/89-8/31/91) at Stanford. Regrettably, Dan developed an opioid use disorder and did not complete his training. He enrolled in California's Medical Board Diversion program, completed rehabilitation, and began a new career in medicine.

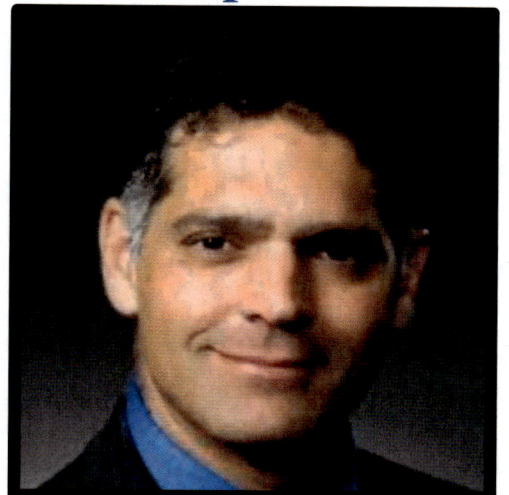

He worked for 2 years as locum tenens in various Bay area urgent care clinics including PAMF and Doctors on Duty. Dan then accepted the position of Lead Physician for Readicare HealthSouth, Santa Clara, CA (1993-1997) and then Lead Physician for US Health Works, Milpitas, CA (1997-2001). He practiced Occupational Medicine and Urgent Care at both positions. Dan then co-founded Alliance Occupational Medicine (AOM), Santa Clara (2001-2011) where he served as Medical Director. AOM was a multidisciplinary medical group dedicated to the treatment and rehabilitation of injured workers in Silicon Valley. During his tenure at Alliance, Dan earned a master's degree (MPH, Public Health) from the Medical College of Wisconsin (2005) and then completed a residency (Occupational Medicine) at the University of Pennsylvania (2007-2008).

After earning his Board Certification in Environmental and Occupational Medicine, he joined Lockheed Martin Corporation, Sunnyvale CA, as a Regional Managing Physician with oversight for the Lockheed clinics within the Western and South-East regions and separately, was the corporation's medical consultant to the Aeronautics Division (2011-2014).

He left Lockheed – and all the travel that entailed - to co-found Access OmniCare, an Occupational Medicine clinic in Fremont, CA (2014-2016) where he again served as the Medical Director providing a broad range of services to local employers including Tesla and the Fremont Unified School District. His mission was to support the health and productivity of employees through preventive care, surveillance, and the efficacious treatment of work-related injuries and illnesses. Dan also served as a California Qualified Medical Evaluator (2009-2019) providing evidence-based medical determinations regarding injury causation, treatment recommendations, and impairment ratings to administrative judges and other stakeholders within the CA Workers' Compensation system. Separately, Dan was an FAA medical examiner for air traffic controllers and pilots and performed immigration examinations for USCIS.

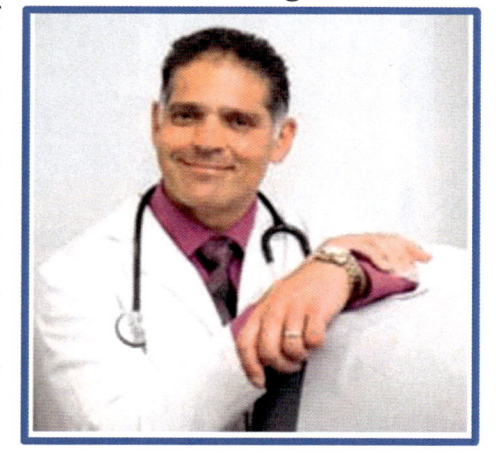

In 2008 Dan started a small side practice providing outpatient care with sublingual buprenorphine (Suboxone) to individuals who self-identified as suffering from opioid use disorder (OUD). Motivated by his personal experience with OUD and the opportunity to make a meaningful difference for his patients and their families, Dan, outside of his full-time work, continues to provide ongoing care to over one hundred patients who remain abstinent and productive.

Dan has worked as the California Site Physician at Sandia National Laboratories, Livermore CA (2017-Present) providing medical counseling and treatment to Sandia's workforce and supporting operations with subject matter expertise in occupational medicine, physical rehabilitation, and public health. Dan was very active (and busy) in supporting Sandia's national security mission during the COVID pandemic.

He served as a medical consultant to the Lab's leadership and to the Livermore CA, and Albuquerque NM, sites in developing de novo processes and operations intended to maintain a healthy workforce and safe workplace including lab-wide informational presentations, isolation policies, on-site PCR testing, and ultimately on-site vaccination. Dan Azar is currently board certified in Occupational Medicine by the American Board of Preventive Medicine, and in Addiction Medicine by the American Board of Preventive Medicine. Dan is a Fellow of the American College of Environmental and Occupational Medicine and a Fellow of the American Society of Addiction Medicine.

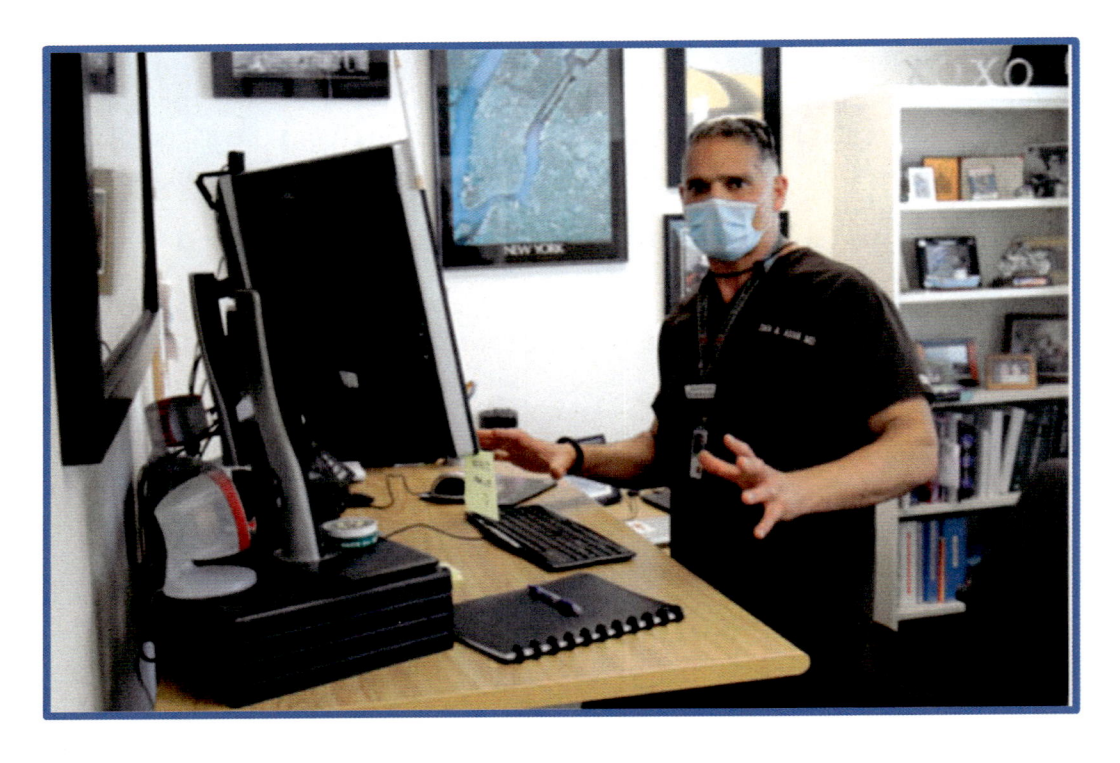

Dan Azar at work in his office at the Sandia/California campus

"Retirement TBD - I still enjoy providing "slow" medicine at Sandia and in my side practice in Addiction Medicine but have already transitioned to part-time at Sandia."

He lists his outside activities as engaged husband and grandfather, resistance training, gardening, home projects, road racing cars (SCCA, spec Miata), road racing motorcycles (AFM, multiple classes), off road motorcycle riding (trails, enduro), hiking and camping.

Memories of Time at Stanford:
- *During my first rotation in anesthesia working with 2 other tall residents and being referred to by the anesthesia techs as "the trees".*
- *While on call at the PA-VAH as a brand new 26-year-old resident I was paged at 2 am to perform an LP in the ER. Coming from Newark, as I am descending the western section of the Dumbarton bridge in my high mileage 1979 Mazda RX-7 at 90 mph I am pulled over by CHP. In a rush to get to the VA I jump out of the Mazda clutching my stethoscope to prove I am a doc on the way to an emergency call. I immediately find myself 30 feet away from young CHP officer, shouting at me to drop my weapon, while simultaneously aiming his unholstered weapon directly at my chest. Needless to say, I am grateful that the only thing he gave me that night was a ticket – and an unforgettable lesson in never getting out of a pulled over vehicle without permission and overtly empty hands. Whew.*
- *At Stanford as a resident, on a daily basis as I set up the meds for the morning's first case, feeling anxious and wondering if this was going to be the day I was to be identified to be an imposter unworthy of my slot at Stanford.*

CHAPTER 10
1990

The reunification of Germany occurred in 1990. Soviet President Mikhail Gorbachev was awarded the Nobel Peace Prize for his efforts to lessen Cold War tensions. Unfortunately, that same year Saddam Hussain ordered Iraq to invade its neighbor Kuwait prompting the US and UK to send troops to Kuwait in Operation Desert Shield the following year. Other Middle East events included a stampede in a pedestrian tunnel in Mecca during the Haj pilgrimage causing 1,426 deaths. NASA launched the Hubble Space Telescope aboard Space Shuttle Discovery in April from the Kennedy Space Center in Florida. Discovery deployed a five-person crew who filmed the process using IMAX cameras. The Hubble telescope was the first space telescope put into orbit that could be repaired by astronauts when maintenance was needed. The mission lasted five days and successfully returned to Earth, landing at the Edwards Air Force Base in California.

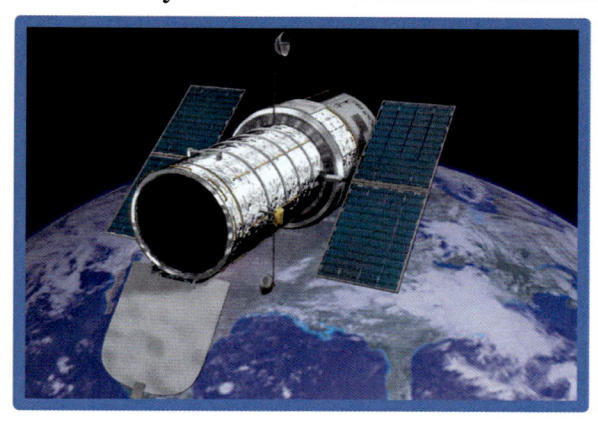

The earliest known portable digital camera was sold in the United States. The Human Genome Project was started in 1990 and was not completed until 2003. In June, Joanne Rowling had the idea for Harry Potter while traveling by train to London. She began writing *'Harry Potter and the Philosopher's Stone'*, which she completed in 1995.

On May 17, 1990, the World Health Organization removed homosexuality from its list of diseases, while on July 26 President George H.W. Bush signed the Americans with Disabilities Act to protect disabled Americans from discrimination. In February smoking was banned on all U.S. domestic air flights lasting less than 6 hours, and in August the very first smoking ban in a bar was enacted in San Luis Obispo, CA.

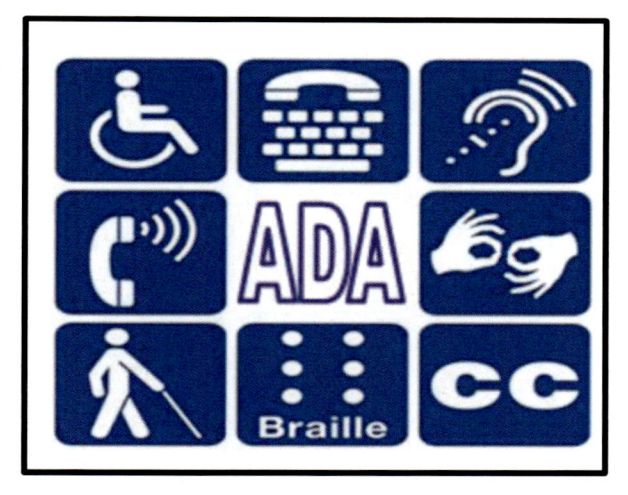

In health-related news, on September 14th American geneticist W. French Anderson performed the first gene therapy on a human when he injected engineered genes into a four-year old child to repair her faulty immune system. Anesthesiologist Nicholas M. Greene at Yale founded *The Overseas Anesthesia Teaching Program* (OTP), which later became the *Global Humanitarian Outreach Program* (GHO). The program encouraged volunteerism, support of anesthesia education and training in low- and middle-income countries, advocated for long-term academic partnerships with hospitals and universities in countries of need, and collaboration with organizations, institutions, and initiatives with common missions and philosophies.

Edward John Bertaccini did his undergraduate training at UCD (BS summa com laude, Biochemistry and minor in Quantum Physics, 1981-1985). He then attended the St. Louis University School of Medicine (MD, 1989). He returned to California to complete an internship (Transitional) at the SCVMC (1989-1990). He trained in Anesthesiology at Stanford (1990-1993) followed by a Fellowship (CCM) (1993-1994). Upon completion he joined the faculty working at the PA-VAH (1994-Present) and is now a Professor of (Anesthesiology and Intensive Care Medicine). He has served as both the Director of the operating rooms and the acting co-director of the intensive care units at the PA-VAH. His research focuses on the molecular structures of drugs related to clinical anesthesia and to biological activity. He frequently collaborated with Jim Trudell at Stanford. Ed is a co-holder of 'United States Patent #62064670 *Novel Methods, Compounds, And Compositions For Anesthesia*' (2019). He is a member of Bio-X, the SPARK program in translational research at Stanford, the Maternal & Child Health Research Institute (MCHRI), and the Wu Tsai Neurosciences Institute.

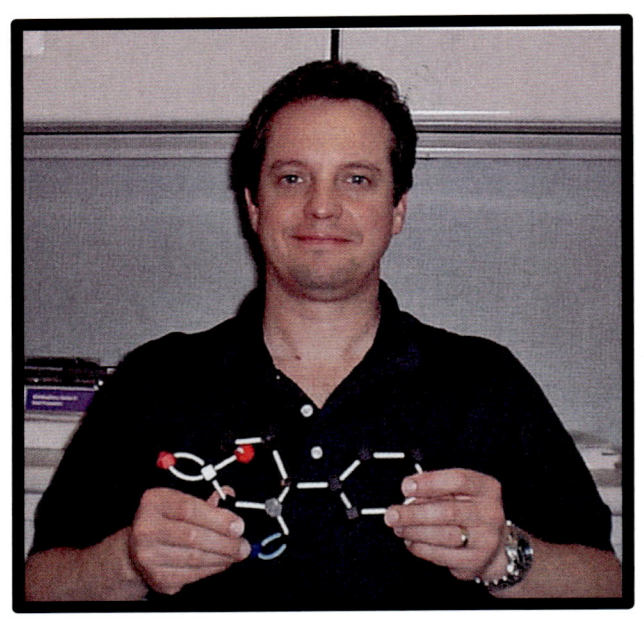

Paul James Elcavage a UCSD graduate (MD, 1988), interned (Transitional) at Atlantic Health System (1988-1989), and did a residency at Stanford (1990-1993). He has worked at PAMF - Sutter at Good Samaritan Hospital, San Jose, and Sequoia Hospital, Redwood City.

Michael Edwin Ennis was born in San Jose and grew up in Tracy, CA. He was an All-American water polo player at the University of the Pacific (UOP) (BS, 1984). He graduated Keck School of Medicine/USC (MD, 1989), interned (Transitional) at USC/LAC Medical Center (1989-1990) and completed a Stanford Anesthesiology residency (1990-1993). He worked at Kaiser – Santa Teresa, SJ (1993-1998), Walnut Creek/Diablo Service Area (1998-2022) and now part time at Sequoia Orthopedic Surgery Center (2024).

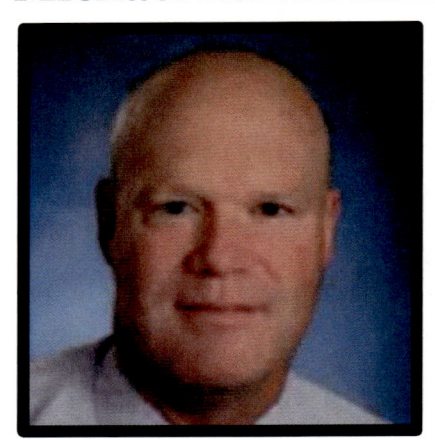

Mike is still involved in coaching, officiating, and playing water polo in age group Masters tournaments around the world. He has won World Championships in every age category from 40 to 60 and numerous National Championships with the Olympic Club in San Francisco. He has helped to coach Monte Vista High School and Diablo water polo teams. His other interests include painting with pastels and working in the yard.

"One Fall afternoon when I was a second-year anesthesia resident, Dr. Rosenthal pulled me out of the OR explaining that he needed me for a special assignment. The Stanford University water polo team need another goalie to practice against. Their current team goalies were both sick and injured so for about a week Dr. Rosenthal made sure I had no cases after 3 pm so I could make it to Stanford water polo practice. I tried to explain to him that I was woefully out of shape and these kids were going to light me up. He just said, "you'll be fine" and then made sure I made every practice I could until the other goalies returned."

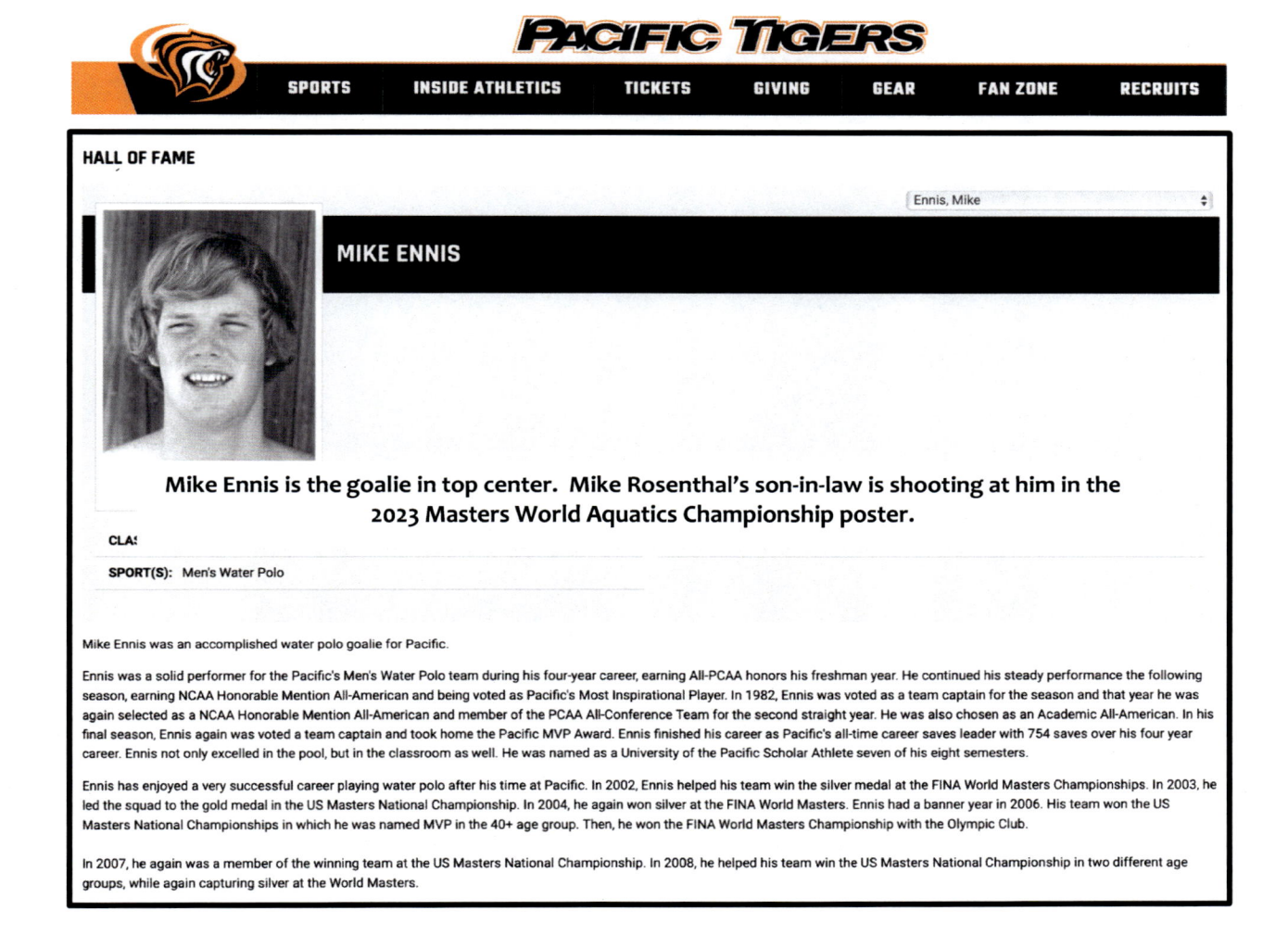

PACIFIC TIGERS

SPORTS | INSIDE ATHLETICS | TICKETS | GIVING | GEAR | FAN ZONE | RECRUITS

HALL OF FAME

Ennis, Mike

MIKE ENNIS

Mike Ennis is the goalie in top center. Mike Rosenthal's son-in-law is shooting at him in the 2023 Masters World Aquatics Championship poster.

CLA:

SPORT(S): Men's Water Polo

Mike Ennis was an accomplished water polo goalie for Pacific.

Ennis was a solid performer for the Pacific's Men's Water Polo team during his four-year career, earning All-PCAA honors his freshman year. He continued his steady performance the following season, earning NCAA Honorable Mention All-American and being voted as Pacific's Most Inspirational Player. In 1982, Ennis was voted as a team captain for the season and that year he was again selected as a NCAA Honorable Mention All-American and member of the PCAA All-Conference Team for the second straight year. He was also chosen as an Academic All-American. In his final season, Ennis again was voted a team captain and took home the Pacific MVP Award. Ennis finished his career as Pacific's all-time career saves leader with 754 saves over his four year career. Ennis not only excelled in the pool, but in the classroom as well. He was named as a University of the Pacific Scholar Athlete seven of his eight semesters.

Ennis has enjoyed a very successful career playing water polo after his time at Pacific. In 2002, Ennis helped his team win the silver medal at the FINA World Masters Championships. In 2003, he led the squad to the gold medal in the US Masters National Championship. In 2004, he again won silver at the FINA World Masters. Ennis had a banner year in 2006. His team won the US Masters National Championships in which he was named MVP in the 40+ age group. Then, he won the FINA World Masters Championship with the Olympic Club.

In 2007, he again was a member of the winning team at the US Masters National Championship. In 2008, he helped his team win the US Masters National Championship in two different age groups, while again capturing silver at the World Masters.

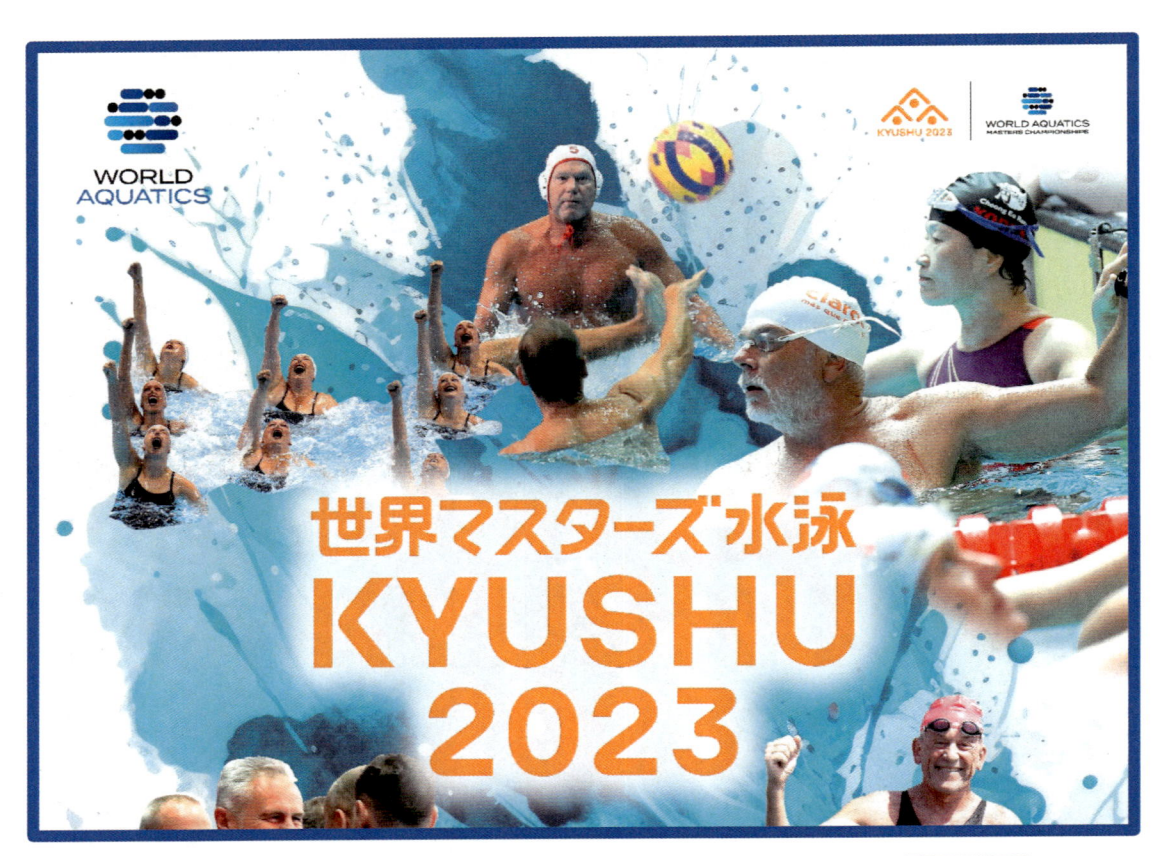

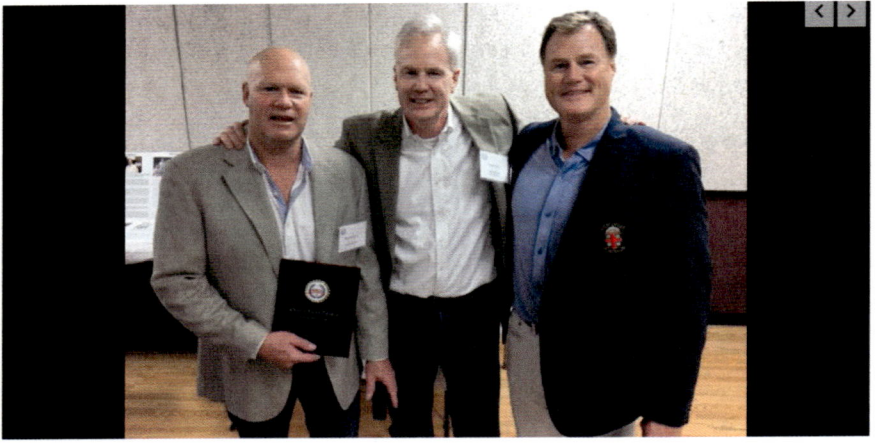

The Ennis brothers, Michael (from left), Greg and Steven, followed the example of their father, Chuck Ennis, a Tracy High coach and teacher, to become athletic standouts in water polo, wrestling and football in their years at Tracy High.
Bob Brownne/Tracy Press

Kimberly Anne Hanson graduated from the University of Nebraska College of Medicine (MD, 1989) and continued there for her internship (Internal Medicine) (1989-1990). She completed her residency (Anesthesiology) at Stanford (1990-1993) and then did a Fellowship (Pediatric Anesthesiology) at Seattle Children's Hospital. She remained on faculty for over a decade in the Departments of Anesthesiology, University of Washington School of Medicine and Children's Hospital and Regional Medical Center, Seattle, WA. She then worked in Omaha, NE, specializing in Anesthesiology and Internal

Medicine as a Pediatric Anesthesiologist affiliated with Children's Hospital & Medical Center. She is now retired.

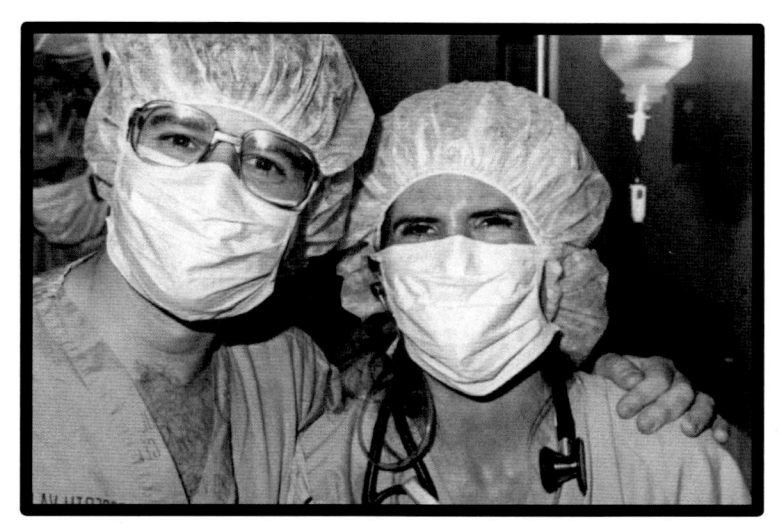

Steve Shafer and Kim Hanson

Thurman Eugene Hunt was an undergraduate at the University of Michigan College of Literature, Science, and the Arts (BS, Cell/Cellular and Molecular Biology, 1978-1982). He attended Stanford (MD, 1988). While in medical school he was a Peter Emge Traveling Medical Scholar at the German Cancer Research Center, Heidelberg (1987-1988). At Stanford he earned Research Honors in both Immunology and Psychiatry. He interned (Transitional) at Henry Ford Medical Center, Detroit, MI (1989-1990) and then completed a residency (Anesthesiology) at Stanford (1990-1993). He was a Fellow (Pain Medicine) at the University of Medicine and Dentistry of New Jersey (1993-1995). He was an Attending anesthesiologist there until 1997. He then joined Karrien Ali as a scientific consultant/ethnobotanical field researcher for Shaman Pharmaceuticals, Inc. (1993-1998).

He was Chair of the Department of Anesthesiology at Hurley Medical Center, Flint, MI (1998-2001). He returned to the SF Bay area as an anesthesiologist and Medical Director of Respiratory Care Services for the Alameda Health System (2002-Present) working at Highland Hospital Oakland, CA. He was Chair of the Department of Anesthesiology, Alameda Health System (2002-2014). In 2017 he earned an MBA (Business of Medicine) at the Indiana University – Kelley School of Business (2015-2017).

George Lederhaas was an undergraduate at the University of Miami - Coral Gables, FL (BS, 1985). He received his medical education at University of Miami Leonard M. Miller School of Medicine (MD, 1989) and interned (Internal Medicine) at the University of Connecticut/Hartford Hospital, Hartford, CT (1989-1990). He was an Anesthesiology resident at Stanford (1990-1993) with a sub-specialty tract emphasis on Pediatric Anesthesia). He initially worked at Nemours Children Clinic, Jacksonville, FL (1993-1998). He then did a Fellowship (Pain Medicine) at the Mayo Clinic College of Medicine and Science - Jacksonville, FL (1998). He worked at the University of Iowa, Iowa City (1998-1999) and has been a staff anesthesiologist with Associated Anesthesiologists, PC, West Des Moines, IA (1999-Present). He was President of the Medical Staff at UnityPoint Health - Iowa Methodist Medical Center, Des Moines (2020-2022). He was an Associate Medical Director for the hospital's hospice program and was Chair of the Surgery Department. He is also a Past President of the Iowa Society of Anesthesiologists. Dr. Lederhaas has board certification from the ABA in Anesthesiology, Pain Medicine, and Hospice and Palliative Care. George has been active in medical missions to Bolivia involving Solidarity Bridge, a group affiliated with Catholic Archdiocese of Chicago.

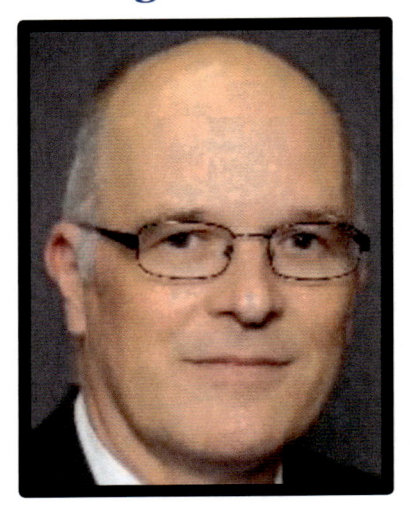

Stanford Memories ... "Excellent teaching from Gordon Haddow, John Brock-Utne, and Robert Buechel on how to practice medicine in resource limited settings. This has been of unbelievable assistance in what I have encountered in Bolivia. Yuan Chi-Lin of Stanford and "Uncle" Terry, Mighty Mo and the rest of the practice at Oakland Children's Hospital in preparing me for the full range of complex pediatric care. Wayne Anderson and Ted Kreitzman as senior residents were phenomenal mentors and took me under their wings to maximize my learning opportunities. Each of the above had the passion and commitment to "sitting the stool" and being actively involved in patient care. They taught me critical thinking and demonstrated compassion to the patients in our care. I give thanks every day for having been taught critical thinking and compassion rather than extremist ideology and virtue signaling which passes for "education" in many places today."

William Cooper Longton

was an undergraduate at the University of Arizona (BA, Chemistry, 1983) and medical student the University of Arizona College of Medicine (MD, 1989). He interned at St. Mary's Medical Center, SF (1989-1990) and then did his residency (1990-1993). and Fellowship (Pain Medicine) at Stanford (1993-1994). He stayed on as an attending Clinical Assistant Professor in the Pain Clinic (1994-1997) before entering private practice pain management at John Muir Health Medical Center. He works at Pain Medicine Consultants in Pleasant Hill, CA. Bill is an avid cyclist, skier, and windsurfer, and is a previous world-class athlete and finalist in the US Olympic Trials in swimming.

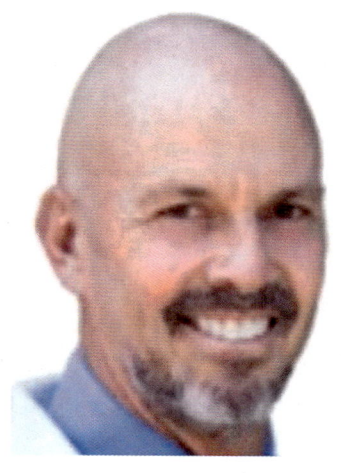

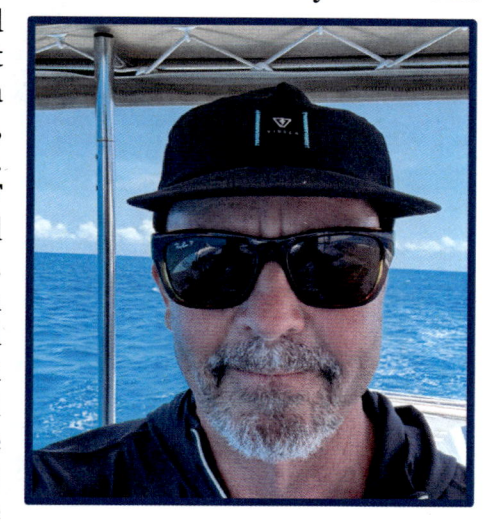

"I am married for 27 years to my lovely wife, who is a gastroenterologist and a Professor of Medicine at Stanford. We have two wonderful children: our daughter is an attorney practicing human rights law in London, and our son recently returned from playing professional water polo in Barcelona after four years of varsity water polo at USC. He is now planning to attend graduate school next year."

Memories:
- *Stanley Samuels lifting up the patient's legs right after induction of anesthesia – "his pressure is in the boots".*
- *Jay Brodsky – numerous wisecracks, classic quote about "nothing makes my heart swell with pride than seeing marginally competent former residents sporting their expensive watches and fancy cars" or something to that effect.*
- *David Gaba talking about solving the Konigsberg bridge problem, or some other arcane topic during a tedious VAH case.*

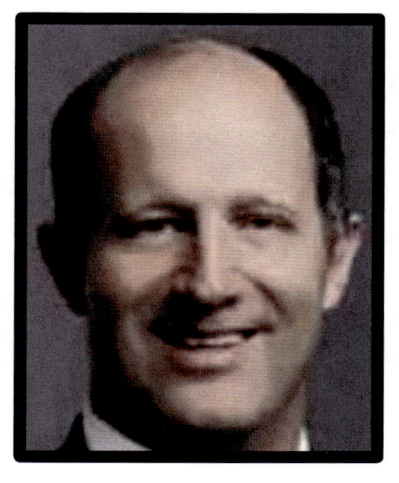

Edward Terry Riley

attended Whitworth University, Spokane, WA (1980) for his undergraduate education. During that time, he worked at as a teacher at a camp for juvenile offenders. He received his medical education at the University of Washington School of Medicine (MD, 1989). He interned at Legacy Health/Emanuel Hospital and Health Center, Portland, OR (1989-1990) and then did his residency (1990-1993) and Fellowship (Obstetrical Anesthesia) (1993-1994) at Stanford. He was Chief Resident his CA3 year. Ed was an Instructor

(Anesthesiology) and member of the Obstetric Anesthesia Division (1994-1996). He remained at Stanford being promoted from Assistant to Associate to full Professor. At Stanford he was the Director of the OB Anesthesia Fellowship program and eventually succeeded Sheila Cohen as the Division Chief of OB Anesthesia for 12 years. His research interests focused on quality improvement and clinical questions relevant to obstetric anesthesia. He is a board member and active clinician with the International Eye Institute and is active with Kybele (an international obstetric anesthesia outreach program). He retired in March 2023, and is now Professor Emeritus in the Department.

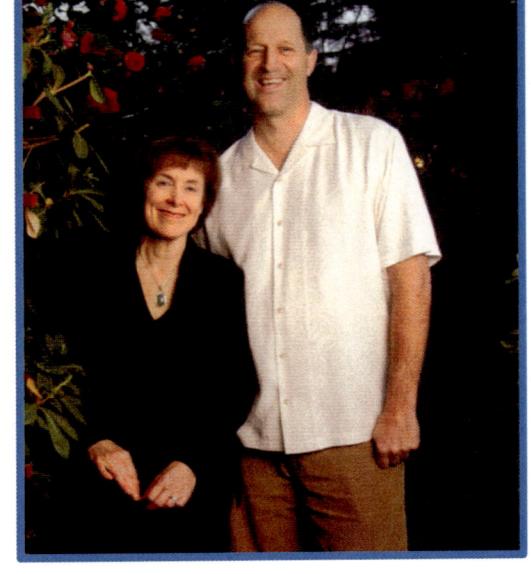

He enjoys bicycle riding, Nordic skiing, fishing, backpacking, hiking, rooting for Eastern Washington University basketball and the Baltimore Ravens.

"When they were cleaning out the old files in one of the offices, they asked me if I wanted any of the files that were relevant to me. In that pile was my application to the residency. Two things popped up out while I read the application. For children I put "pending". My wife was pregnant with my now 35-year-old son at the time. Second, I listed my future interests as: Obstetric anesthesia, ICU, research, and international medicine. I did not go into ICU, but Stanford gave me the springboard to accomplish all my other goals. It was a great place for training and a career."

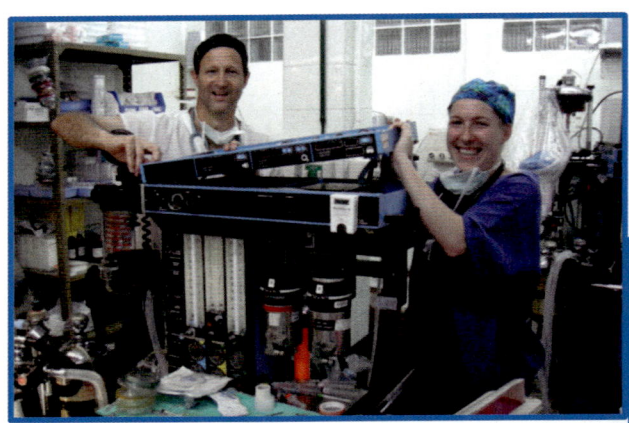

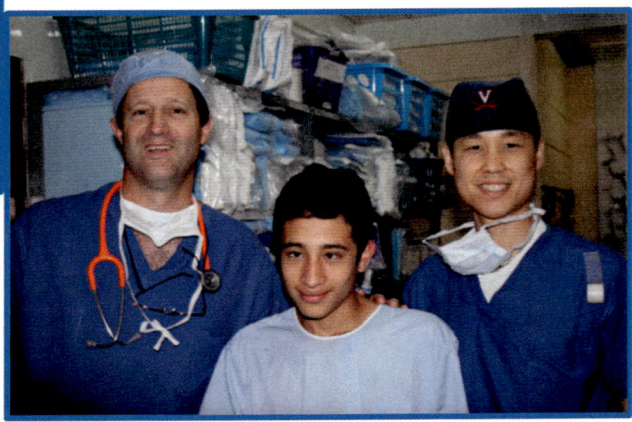

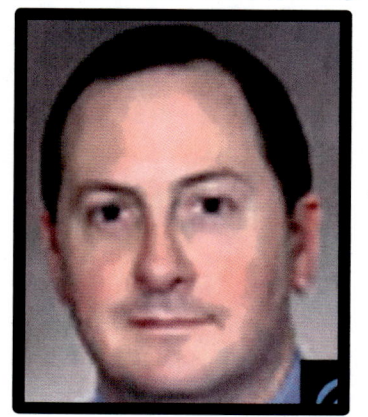

Berklee Robins was born in Rochester, NY. He attended the University of Rochester (BA, Biology) and trained at the Mt. Sinai School of Medicine (MD, 1989). He did an internship (Transitional) at Overlook Hospital/ Columbia University, Summit, NJ (1989-1990) and a residency at Stanford (1990-1993). He was an Assistant Professor (Anesthesiology) at Stanford for a short period. He then was a Fellow (Pediatric Anesthesiology) at Boston Children's Hospital (1995). Following a year on the anesthesia staff at Vanderbilt University as an Assistant Professor (1995-1996) he moved to Portland as an Associate Professor (Anesthesiology and Pediatrics) at OHSU (1996-Present). He works at OHSU Doernbecher Children's Hospital, Marquam Hill. Berklee received a master's degree (MA, Bioethics and Health Policy) from Loyola University Chicago (2013-2016) and is a Senior Scholar in the OHSU Center for Ethics in Health Care (2017-Present). He volunteers on humanitarian trips overseas, mainly working with children with cleft lips and palates.

"I have great memories of my time at Stanford. Only in retrospect do I realize how fortunate I was to match ... it was indeed my first choice, even though I lived in NY. I was offered a job back East after Fellowship and again a year later, but I realized I could never go back to the way it was."

"Great memories of the camaraderie, starting a ruptured AAA at the VAH with Steve Shafer running into the OR in his street clothes, many hilarious OB tales, and summer coed softball (who knew Fred Mihm was such a slugger!). I still teach residents "MS MAIDS" that Emily Ratner taught me on my first day of residency."

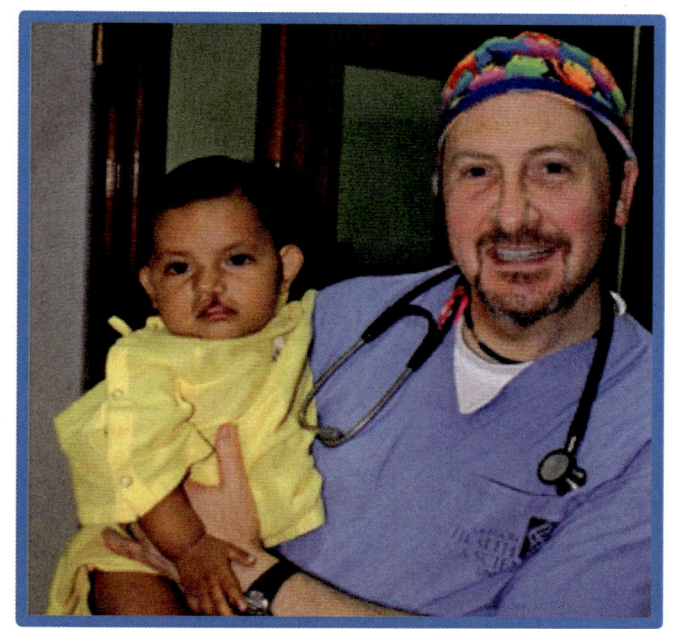

Clinton Lee Warne studied at Cornell University (BA, Economics, 1977-1982). He spent his junior year abroad at the London School of Economics. He graduated from the New York University School of Medicine (MD, 1986). He interned and did a residency (Internal Medicine) at the University of Pennsylvania (1986-1989). He worked as an emergency room physician at Pennsylvania Hospital/University of Pennsylvania (1989-1990). He then did his Anesthesiology residency at Stanford (1990-1993). He served as an Adjunct Assistant Professor (Anesthesiology) at Stanford from 1998-2008.

Clint worked in private practice in Sacramento (1993-2001), in Portland (2001-2007), and in Eugene, OR (2007-2020). At each, at various times he was in charge of Recruiting, Quality Assurance and Chief of the Anesthesia Department. He retired in 2021.

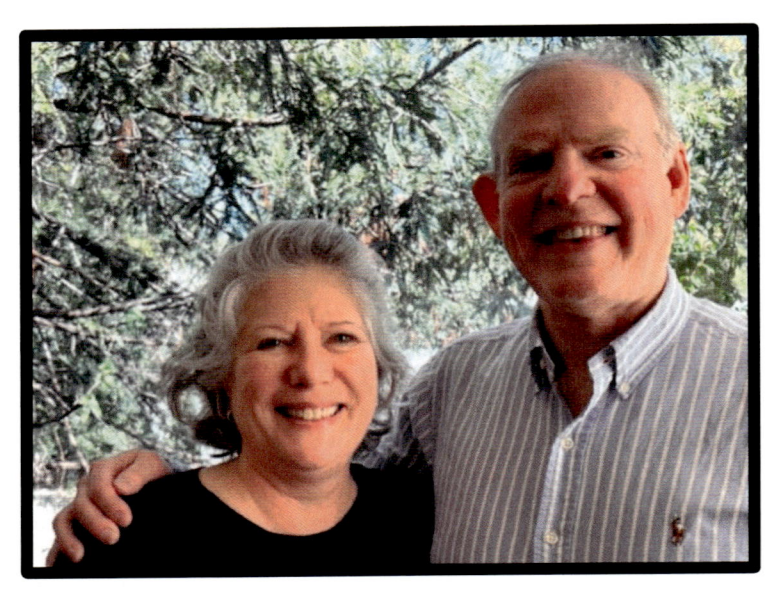

Clint and wife Kim, a nurse he met while a resident at Stanford. Their wedding reception was at the Stanford Barn.

"I appreciated the excellent training I received at Stanford, especially after I started in private practice when I saw how carelessly some of my partners who had trained at other programs did things compared to the way I had been taught. I remember Phil Larson teaching me how to "stand up straight and intubate like a professional, instead of bending over like an amateur" and John Brock-Utne teaching me to let a small child wrap their tiny hand around my finger during a mask induction to make the experience less frightening for them."

"My parents were both college professors, and I have always enjoyed teaching. I was a member of the Stanford Adjunct Clinical Faculty from 1998-2008. I enjoyed teaching the residents how to do smooth, safe, efficient anesthesia the way they would someday if they went into private practice. With my Internal Medicine and Emergency Room background, I had an extensive medical knowledge beyond anesthesia, which helped me add an extra element to teaching the residents."

" I have been fortunate to have made good friendships through each part of my career, and one piece I really enjoyed about teaching at Stanford was the opportunity to go visit with Rich Jaffe or Alex Macario, and the other people who were my close friends while I was there."

"During the course of my career, medicine became corporate, with giant hospital systems, the government, and insurance companies controlling everything and physicians becoming a cog within the corporate system. Doctors and nurses are turned into "providers" while administrators pay themselves enormous, outrageous salaries. This is a very unfortunate development that occurred during my career."

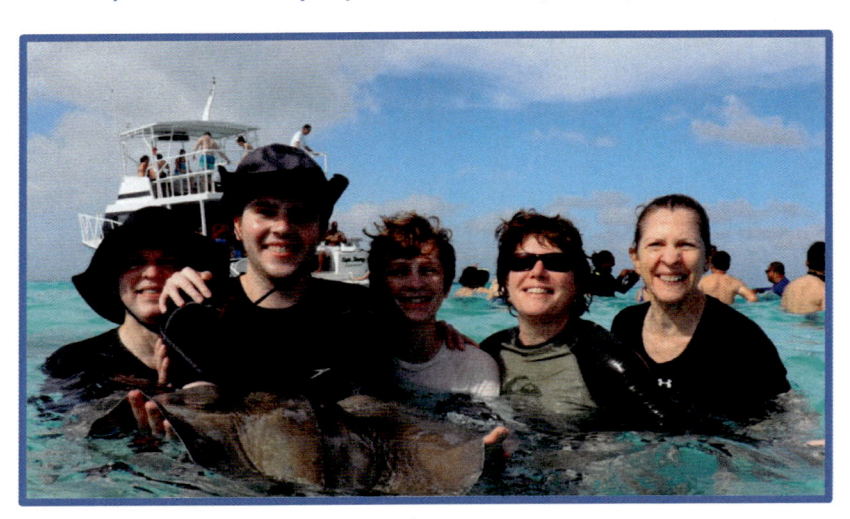

Warne family on vacation in the Cayman Islands

Matthew Francis White is a native of San Francisco. He attended UCD (BS, 1984) and then UCSD (MD, 1989). He interned (Transitional) Scripps Mercy Hospital (1989-1990) and was a Stanford Anesthesiology resident (1990-1993). He went to work as a staff anesthesiologist for PAMF (1993-1998) but had a substance abuse problem. After successful rehabilitation he returned briefly to Stanford on the faculty (1999-2000). After that he worked in Daly City with AMG (2000-2015) (MAC/Sheridan/Envision, (2015-2022). He is currently with Menlo Anesthesia Physicians (2023-Present). Matt enjoys spending time in the outdoors with road and mountain biking, hiking, and traveling.

"Upon reflection, I think of the nice relationships forged by working one-on-one with faculty members. I think the education I received was excellent. My style of practice is clearly based on that of my Stanford Attendings. From talking to many colleagues over the years, I think the atmosphere of respect and collegiality in our program at Stanford was pretty unusual. And I will always be grateful for the kindness and support offered to me during very difficult times."

Elizabeth Joricia Youngs attended Bryn Mawr College (AB, 1984). She was a UCI medical graduate (MD, 1989), and an intern at Pacific Presbyterian Medical Center (1989-1990). She completed her residency (1990-1993) and Fellowship (Clinical Pharmacology) at Stanford (1994). She continued as a Clinical Instructor at the PA-VAH (1994-1998), then worked at St. Rose Hospital, Haywood, as a staff anesthesiologist and Chief of the anesthesia group (1998-2001).

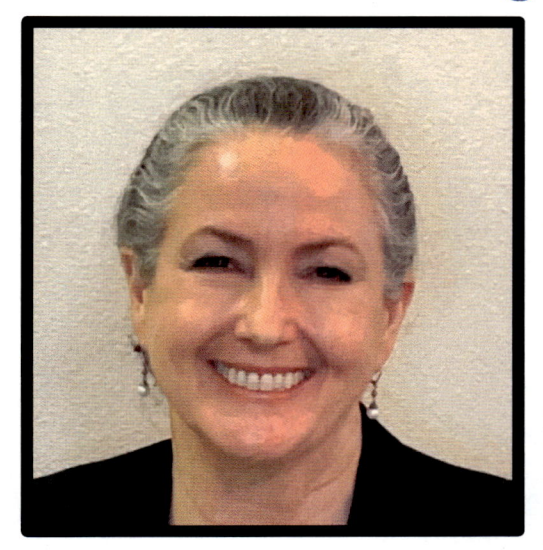

"I spent many years taking care of my family, including my special-needs daughter, who passed away in 2019. Probably the most life-changing story is that 15 years ago, Dr. Ron Pearl welcomed me back to Stanford after I had spent 7 years at home, taking care of my family. Returning to anesthesia was mostly like riding a bike, but I did have to learn about all the new developments that had occurred during my absence. I truly appreciate the support of the attendings who figuratively held my hand while I returned to clinical work. I am so grateful that being part of the Stanford community made it possible to return to the profession that I find so fulfilling."

She has worked per diem as a Clinical Instructor at Stanford (2009-2019) and has been associated with the Empire Anesthesia group (2011-Present). Outside of work she enjoys sewing and "making things out of various materials."

Interesting Anecdotes/Memories of Time at Stanford:

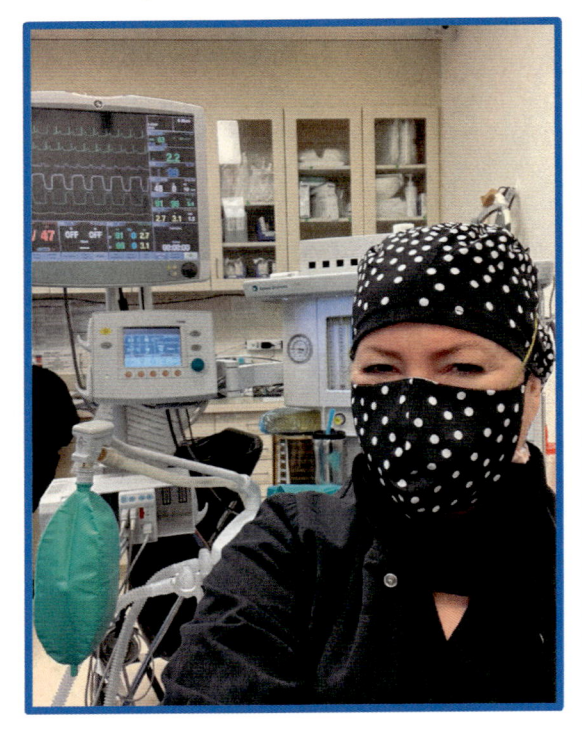

- I fondly remember many faculty members (including the two authors of this book) spending time with me in the OR and teaching me about their favorite topics in depth (mostly anesthesia topics, but also Leonard Cohen).
- I had an interesting trip to Honduras with Interplast, taking care of children who needed plastic surgery, with limited equipment, while being sick myself the whole time and getting intravenous antibiotics before and after each workday.
- I attended a WARC meeting, where I met the famous Dr. Ted Eger, who kindly spoke with me about water models and pharmacokinetics, which led to a whole journey into research in pharmacology with Dr. Steve Shafer.
- I was able to participate in anesthetizing a few gorillas at the San Francisco Zoo, thanks to Dr. Fred Mihm.

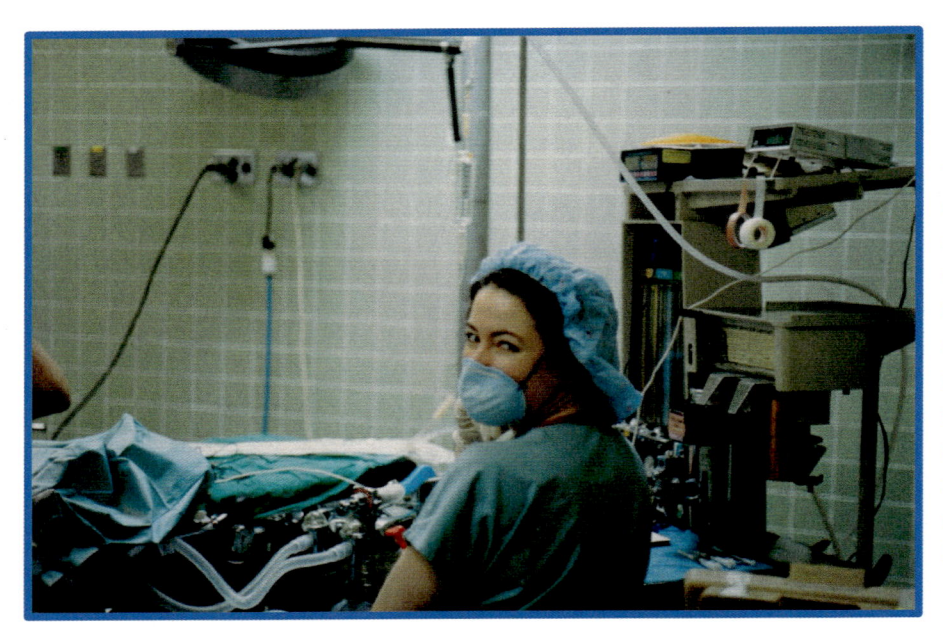

"I don't have any photos of myself at Stanford during residency. This is a photo of me during my Interplast trip to Honduras. The "wall oxygen" came from a big tank on the floor behind the machine. There was no ventilator and no EKG monitor, and I don't remember what we did for blood pressure."

Kenneth Paul Zuckerman was born in Cleveland, OH. He received his undergraduate education at the University of Chicago (AB with honors, 1984) and graduated from Tulane University School of Medicine (MD, 1989-1990). He interned (Surgery) at UCSF (1989-1990) and was a Stanford Anesthesiology resident (1990-1992). He completed the final 6-months of his CA3 year at Children's National Medical Center, Washington, DC, doing Pediatric Anesthesia (1993).

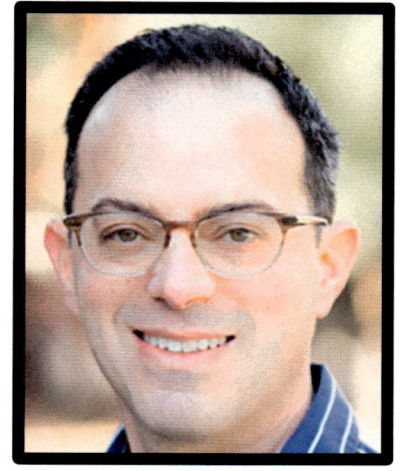

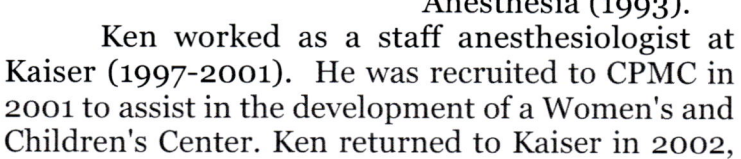

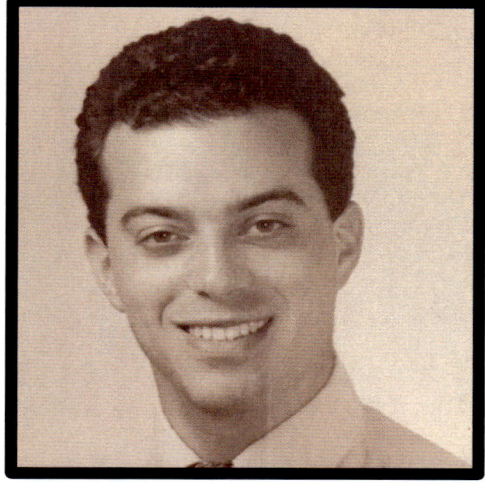

Ken worked as a staff anesthesiologist at Kaiser (1997-2001). He was recruited to CPMC in 2001 to assist in the development of a Women's and Children's Center. Ken returned to Kaiser in 2002, where he was the Chief of Pediatric Anesthesia, as well as the Chair of regional committees on sleep apnea and the centralization of pediatric care (2003-2006). He then returned to Oakland Children's Hospital (2006) and was Director of the Anesthesia Department (2013-2016). While working at Oakland Children's, he and others including former Stanford anesthesia resident Kristen Johnson cared for patients at the Pediatric Dental Initiative (PDI) (2009-2023). He served as Medical Director at PDI in 2019 and 2020.

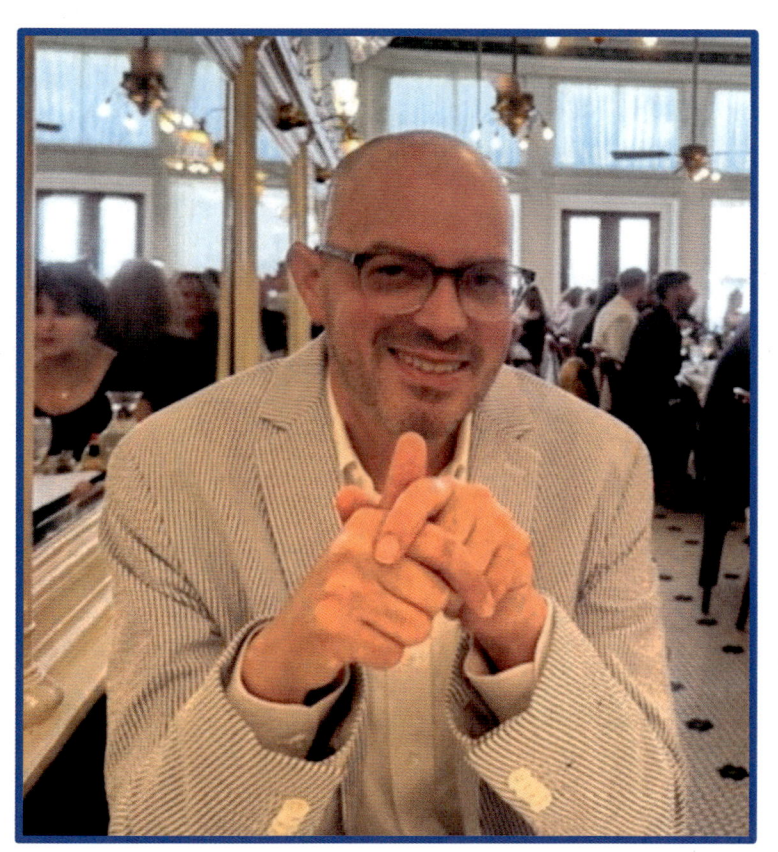

He completed another Fellowship (Medical Acupuncture) at Helms Medical Institute (2017) and trained as an apprentice in Sports and Orthopedic Acupuncture (2019).

He has participated with the Hospital de la Familia program in Guatemala on several medical missions.

In his free time, he enjoys skiing, swimming, and gardening. He is also an avid baker who completed an internship at the San Francisco Baking Institute (2018).

"I remember Dr. Larson's mentorship, especially his skill at making fiberoptic intubation a matter of routine and Dr. Cohen's thoughtful and collaborative approach caring for complex OB patients."

"When I wrote the referral criteria for pediatric patients within the Kaiser system, I was strongly influenced by the work that Al Hackel had previously done with the Bay Area Pediatric Anesthesia Consortium."

Talmage Dan Egan completed his undergraduate education at Brigham Young University (BA magna cum laude, Humanities Studies, 1978-1982). He graduated from University of Utah School of Medicine (MD, 1986) and did a residency (Surgery) there (1986-1988). He switched to Anesthesiology and completed his CA1 and CA2 years at the University of Utah (1988-1990) before transferring to Stanford for his CA3 year (1990-1991) and a Fellowship (Clinical Pharmacology) (1991-1993). He worked at the PA-VAH with Donald Stanski and Steven Shafer. He had an appointment as Clinical Instructor (Anesthesiology) (1991-1992) then Assistant Professor (1992-1993) at Stanford.

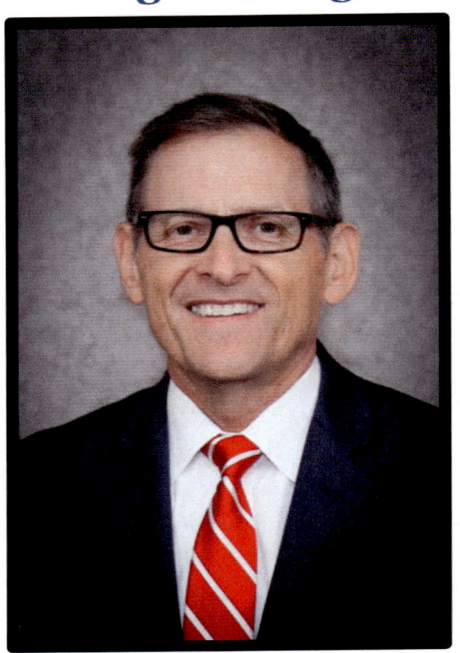

He returned to the University of Utah initially as an Assistant Professor and staff physician (1993). He is holder of the K.C. Wong Presidential Endowed Chair in Anesthesiology there since 2004. Dr. Egan was appointed Chair of the Department of Anesthesiology at the University of Utah Health Sciences Center (2015-Present). He is also an Adjunct Professor in the Departments of Pharmaceutics, Bioengineering, and Neurosurgery at the University of Utah School of Medicine.

In 2002 he spent a sabbatical as a Visiting Scientist in Clinical Pharmacology at the Imperial College in London, UK, where he studied the effects of dexmedetomidine using functional magnetic resonance techniques. He worked at the Chelsea and Westminster Hospital and Imperial College with Professor and Chair Mervyn Maze. Egan has also completed intensive physician executive training at the Harvard School of Public Health.

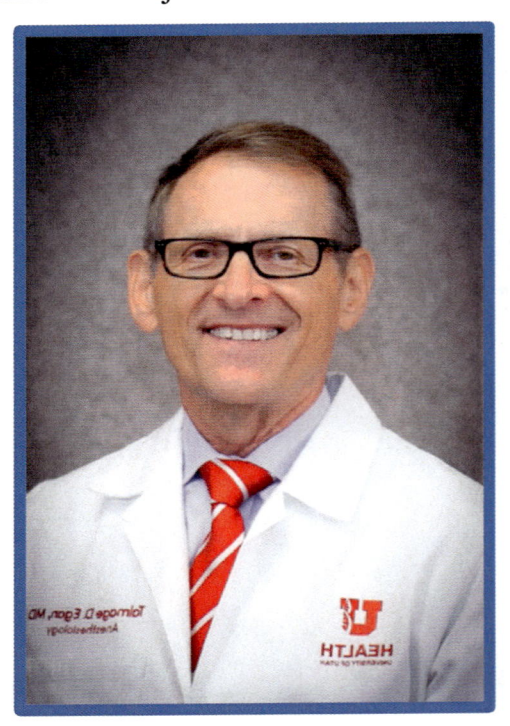

His clinical practice focuses on neurosurgery and obstetric patients. He is past President of the Medical Staff and Chairman of the Medical Board (2006-2008) and served for over a decade as the Chief of Neuroanesthesia. His research interests include the clinical pharmacology of sedatives and analgesics, the development of novel intravenous anesthetics and alternative propofol formulations, the development of optimal drug administration regimens based on pharmacokinetic-pharmacodynamic concepts, the identification of factors (i.e., gender, body weight, shock, etc.) that influence drug behavior, and computer-controlled drug delivery technology. Dr. Egan is a pioneer in the development of total intravenous anesthesia techniques, particularly the clinical application of the short acting opioid remifentanil, and the characterization of the interaction between propofol and opioids.

These interests have resulted in successful entrepreneurial ventures, patents, and trademarks. He is a founding owner of a medical education and consulting company called Applied Medical Visualizations (Medvis).

Applied Medical Visualizations (Medvis) is a consulting/contracting company that specializes in transforming the user experience for your medical device or medical technology:
- *medical device design: user interfaces, visualization, and industrial design*
- *medical technology prototyping: software*
- *medical technology usability and user experience evaluation*
- *interactive medical education: educating clinicians on best practices and on your medical technology*

They collaborate with companies on bringing innovative technologies and designs into medical devices. The technologies that they have developed are scientifically demonstrated to improve medical comprehension. They have developed and tested state of the art solutions for education, information presentation, patient monitoring, and information management incorporating a user centered design approach that simplifies user interaction with intuitive presentation and visualization of information. Their products allow our customers to better manage patient care and improve patient safety while minimizing cost.

Dr. Egan served for many years as a board member, treasurer, and president of the International Society for Anaesthetic Pharmacology. He served as an Associate Editor for the British Journal of Anaesthesia (2013-2023) and has served as Associate Editor for Anesthesiology (1999-2005). For many years Dr. Egan was a member and Chair of the ASA Subcommittee on Drug Disposition. He is a co-editor of the very well-received pharmacology and physiology textbook published by Elsevier entitled *'Pharmacology and Physiology for Anesthesia: Foundations and Clinical Application'*. That book is now in its 3rd edition.

He is the principal creator of Safe Sedation Training (SST), a virtual preceptorship for training non-anesthesia professionals in procedural sedation. This course has been taken by more than 20,000 students worldwide.

Dr. Egan was the inaugural recipient of the IARS Teaching Recognition Award (1997), the FAER/Roche Pharmaceuticals Clinical Research Award (1998), the Jan Kukral Distinguished Lecturer Award from Northwestern University School of Medicine (2001), a Lifetime Achievement Award from International Society for Anaesthetic Pharmacology (2016), and numerous other honors.

"On John Brock-Utne: "I am fond of saying that I can't think of a Norwegian from South Africa living in California that I like more!"

On Jay Brodsky: "Thanks so much for all that you taught me Jay. I did a lot of thoracotomies for neurosurgical spine cases over 30 years, and I always relied on what I learned from you. You were a very memorable part of my time at Stanford, even though you made fun of my provincial Mormon roots from time to time (I knew it was all in good fun …). My favorite thing was what you wrote inside the cover of a monograph you had edited on thoracic anesthesia that you gifted to me: "Dear Talmage, Think what I could have accomplished in thoracic anesthesia if I had known you first!" Classic Jay Brodsky!"

Jay Brodsky, "I remember being in Mormon Square in Salt Lake City with Talmadge. We saw a bewildered young Japanese woman standing alone at a street corner. Talmadge, who had done his mission in Japan went over to see if he could help her since he spoke fluent Japanese. Much to our amazement we discovered that she was actually a LDS missionary from Japan assigned to Salt Lake City

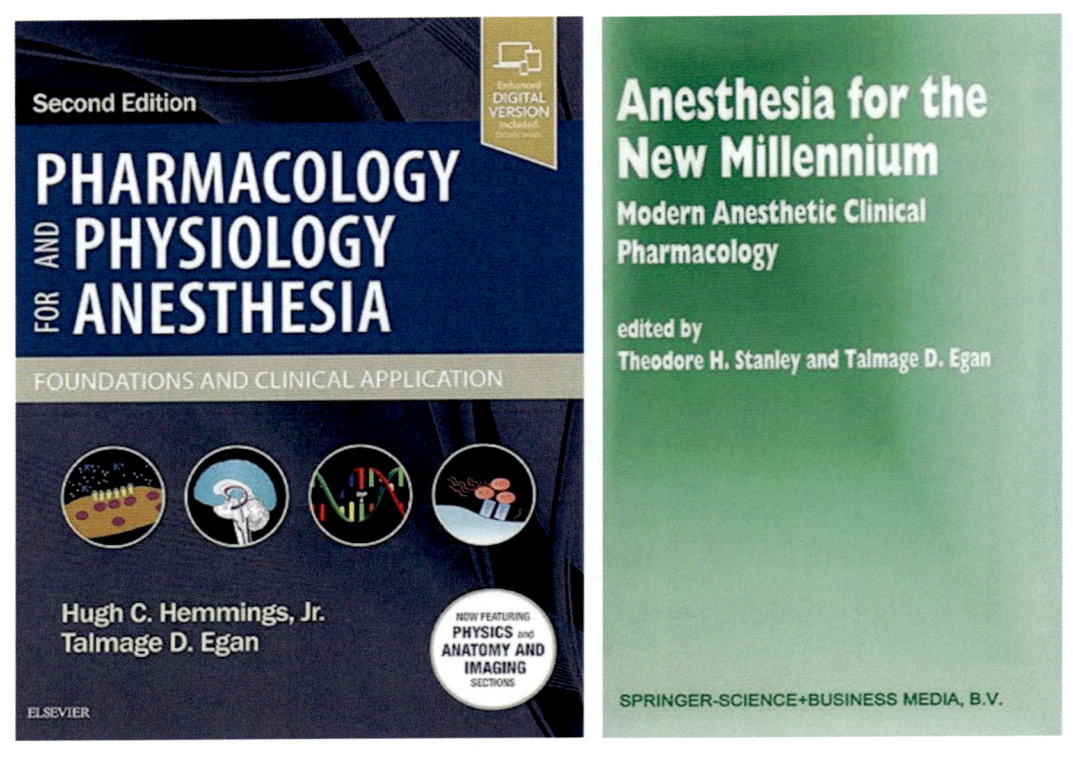

Stephen Douglas Glacy graduated from the University of Kansas School of Medicine (MD, 1986) and did an internship (Transitional) there (1986-1987). He then began residency in Anesthesiology at Washington University (1987-1990) and completed his CA3 year at Stanford (4/1/90-3/30/91). While at Stanford he was placed on probation for abusive behavior and suspected drug use. He practiced in Scottsdale, AZ (1991-2008) doing interventional pain management. In 2008 he was found guilty of professional misconduct. He admitted to writing and filling prescriptions under a pseudo-patient name for himself. He then failed to follow the treatment facility's recommendation to undergo a psychiatric evaluation. He surrendered his license to practice medicine in Arizona to the state's Medical Board.

John Mark Schwab University of Texas Southwestern (MD, 1987) was an Anesthesiology resident at University of Texas Southwestern Medical Center (1988-1990). He completed his CA3 year at Stanford (1990-1991). He practices anesthesiology in Newport Beach, CA.

Karriem Hakim Ali holds a degree in Chemistry (Organic/Medicinal) from Harvard College. He received his medical degree from Stanford (MD, 1988) with Distinguished Honors in Research for work as a Stanford-NIH Cancer Biology Fellow. As a Year IV medical student, Karriem was also awarded an American Heart Association Critical Care Cardiology - Immunology Research Fellowship and conducted a successful, proof-of-concept, pre-clinical trial of an anti-Lipid A monoclonal antibody for mitigation of septic shock in the ICU, under the guidance of Professor Thomas Feeley.

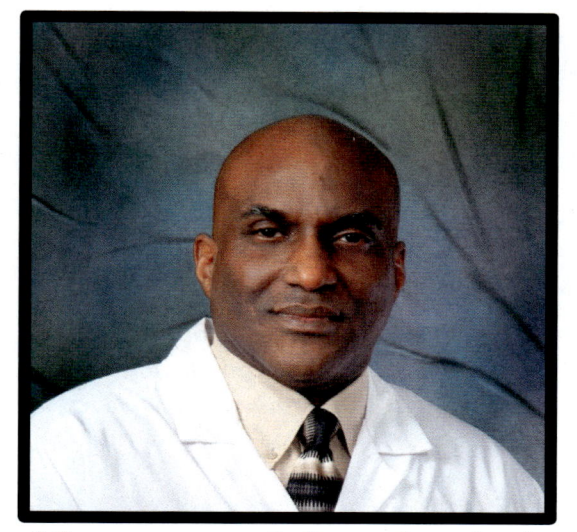

When he began his Stanford Anesthesiology residency three years later in January 1990, Karriem entered in the pilot year of the new research-focused track where residents were to spend the final six months of their 3-years conducting biomedical research. Not wanting to wait around for two years, Karriem conducted a small pilot study with John G. Brock-Utne to identify an anesthesia delivery modality that would be suitable to use under disaster conditions.

"This study was motivated by the devastating magnitude 6.9 Loma Prieta earthquake that shook San Francisco in October 1989 during the World Series game at Candlestick Park. The collapse of the of the Bay Bridge and other structures required emergent surgical care, including several amputations in order to free trapped survivors. Unfortunately, on-site anesthesia delivery was severely limited due to the lack of access to A/C power needed to run standard anesthesia machines. Serendipitously, Dr. Brock-Utne was deeply familiar with the delivery of "Anesthesia in Difficult Situations" from his own residency training at the University of Natal King Edward VIII teaching hospital at the KwaZulu Nelson R. Mandela School of Medicine in South Africa. As a team, Brock-Utne and I devised simulations to mimic various adverse conditions, and the resulting publication earned them the Stanford Resident Research Award and the CSA Outstanding Clinical Research Honor."

In October 1992 Karriem resigned from the residency program to pursue his research interests full-time.

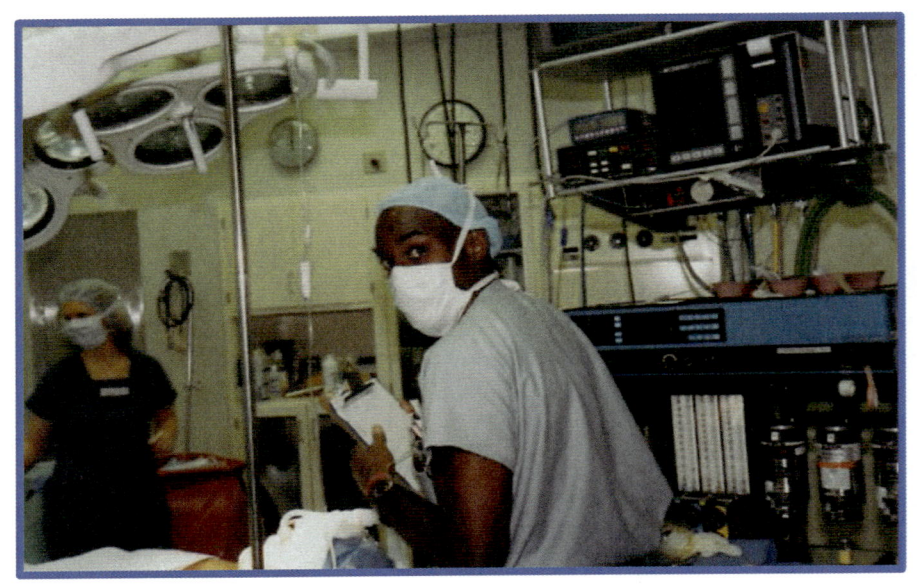

"I really loved anesthesia, but wasn't into the socio-politics of it all ... I was fascinated by the neuroscience and neuropharmacology, so I preferred MAC anesthesia and other scenarios that involved the awake patient, while everyone else was into the other end of the spectrum of care where patients are bound for the ICU. I still have this interest and perspective, albeit outside of the context of surgical procedures. I was hoping to pursue investigations of cannabinoids and their effects on humans via the "Endocannabinoid System" by modelling the several compounds and pharmacologic effects involved as being analogous to multimodal, or balanced, anesthesia; however, that space is even more deeply embroiled in shortsighted politics ...👲"

He was recruited to join Shaman Pharmaceuticals Inc, a start-up biotechnology company in South San Francisco. He was a Medical Director of field research teams plying similar trails as the Interplast surgical teams.

"Shaman pursued natural product drug development leveraging a bioprospecting model across several disease platforms, most notably diabetes and metabolic syndrome working with Stanford Medical School professor Gerald M. Reaven."

Shaman was a great opportunity to apply his background in clinical pharmacology, organic and medicinal chemistry, while at once observing the delivery of health care in difficult situations. Later, Karriem wrote a book based upon his many life-changing experiences working in the Amazon Rainforest and Shaman Pharmaceuticals R&D, titled "Axícala Alíqu: The Sacred Song of Life".

Book description: Welcome to a great journey. You will enjoy meeting the Shaman Axícala Alíqu (Ah-shee-ca-la Ah-lee-coo, meaning 'Sacred Song of Life'), and exploring the rainforest realm of his people, who are commonly referred to as 'the Unknown'. As we trek page-by-page, this realm will beckon your mind to open and explore the unknown under the guidance of the ayahuasca 'vision vine'- the yajé (ya-hay)- that grows each chapter along the way.

In a later incarnation, Karriem worked as Medical Director at Aradigm, a start-up company founded by another colleague from Stanford Medical School and Stanford Anesthesia Department research, Reid Rubsamen. In today's world of global collaboration and remote working, Karriem seems to have found his niche, consulting in natural product-driven therapeutics development. At present, bis principal area of research is focused on the development of oligosaccharide immunomodulator

"I always liked Dr. Larson, and even worked with him as the medical student representative to the CMA Scientific Advisory Panel on Anesthesiology in the mid-1980s. He was the kind of person that I thought academic physicians would be~ forthright and knowledgeable, of a mind toward advancing the quality of patient care/ outcomes. I was naïvely mistaken, of course, and that was a bit of a shock as a resident. Fortunately, there were a few other faculty members, like you Jay, Drs. Feeley, Brock-Ütne, Carter Cherry, Lawrence Siegel, Mike Rosenthal, Lorne Eltherington, and a few others whose names don't readily come to mind after three decades ... I was in touch with Tom Feeley a bit back during the first years of COVID~ 2021, I think. He was my faculty advisor as a Stanford Medical School student, and also the faculty investigator on the research that we published on anti-Lipid A monoclonal antibodies in gram- septic shock. It was good to catch up via Zoom and hear his war stories from moving to Texas and MD Anderson."

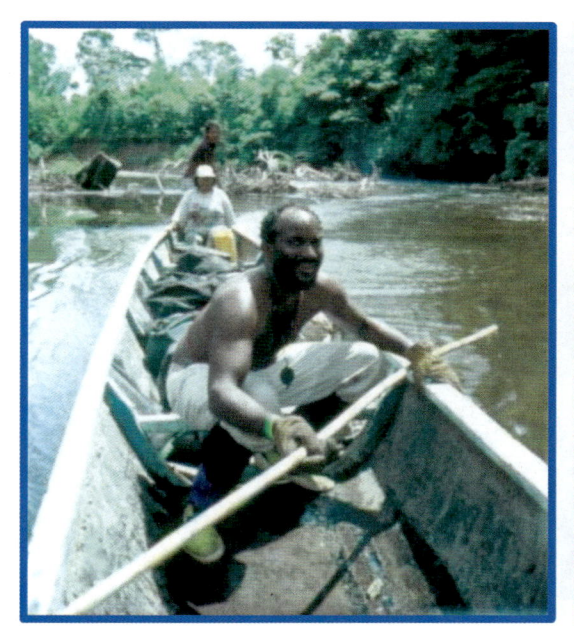

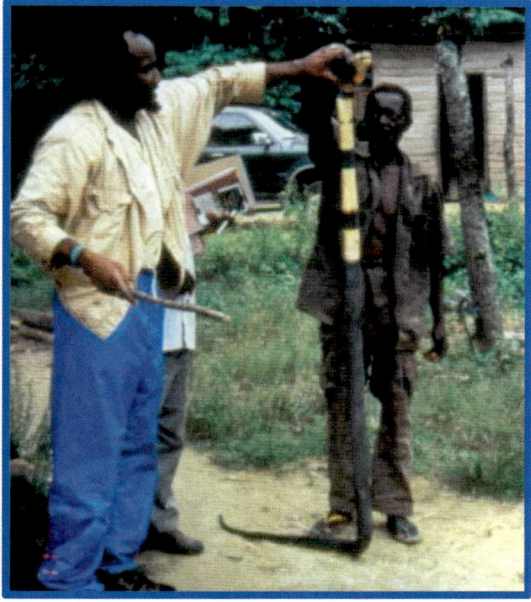

Dr. Ali has worked in the rain forests of Columbia and the Congo

"A lot has changed everywhere since I was a resident, mostly in unanticipated ways with more change coming every day. Back then, the Apple Mac computer was novel, and the iPhone/iPad were unimaginable devices beyond the world of Star Trek."

John Brock-Utne, "Karriem was in my opinion and excellent researcher. He asked the right questions and never got side-tracked. I am very proud of his research achievements, which have been cited many times. I was disappointed when he chose to leave our specialty, but Karriem followed his dream and won."

CHAPTER 11
1991

A major event in 1991 was the dissolution of the Soviet Union. Although 77% of voters in a national referendum were in favor of keeping the 15 Soviet republics together, 6 of the Union's republics boycotted the vote. The first republic to declare its independence in August was Ukraine, followed by Belarus, then Moldova, Azerbaijan, Kyrgyzstan, Uzbekistan and finally Tajikistan on September 9th. Yugoslavia also dissolved when Slovenia and Croatia each declared independence. Fighting between Serbia and the other former republics of Yugoslavia led to a war that lasted for the rest of the decade. That same year the lifting of trade restrictions within the European Economic Community (EEC) and the Maastricht treaty led to the eventual creation of the European Union (EU) in 1993. On January 12th Congress passed a resolution authorizing the use of military force to expel Iraqi forces from Kuwait. On January 15th the U.N. deadline for the withdrawal of Iraqi troops from occupied Kuwait expired, preparing the way for the start of Operation Desert Storm. A U.N. authorized coalition force from 34 nations fought against Iraq which had occupied Kuwait the previous year. Although President Bush declared victory and ordered a cease-fire in February, the Gulf War marked the beginning of the since-continuous American military presence in the Middle East. President George H.W. Bush and Soviet leader Mikhail Gorbachev signed the START I Treaty during July 1991 agreeing to reduce the number of nuclear warheads in each country to a miniscule 7,950. START I came into effect in 1994 with both sides initially adhering to the limits, but it expired in 2009. In 1991 the 911 Emergency Number was first tested in several cities. Fires in the Oakland hills burnt thousands of homes and killed 25 people. At Stanford University "Touchdown Tommy" Vardell set the school record for most rushing yards in a season by a Cardinal running back with 1084 yards. The record was broken by Toby Gerhart (2009) and subsequently by Christian McCaffrey (2015). The current 49er General Manager John Lynch was the starting strong safety on the

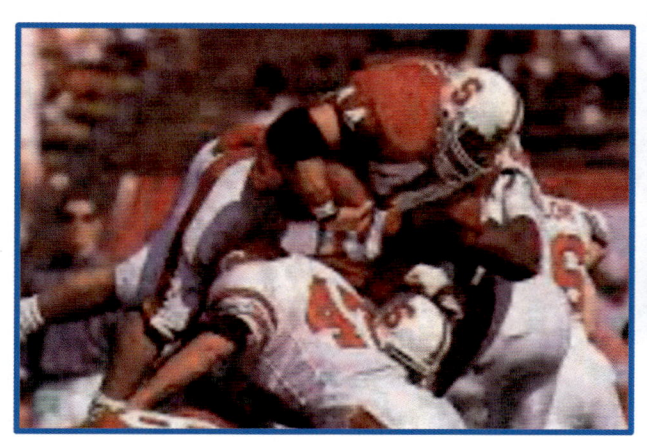

"Touchdown" Tommy Vardell in action

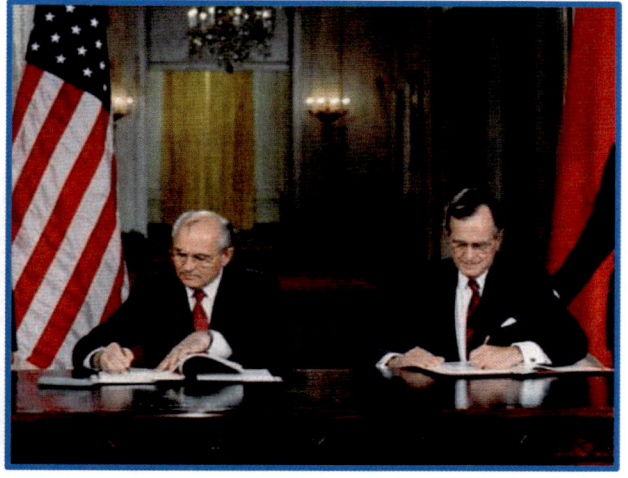

Mikail Gorbachev and George H.W. Bush sign the START I Treaty

Stanford football team that year. In 1991 the Lucile Packard Children's Hospital opened to patients.

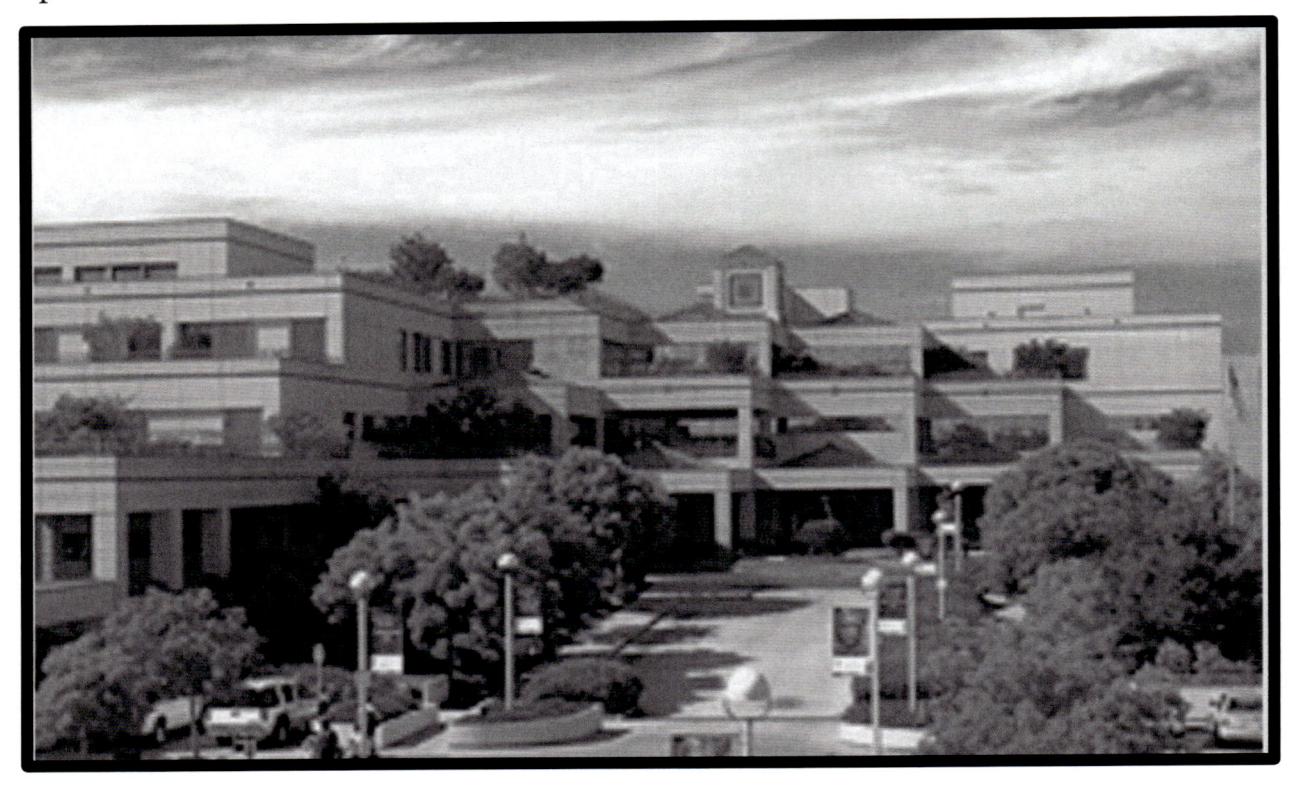

Lucile Packard Children's Hospital at Stanford opened in 1991.

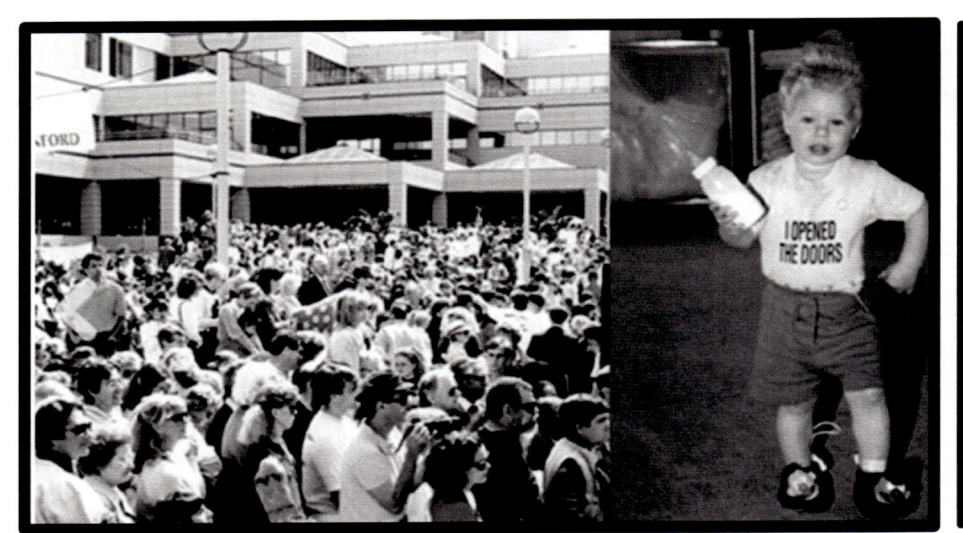

Lucile Packard Children's Hopital on opening day

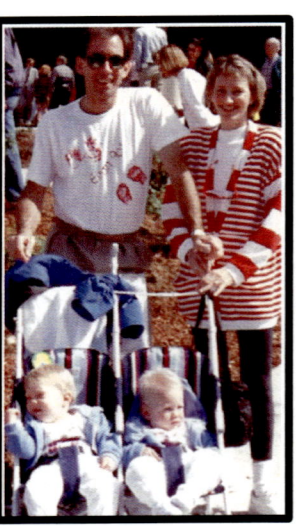

The Fischell family in attendance

Gregory Harnett Botz attended UC-Riverside (BS, Biology, 1984). He graduated from the George Washington University School of Medicine (MD, 1990). He interned (Internal Medicine) at Huntington Memorial Hospital, Pasadena, CA (1990-1991) and then completed his Anesthesiology residency at Stanford (1991-1994). His residency was followed by Fellowships (Medical Simulation) (1994) and CCM (1994) both at Stanford. In 2004 he also completed the Advanced Training Program in Healthcare Delivery Improvement at Intermountain Healthcare, Salt Lake City, UT.

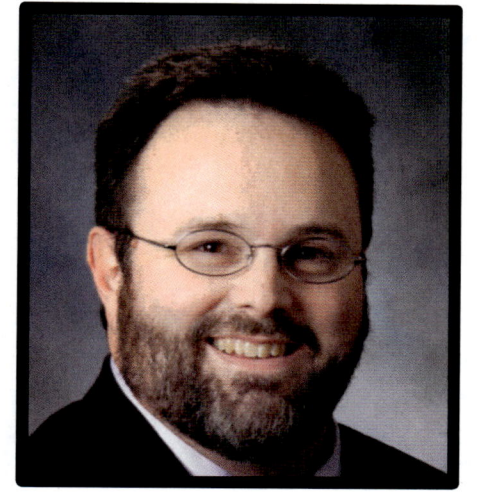

Greg was appointed Clinical Instructor (Anesthesiology) at Stanford University Medical Center and Lucile Packard Children's Hospital (1994-2000). He left for Duke University Medical Center as an Assistant Professor in the Departments of Surgery and Anesthesiology. He subsequently moved to Houston to the Department of Critical Care Medicine in the Division of Anesthesiology, Critical Care Medicine and Pain Medicine at The University of Texas M. D. Anderson Cancer Center, Houston, TX. He started as Assistant Professor (Anesthesiology and Critical Care Medicine) and was eventually promoted to Professor. He is Associate Medical Director, Intensive Care Unit, at the University of Texas, M.D. Anderson Cancer Center, Houston, TX (2003-Present). He has led education programs using simulation as Medical Director of the Life Support Training Center (2009-2013) and then Clinical Medical Director of the Simulation Center (2013-Present).

He was Program Director, Anesthesiology Critical Care Medicine Fellowship, University of Texas Health Sciences Center (UTHSC) - Houston (2008-2014). During the nearly 3 decades he has been at M.D. Anderson he has served as a member of the Educational Role Recognition Committee, Perioperative Critical Incident Response Task Force, Advance Care Planning Committee, Perioperative Enterprise Safety Council, Graduate Medical Education Committee, Patient Safety Committee, DNR Revision Task Force, Mobile Computing Device Advisory Group, Clinical Research and Information Systems Committee, Clinical Safety and Effectiveness Training Steering Committee, Critical Care Research Group, and is currently a member of the ICU Operations Committee (2003-Present). He has served as the University of Texas Chancellor's Health Fellow in Quality of Care and Patient Safety. He leads the University of Texas System Fellowship in Clinical Safety and Effectiveness. In 2012, he was elected to the University of Texas Kenneth I. Shine Academy of Health Science Education.

Dr. Botz is a pioneer in the field of Threat Safety Science. He and his colleagues at M.D. Anderson developed techniques of deliberate practice through immersive simulation of real-life scenarios to accelerate the development of life saving competencies. The work has targeted improvement of threat safety management by professional caregivers, law enforcement professionals, and the public. His research and development work has focused on prevention, preparedness, protection, and performance improvement related to man-made threats such as terrorism and natural threats (e.g. storms and earthquakes). He is the Medical Director for the University of Texas at Houston's Police Department, a center of research and development for threat safety management. Greg is also a founding contributor to the global bystander care training program, called Med Tac, that combines professional expertise and evidence-based techniques from the medical and tactical communities to train people with lifesaving behaviors that can be used in the first few minutes after a life-threatening event and before professional first responders arrive. He and his team were awarded with the Pete Conrad Global Patient Safety Award (2018) for their work in this area. They lead ongoing training and R&D in Texas, California, Florida, and Hawaii, and the programs have expanded to lifeguards, diving programs, and commercial air travel.

The Medical Tactical Certificate Training Program, also known as Med Tac, was founded in 2015 by Dr. Botz and William Adcox at MD Anderson and Charlie Denham and Dr. Charles Denham in California when they were developing an active shooter training program for the Texas Medical Center and schools in Texas and Orange County CA. It is a global bystander rescue care training program that focuses on life-saving actions that can be performed by non-medical bystanders for the eight leading preventable causes of death to children, youth, and adults. In urban areas in the United States, professional first responder response time to the scene of an emergency averages 8-10 minutes. Immediate bystander rescue care has been found to have a significant effect on survival rates and permanent harm. Created and expanded upon after the dramatic increase in active shooter and terrorism events, Med Tac integrates the American Heart Association HeartSaver CPR/AED Training Program, the American Red Cross equivalent training, and the Stop the Bleed Program sponsored by the US Department of Homeland Security and the American College of Surgeons.

Dr. Botz serves as a national consultant for the SCCM's Fundamentals training programs. He was a senior editor for the ABA Joint Council on Anesthesiology Examinations, the program director for the UTHSC-Houston Anesthesiology CCM Fellowship, the Regional Faculty for the American Heart Association Emergency Cardiovascular Care training programs, and a member of The University of Texas System Health Care Components ICU Quality Improvement Collaborative. He has participated in SCCM education programs in collaboration with the Japanese Society of Intensive Care Medicine, the Saudi Critical Care Society, the Indian Society of Critical Care Medicine, and the Association of Intensive Medicine in Brazil. He is a Fellow of the American College of Critical Care Medicine.

He remains active at Stanford as an Adjunct Clinical Professor. He is currently a University of Texas System Distinguished Teaching Professor and Professor of CCM at the M.D. Anderson Cancer Center, Houston, TX.

Grace Chun (Meng)

attended the University of Pennsylvania (BA, 1986) and the Albert Einstein College of Medicine (MD, 1990). She interned (Internal Medicine) at Jacobi Medical Center/Albert Einstein College (1990-1991). She was a resident in Anesthesiology at Stanford (1991-1994). After finishing her anesthesia training, she worked in private practice in Gilroy, CA, before moving to Minnesota.

Memories of Time at Stanford: "I still remember the first day of my residency at Stanford like it was yesterday. Having reviewed the anesthesia machine checklist in the Miller textbook, I decided it will take me at least one hour to check the machine out prior to evaluating my patient preoperatively. I got to the operating room very, very early (earlier than the cardiac anesthesia resident who was surprised to hear that I was trying to use the machine checkout list in Miller), only to find I still had to rush through the checklist because I wasn't done after an hour. Needless to say, I felt very unprepared for the day. My entire first day in the OR with Dr. Jaffe was essentially spent trying to figure out which monitor was alarming. I never felt so distracted, while being so simultaneously lost, in my life. Luckily, this meant that things could only improve over the next three years. I absolutely enjoyed my time at Stanford, interacting with my classmates, teachers, and the OR staff. Every day I feel very lucky to have chosen a profession that is so rewarding and, most of the time, fun, especially now that I can sleep in my own bed each night!"

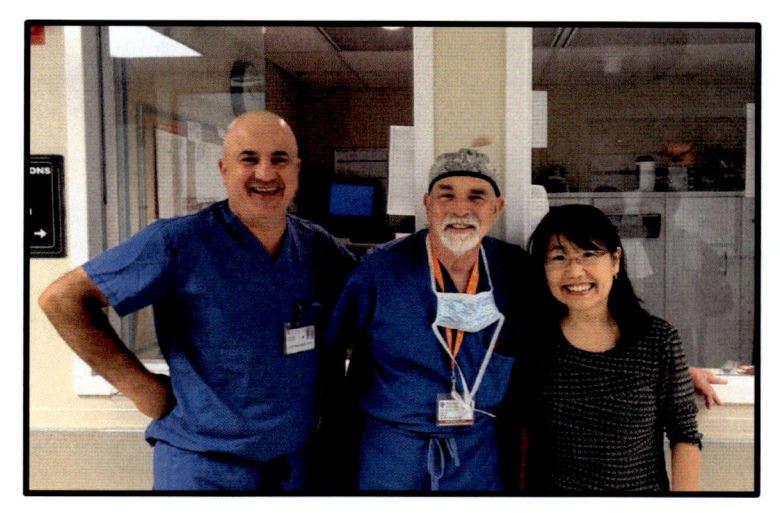

"After finishing my residency, I joined a private anesthesia practice in Gilroy, the "Garlic Capital of the World", where I spent two years either commuting 3 hours to/from work or taking overnight calls every two or three days. After realizing this lifestyle wasn't meeting any of my bucket list goals in life, I traded sunburn for frostbite by moving to MN in 1996. Over time, I learned to speak Minnesotan, with phrases such as "You betcha!", "Uff da!", and "hot dish" creeping into my vocabulary! This, of course, makes my patients laugh in shock! Despite living here for over 20 years, I still can't understand people voluntarily choosing to sit in a shed over a hole in the ice to fish when the temperature feels like it's approaching absolute zero, when one is simultaneously paying a mortgage on a nice, heated house."

Grace practices anesthesiology in Minneapolis – St. Paul, MN. She has worked at Phillips Eye Institute, Mercy Hospital - Unity Campus, and Mercy Hospital and is now affiliated with the both the High Pointe Surgery Center and Surgical Specialty Center of Minnesota.

- *I enjoyed practicing in a hospital-based private practice, which included Mercy and Unity Hospitals in the northern suburbs of the Twin Cities for over 20 years. In 2017, lured by the siren song of no more overnight-call, I moved to an outpatient-only anesthesia practice. Our current group of ten anesthesiologists covers two surgery centers, providing anesthesia for orthopedics, ophthalmology, ENT, plastic surgery, and urology cases. Until I started working in outpatient surgery, I didn't know that seasoned surgeons would voluntarily REQUEST 6:30 AM start times! While I have always been a morning person, a downside of driving at 5 AM in the winter darkness is seasonal 'fear'. If your morning coffee hasn't kicked in yet, a deer popping out in front of your car will definitely wake you up and test your coronary artery patency in a hurry!*
- *Of course, I truly miss the academic setting, especially when new techniques, technology and medications appear on the scene. Soon after ultrasound-guided nerve blocks became popular, I was so excited to move on from "poke and hope" to "seeing is believing." I even once had a fleeting thought that maybe I should go pursue a regional anesthesia fellowship. It is often difficult to get my hands on new advancements in private practice due to the omnipresent cost containment goals. Working as a volunteer anesthesiologist at Stanford soon after I graduated allowed me to maintain an academic connection for a while, but it became challenging once the household census count was more than just me and my husband.*

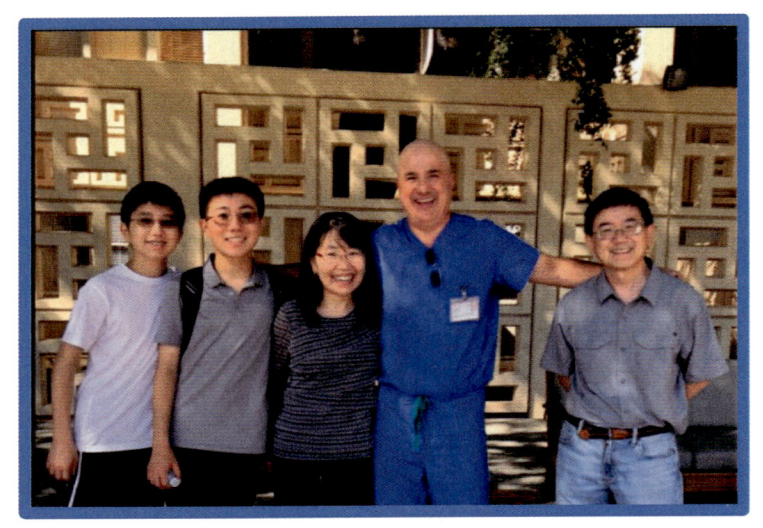

- My husband and I have two children, both currently in college and who are seriously contemplating postgraduate work. Thus, neither will be financially independent anytime soon. They seem to really embrace the concept of education, thus keeping my husband's and my need to remain gainfully employed for yet some more years. Luckily, we both love our current work arrangement, especially my husband who has been working from home since 2020 and tries to avoid going into the office as much as avoid eating lutefisk!

Jenifer Jo Damewood was an undergraduate at the University of Texas - Austin (BS, Nursing, 1983). She worked as an RN before attending medical school.

"Prior to medical school, I worked as an RN in a busy surgical ICU which included pediatric and adult cardiac patients as well as trauma. The SICU Chief was Harry Wallfisch, an anesthesiologist intensivist. He was my inspiration that led me to medical school and anesthesia."

She graduated from the University of Texas Medical Branch School of Medicine, Galveston (MD, 1990). Jennifer interned (Internal Medicine) at Good Samaritan Hospital/University of Arizona College of Medicine, Phoenix (1990-1991), and was a Stanford Anesthesiology resident (1991-1994).

"After Stanford, permanent jobs were scarce in the Bay Area given the changing economics of health care in 1994. I took it as an opportunity to look around, and I was thrilled to fill in for Kent Garman and practice with Vicky Coe in their cardiovascular practice at Sequoia Hospital, Redwood City. At the time Kent was taking time off while he served as President of the CSA. As a new full-fledged anesthesiologist, I was particularly keen to do the "big" cases."

Jenifer practiced at Kaiser - Santa Clara.

"After my intensive cardiac and aortic experience at Sequoia, I was offered a job at Santa Clara Kaiser where I happily spent the remainder of my anesthesia career. My colleagues were tremendous, and the case mix was like an academic institution."

She took early retirement on January 31, 2022.

"Kaiser and TPMG offer a full early retirement at age 60 that is impossible to pass up. I wasn't sure that I was ready, but the pandemic had a way of disrupting life and work as we knew it. I have missed the people but interestingly, I haven't really missed anesthesia. I have been busy with family and "activities of daily living" like exercise, cooking healthy meals, reading A LOT, and making time for friends."

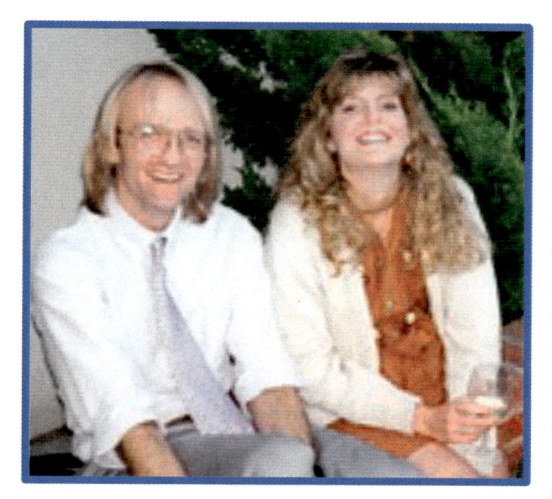

She is married to Stanford anesthesiologist Steve Howard, and they have one daughter.

"I remember secretly dating my husband (now of almost 30 years) while serving as Chief Resident at the PA-VAH the last 2 months of my residency. There really wasn't anything clandestine about our relationship (unless considering going to a Grateful Dead concert), but his colleagues David Gaba and Kevin Fish were quite concerned, and we are well aware that this would be a definite NO now! We had been trying to keep our relationship a secret. Then on Memorial Day 1993 we were out minding our own business in Mountain View looking for a sushi restaurant when we crossed Castro Street only to run into Dr. Fish - Chief of the department at the PA-VAH at the time - and we were holding hands, and I was wearing Steve's tie dye t-shirt. Dr. Fish was shaking his head but had a big smile on his face."

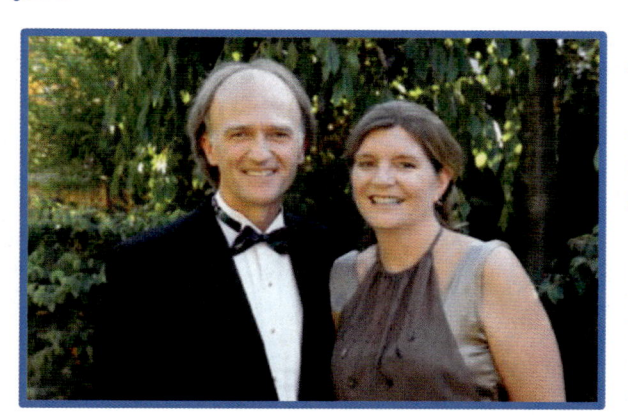

Steve and Jenifer at Department's 50th Anniversary

Anecdotes/Memories Of Time At Stanford include:

- *How John Brock-Utne, Stanley Samuels, and Jay Brodsky all stayed so thin after hanging out in the basement with the pastries day after day.*

(Ed note: In those days there was no breakfast nook in the Department, but Medical Records in the hospital basement provided breakfast as an enticement to sign delinquent medical records. Resident and faculty anesthesiologists spent every morning eating in the hospital basement.)

- *A case with Gail Boltz- tonsillar bleed in the middle of the night. Gail insisted on having blood available and good thing - just after a very careful intubation the bleeding became a waterfall. The patient had HIV and I stood there and held the tube while the ENT surgical chief tied off the external carotid artery. Dr. Fee was not present but in the change room.*
- *Many memories of Jay Brodsky either in the thoracic room or directing air traffic control from the OR hallway.*
- *My close friend and co-resident was the first woman to become pregnant while in the Stanford anesthesia residency program - EVER! Sheila Cohen always took the female residents under her wing and in addition to teaching anesthesia obstetric care, she made sure she discussed self-care including talking calcium supplements to prevent osteoporosis. I always chuckled in that many of the women that she counseled were Amazonian-like compared to Sheila's small slight stature.*
- *The lockboxes that we carried around OB with our syringes of bupivacaine 0.0625% and 0.33 mcg sufentanil. Now we know that the access then was far too easy.*
- *The days of pre-op(ing) the night before the patient's surgery - when patients were admitted to the hospital the day before AND when residents actually did the pre-op.*

- The ICU call room (remember every 3rd night call) with multiple bunkbeds - residents climbing up and down all night as multiple pagers going went off- after all, sleep isn't that important.
- The good old days of voice pagers- V tack, V tack, V tach - WHERE?
- Trip to the SF Zoo with Fred Mihm, George Wakerlin, and Wayne Anderson to anesthetize a baboon for a blood draw. The baboon was tranquilized by a blow dart of ketamine and hauled on a wagon into the veterinary clinic.
- Years later I reunited at Kaiser with Gordon Haddow and (surgeon) Mario Pompeli. Gordon had been my attending for many a cardiac case and a few liver transplants at Stanford while Mario was a cardiac surgery fellow at that time.
- Neuro rotation where Phil Larson had the residents intubate patients awake and then have them position themselves on the OR table ala tincture of demerol 100 mg and glycopyrrolate. Patients were nicely stoned and did not seem to mind. Certainly, a big resident benefit to get so skilled with awake fiberoptic intubations.
- During my rotation at the PA-VAH, residents had the opportunity to work with Dr. Mervyn Maze. He was doing research on alpha agonists, and he would insist that we premed the patients with clonidine - those veterans slept for days. The residents always tried to avoid it, or reduce the dose but Mervyn was adamant that we give it. Little did we know that dexmedetomidine would be such a universally important anesthetic adjuvant in today's practice.
- Traveling to Oakland Children's Hospital for a 3-day stint of call as there weren't enough pediatric cases at Stanford at the time.

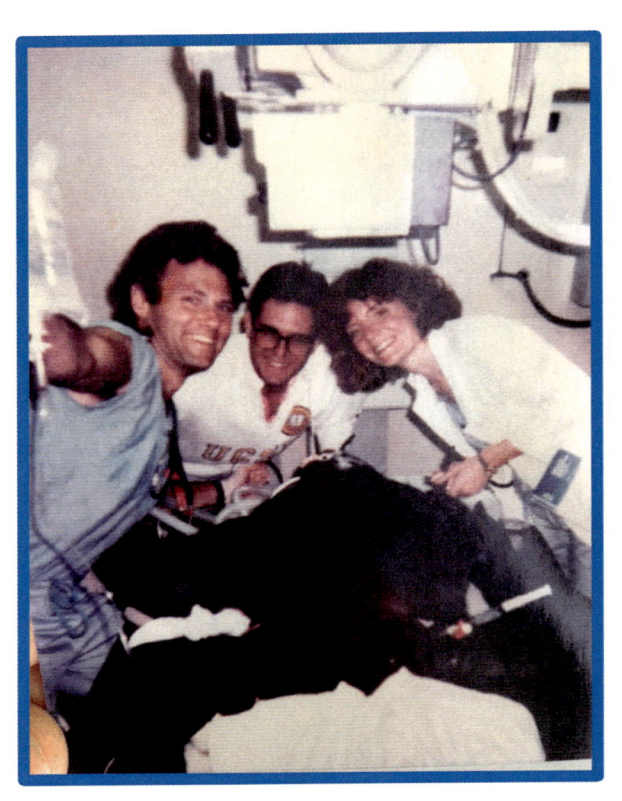

(L-R) George Wakerlin, Wayne Anderson, and Jenifer Damewood anesthetize a gorilla under Fred Mihm's direction

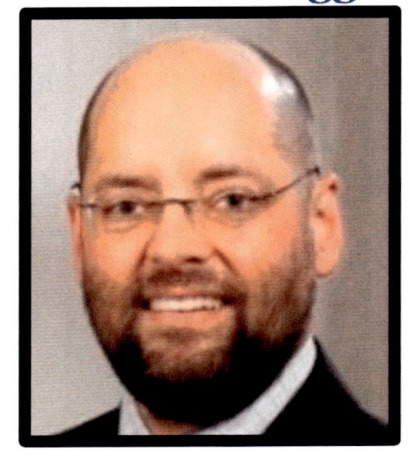

Mark Allen Eggen did his undergraduate work at the University of Minnesota (BS, 1986) and then trained in medicine at the University of Minnesota Medical School (MD, 1990). He interned (Transitional) at Marshfield Clinic (1990-1991). He completed his Anesthesiology training at Stanford (1991-1994) and has been associated with the St. Cloud-VAH, MN, and Abbott Northwestern Hospital, Minneapolis, MD. He was a member of Midwest Anesthesiologists (1994-2013). He was President of Health Billing Systems, Inc. and a principal of Analytical Instruments, a company that sells and services used biomedical research instruments. Dr. Eggen is also on the board of directors of the Federation of State Medical Boards and was on the Minnesota Board of Medical Practice for 8 years. He retired from clinical practice at the end of 2013 but remains active on medical missions to Guatemala. He is a licensed bush pilot.

Memories of Stanford, "It was a lovely party!"

- *We lived in the Welch Road apartments, on campus, a block from SUH. One night, the phone rang. I answered it. There were 13 GSW casualties in the ED coming to the OR and they needed all hands-on deck. That was a crazy night, I was a CA2 and had to do my own case. It was a bleeding out chest wound. Thankfully, the surgery resident and I got the bleeding controlled and it ended well. It's amazing the trauma that a young individual can sustain.*
- *John Brock-Utne and I wrote a paper on A-line stopcock.* (Eggen MA, Brock-Utne JG. Artifactual increase in the arterial pressure waveform: remember the stopcock. Anesth Analg (2005) 101:298-299) *I had another identical incident in the past month. I was directing an endovascular cerebral aneurysm coiling case with an arterial line for rapid close BP management. The nurse anesthetist inadvertently bumped the stopcock, and the tracing was artifactually elevated. I received an urgent call to the Cath lab where a distressed nurse anesthetist was busily administering nicardipine. After recognizing the issue and zeroing the A-line, we discovered significant hypotension from the nicardipine. A tincture of time and that resolved. All ended well.*
- *Jay Brodsky and I wrote a paper on instilling lidocaine into chest tubes to improve post-op analgesia.* (Brodsky JB, Eggen M, Cannon WB. Spontaneous pneumothorax in early pregnancy: successful management by thoracoscopy. J Cardiothorac Vasc Anesth (1993) 7:585-587) *The surgeon, Dr. Cannon was super helpful in that work. We didn't pursue that idea further. My concern was systemic absorption of lidocaine. The concept was simple, but the side effects could be problematic. At the time, we placed epidurals, typically lumbar and ran morphine. It wasn't that effective. Using thoracic epidurals improved analgesia but increased risk of procedure related complications. My practice has evolved to paravertebral blocks using bupivacaine and Exparel. Three days of analgesia with no catheter to manage.*
- *Another significant change in cardiac surgery has been the off-pump CABG. CPB runs have become much less common. Valve surgery has moved into the field of cardiology with TAVR and mitral clips. Aortic and cerebral aneurysm have gone endovascular. The aortic dissections are still CPB cases, typically circulatory arrest, then the bleeding is miserable. Aprotinin was a great drug to control this type bleeding, unfortunately, aprotinin is not currently on the market. Stanford did a bunch of the original aprotinin studies when I was a resident there. I question the validity of that research. I recall being instructed by the CV Fellow to "pick" the envelope with the key to the aprotinin over placebo late at night when one of these aortic dissection cases was booked. Pharmacy staff weren't on duty, and it was my job to get the study drug from the pharmacy. The night cases likely got more aprotinin and the day cases got less.*
- *I had 3 OR fires while a resident!* (Eggen MA, Brock-Utne JG. Fiberoptic illumination systems can serve as a source of smoldering fires. J Clin Monit (1994) 10:244-246) *That was BAD not to mention dangerous. I think I was secretly called a pyromaniac by my anesthesia colleagues. The first one was a case of the 32-year-old woman. The surgeon introduced a trocar and a pneumoperitoneum. Before endoscopy the unprotected illuminated end of FIS was placed on the drapes at xiphoid level. The FIS was at maximum intensity. Within one min burning smell and smoke smolder fire was seen. The surgeon was informed and removed the light source. The smoldering fire stopped immediately. The second was an electrocautery unit not holstered during a total hip replacement. The surgeon leaned on it, it arced to the table rail at waist level and started a fire on the surgeon's paper gown. The scrub tech had a major basin of water and used it to douse the fire. The surgeon danced all over the room. He wasn't a well-loved character. Later, the scrub tech said she had been fantasizing about dumping a major basin of water on him and she finally had the opportunity! A third was at the PA-*

VAH. The senior urology resident was on vacation and a junior resident was called up from the lab to replace him for a week. The new resident didn't have much experience doing urology cases. He was struggling with a ureteroscope and removed the light source, setting it energized on the drapes which then caught fire. In my private practice life, fires continued. A surgeon doing a laparoscopic tubal ligation set an energized light source on the drapes which left a burn on the patient's chest that looked like a cigarette butt burn.

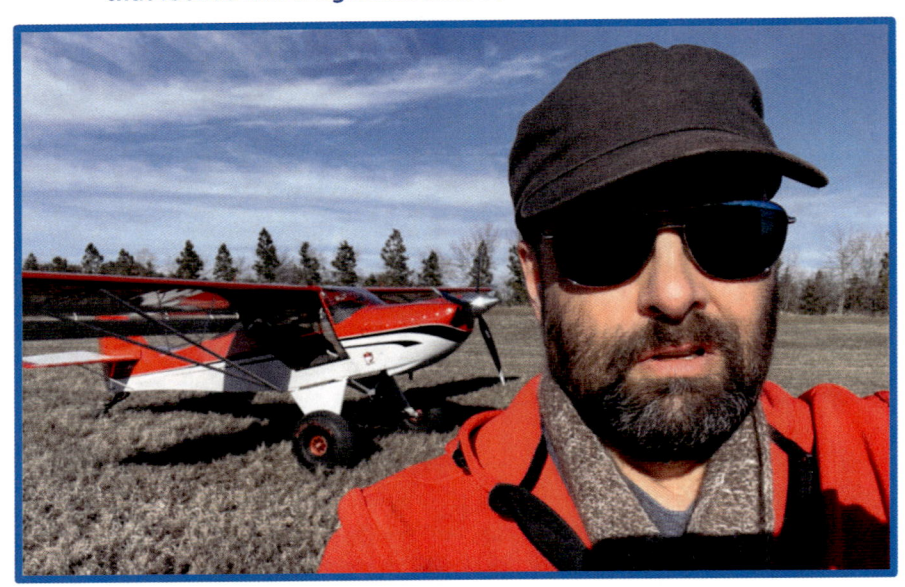

- *Looking down the line in Guatemala, we are running out of surgeons who can do typical procedures like TAH, open chole and open hernia repairs using old school techniques. The new generation of surgeons are dependent on a level of technology that can't be supported in a field hospital setting where the electricity is sometimes working and when it is the voltage varies between 100VAC and 140VAC making use of any electronics impossible. Our youngest surgeon is 60 and they are aging out. I can't see how to support laparoscopic much less robotic surgery for lots of reasons, particularly the price of equipment and disposables. Plastic surgery is different. They haven't adopted all the technology. Doing cleft lips and palates is the same as 50 years ago. The plastic surgeons don't get much opportunity to hone those skills stateside, so they are lined up to join our team in Guatemala.*

Lauren Anne Elliott was an undergraduate at Stanford University (BS, 1986) and a graduate of UCI Medical School (MD, 1990). She was an Anesthesiology resident and Fellow (Adult and Pediatric Cardiac Anesthesia)(1991-1994). She worked at Kaiser after completing her training (1995-1996) and was a Clinical Instructor (Anesthesiology) at Stanford (1997-1998). She no longer practices anesthesiology.

Catherine Lee Hamilton attended Santa Clara University (BS, Combined Sciences, 1974-1978) and then Northwestern University (MA, Counseling Psychology, 1978-1979). She then attended the UCLA School of Dentistry (DDS, 1979-1983). She graduated from the Keck School of Medicine/USC (MD, 1990), interned (Internal Medicine) at CPMC (1990-1991), and then completed her Anesthesiology residency (1991-1994) and Fellowship (Obstetrical Anesthesiology) (1994-1995) at Stanford. She worked as an anesthesiologist in the SF Bay area.

Martha Cox Ho was an undergraduate at Iowa State University (BS, Economics, 1981) and then graduated from UCSF (MD, 1990). She interned (Transitional) at SCVMC and was a resident at Stanford (1990-1994). After training she briefly worked at Seton Medical Center, Daly City (1994) and then at Hennepin County Medical Center, Minneapolis, MN (1995-2001). She later worked at Mercy Hospital, Coon Rapids, MN (2001-2016) and then at Philips Eye Hospital, Minneapolis from 2016 until retiring in 2019. Post-retirement she enjoys bicycling, does AARP tax counseling and instruction, travelling, tutoring, learning Spanish, and resuming piano lessons after a 50-year break.

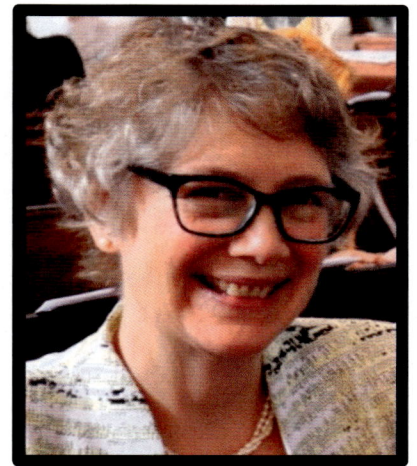

- *My training at Stanford prepared me well for a busy, full career after coming home to the Midwest. For several years I was the pediatric point person at a busy trauma hospital where I was happy to do a wide range of adult cases too. I then took the opportunity to join Stanford residency colleagues Mark Eggen and Grace Chun in a busy private practice where I enjoyed cardiac cases and maintained skills with plenty of ortho, OB and pediatrics. The last 3 years before retiring, I worked with a slower paced group at an eye hospital and two surgery centers (no more 4 am ruptured aneurysms!) Family life was sweet for my husband Fred, children Matt, Kristin (Stanford baby), Marc, and me in Minnesota.*
- *I learned so much from so many faculty members at Stanford, the PA-VAH and SCVMC ... I could fill the page with names ... Sheila Cohen, Jay Brodsky, Richard Jaffe, Gail Boltz, Rona Giffard, Ron Pearl, Stanley Samuels, Emily Ratner, Pam Fish, Kevin Fish, Dave Gaba, Harry Lemmens, Steve Howard, Steve Shafer, Frank Sarnquist, Mike Rosenthal ... it's amazing how easily all those names come to me so quickly. What a great program Stanford was and I'm sure it continues to be!*
- *I greatly appreciated the perspectives of poet/anesthesiologist/parent/ Audrey Shafer.*
- *I do have fond memories of John Brock-Utne and of my years at Stanford. I first met him when he interviewed me prior to my entry to the match. Happily, I was able to come to Stanford as my first choice in the match and enjoyed working with him and a lot . I learned so much from both of you. Jay, I was always grateful that he wouldn't let me use the fiberoptic scope when we placed double lumen tubes ... he taught me so many tricks to get the tube into good position ... skills I used many times over the years helping colleagues fine tune tube placement when the fiberoptic just didn't help!*

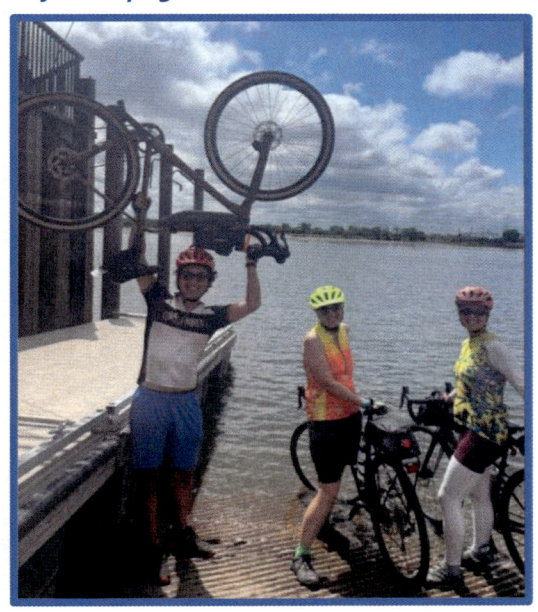

Martha Ho with her children dipping the front tires of their bikes in the Mississippi River after completing the Ragbrai tour across Iowa.

Ed Note: RAGBRAI, short for Register's Annual Great Bicycle Ride Across Iowa, is a non-competitive bicylcle tour across Iowa from the western to eastern border. First held in 1973, RAGBRAI is the largest bike-touring event in the world.

- *I was a little chagrined to learn from Grace Chun that my retirement predated Dr. Brodsky's! I retired at 60, just before the pandemic. I did brush up on ICU knowledge/skills but Minnesota avoided the worst of the pandemic, so my volunteer work involved simply giving Covid vaccinations. Turns out, early retirement gave me more precious time with my beloved husband of nearly 40 years, Fred. He suddenly became ill and died 9 weeks later of pancreatic cancer in early 2023. Life changes quickly. My kids and friends have been so helpful, and I try to keep busy with AARP tax volunteering, English language tutoring, reading, and biking.*

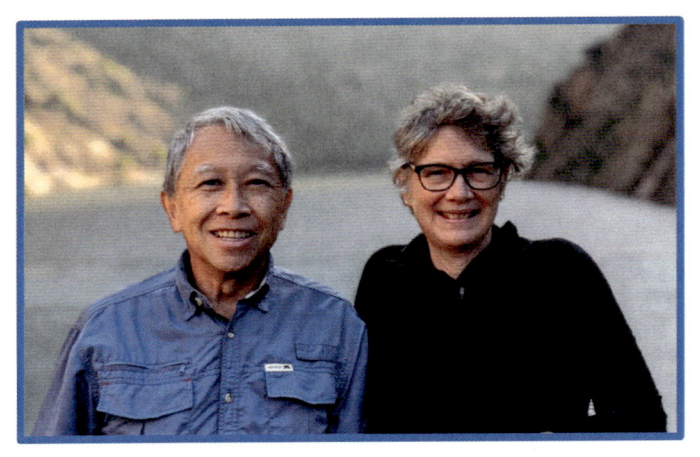

With my beloved Fred.
My kids, family and friends keep me going.

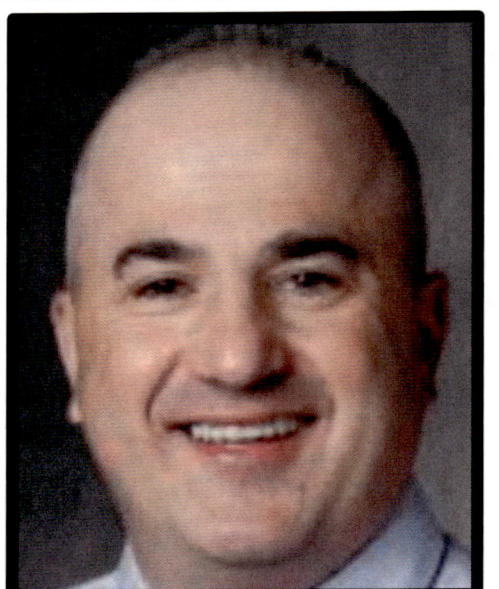

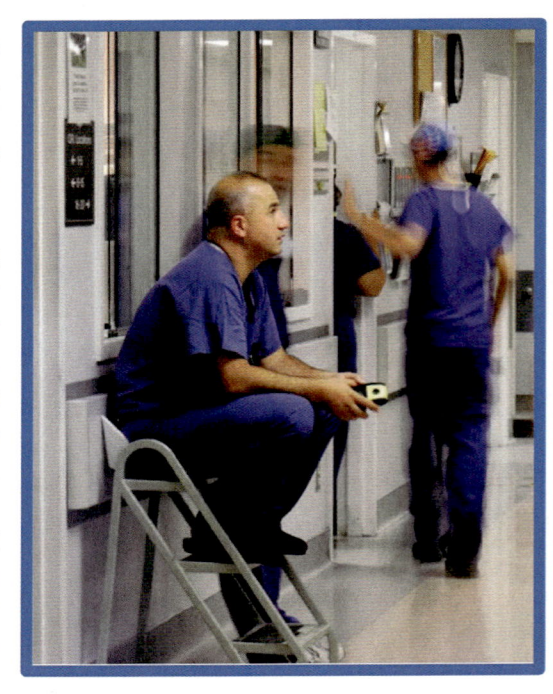

Alex Macario was in Buenos Aires, Argentina. His family moved to the US when he was 10. As an undergraduate he attended the University of Rochester (BS, Sociology, 1986) and then was a graduate student majoring in health care organizations and markets (MBA, Health Economics, 1988). He received his medical education at the University of Rochester (MD, 1990). He interned at the Graduate Hospital, Philadelphia, and completed his Anesthesiology residency at Stanford (1991-1994). He was Chief Resident in 1994. He did a Fellowship (Health Services Research) at Stanford (1995). Dr. Macario began his academic career as Clinical Assistant Professor in 1995, and was promoted to Assistant Professor (Anesthesiology) in 1996, to Associate Professor (2001), and then to Professor (2006-Present). Dr. Macario has been a member of the multi-specialty group (MSD) formerly known as the Gen-OR group.

Alex was the Department's Vice-Chair for Education (2006-2024). He established an academic program in operating room management. He is the Program Director for the Department's Management of Perioperative Services Fellowship (1996-Present) which has trained dozens of physicians from the US and other countries. He was Program Director for the Anesthesiology residency (2006-2023). He designed and led other innovative educational programs, including the Fellowship in Anesthesia Research and Medicine track for anesthesia residents who want to pursue research-intensive careers, many of whom have gone on to obtain NIH funding. He also served as program director for the Combined Internal Medicine - Anesthesiology Residency (2013) and the Combined Pediatrics -Anesthesiology Residency (2010). He was the founder of the Department's Faculty Teaching Scholars Program (2007- 2017).

Dr. Macario was a member of the Executive Committee of the Stanford University School of Medicine Faculty Senate (2007-2012). He also serves on the Board of Directors for the ABA and is currently its Secretary (2017-Present). He will serve as ABA President at the end of his term. He is a member of the Anesthesiology Review Committee for the Accreditation Council for Graduate Medical Education which aims to improve health care and population health by advancing the quality of resident physicians' education (2019-Present).

His numerous awards and honors include Ellis N. Cohen Achievement Award (2009), the inaugural Outstanding Contribution to Graduate Medical Education as Program Director, at Stanford University (2015), the Faculty Mentor Award from the ASA Committee on Professional Diversity (2012 and 2013), and the Excellence in Education Award (ASA, 2018). The Excellence in Education Award is given to one anesthesiologist per year for extraordinary contributions to graduate medical education.

Dr. Macario's research career has been dedicated to the economics of health care, helping develop the scientific study of the management of the operating room suite including pioneering work related to efficiency and scheduling. Dr. Macario's research team also studies medical education and board certification. He has 400+ peer reviewed publications which have thousands of citations. His publications focus on the economics of health care, with particular attention on the tradeoffs between costs and outcomes for patients having surgery and anesthesia. He has also investigated predictive methods for duration of surgery and the importance that the correct surgical procedure is booked, and that accurate time stamps are collected.

Dr. Macario authored "A Sabbatical in Madrid: A Diary of Spain," an award-winning travel memoir In his free time, Dr. Macario enjoys rooting for Stanford sports, biking up the local hills, & playing tennis.

"A Sabbatical in Madrid" summary: In August 2001, Alex Macario, an anesthesiologist at Stanford Medical School, moved his family to Madrid for a ten-month sabbatical. In the tradition of Peter Mayle's A Year in Provence, they discover Spain, as warmly chronicled in their diary. You will live with them as expatriates during 9-11, and travel with them as they encounter dinero negro, settle in at Balear Dos, try to win El Gordo, examine the masterpiece Guernica, participate in Easter week in Sevilla, admire the

last dance of the honorable bull Guitarrero, and learn to love fztbol and jamsn iberico. Facts and delightful personal observations carry the reader along on a story that promises emotional payoff.

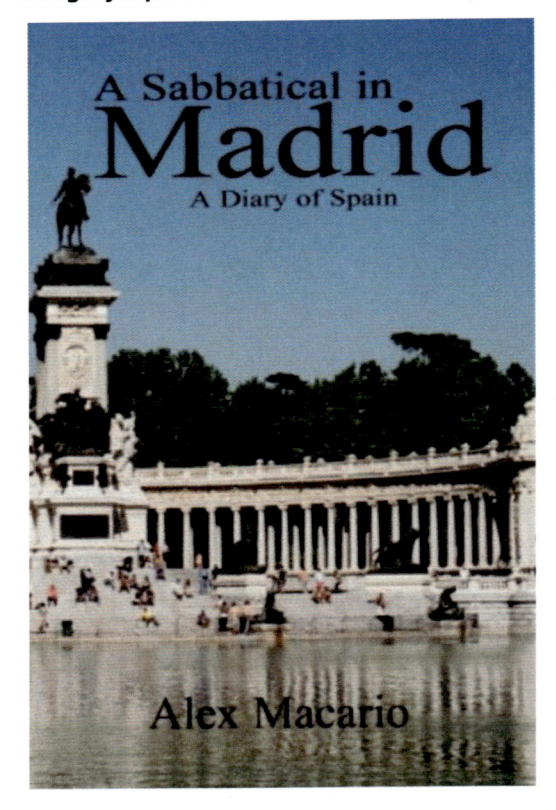

"Memories ... going to the deGuerre swimming pool (now the Avery Aquatic Center) with Rick Ronquillo and Jeff Clayton to do laps in the 50-meter pool."

"Flying in the helicopter to remote areas in California to help with organ harvests."

"One of my fondest memories is breakfast at medical records with my classmates."

John Brock-Utne ... "I knew from the start of his residency that Alex was going to have an academic career, especially in economics. One day he asked me: "Why do we have so many different esophageal stethoscopes?" He wondered if there was an acoustic difference between them. So we did a study and found no differences. Stanford eliminated both the 12 Fr and 24 Fr saving lots of money."

(Macario A, Brock-Utne JG. Elimination of 12 and 24 Fr esophageal stethoscopes from anesthetic practice (an attempt at cost containment). Anesth Analg (1994) 79:393.)

Fernando Fabian Okonski was born in Buenos Aires, Argentina. He began his undergraduate education at UCI (1982-1983) and then graduated from UC-Berkely (BA, Biochemistry, 1983-1986). He received his medical education at USC (MD, 1990), interned (Internal Medicine) at SCVMC (1991), and trained in Anesthesiology at Stanford (1991-1994). He worked as a Pediatric and Cardiac Anesthesiologist at Vituity, San Jose/Los Gatos (1995-2018). He was an Adjunct Clinical Instructor of Anesthesia at Lucile Packard Children's Hospital (2009-2017) and was

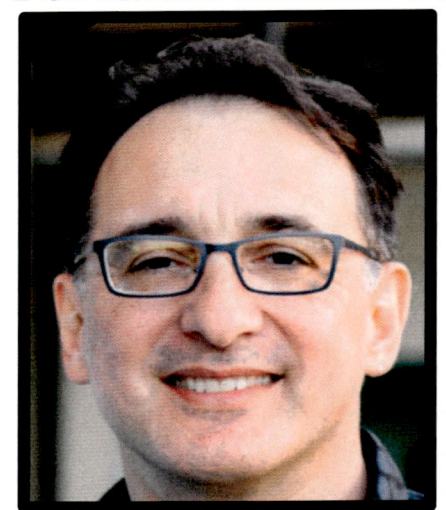

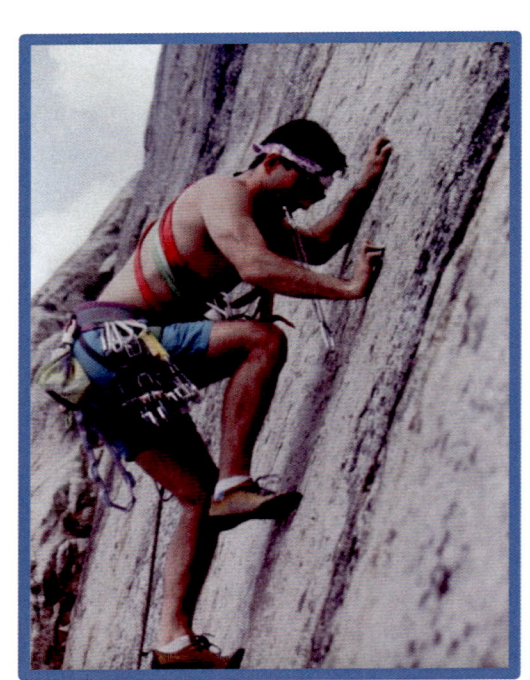

**Fabian Okonski at Donner Summit
(Photo by Jeff Clayton)**

184

promoted to Clinical Assistant Professor (Anesthesiology) at Stanford Children's Health and Lucile Packard Children's Hospital (2018-Present).

He has a special interest in marine mammal medicine, and he works regularly as an anesthesiology consultant (Clinical Science Researcher) with veterinarians at the Marine Mammal Center in Sausalito, CA, providing anesthesia and research support for perioperative care of pinnipeds and cetaceans (2015-Present). He has travelled extensively on medical missions around the globe including Vietnam, Nepal, Guatemala, and Bolivia, often with Resurge (formerly Interplast) (1994-Present). He is also a volunteer pediatric anesthesiologist with the HUGS Foundation Inc. (2019-Present).

The mission of HUGS (Help Us Give Smiles) is to deliver free medical care to children and adolescents challenged by microtia, cleft lip, cleft palate, and other facial deformities. Since its establishment in 2003, HUGS has accomplished more than 30 missions around the world.

Fabian lives in Palo Alto and enjoys sports car racing, rock climbing, snowboarding, and cycling.

Beemeth Tzaraoh Robles

was born in Los Angeles. He attended UC-Riverside as an undergraduate (BS, Biology) and then Stanford (MD, 1988). He was an intern and resident (Surgery) at Stanford (1988-1991). He then completed his Anesthesiology residency (1991-1994). During residency he worked in the Department of Emergency Medicine, Life Flight (1991-1994). He was a Founding Partner of Visalia Anesthesia Medical Associates (1994-2002) and Co-Founder of the Kaweah Delta Healthcare District Cardiac Anesthesia Division and is the former Chief of the Department of Anesthesia there.

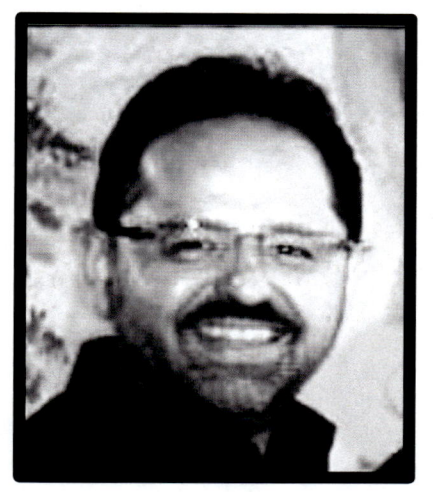

"I started my career in Visalia in 1994 after leaving Stanford. I would say that my time in Visalia was probably my best years in regard to building a Department, an anesthesia group and a Division of Cardiac Anesthesia. Had a great run in Visalia but the realities of medicine and the business of Medicine were slowly undoing the happy person I had been. It's a long story, but in 2002 I left. I was definitely needed in Visalia but with all the hats I wore, I was worn down and needed a change. Eventually Ted Kreitzman recruited me to Phoenix where I have been since August 2002."

He was Medical Director for North Valley Surgery Center, Phoenix, AZ, for 9 years and is a Partner of Metro Anesthesia Consultants PC (2002-Present). He works at Banner-University Medical Center and St. Joseph's Hospital and Medical Center, Phoenix. He plans to continue working into his 70's and retire in 2033.

"Phoenix has been good to us and it's been a great run. I hope to have another 10 to 12 years as the practice evolves. I think retiring at 72 to 75, assuming my health holds up, which so far is great, will allow me to continue to enjoy what I do."

His lists his outside interests as woodworking, construction, wine and fine food. He enjoys traveling in Europe and supporting "second amendment rights".

"When I look back on my career, I will be able to say that I made Stanford proud. Stanford prepared me for the challenges that would come with anesthesia, and it gave me the courage to take on the challenges that came from the Business of Medicine."

Adam Jon Rubinstein was born in East Lansing, MI. He attended the University of Michigan – Ann Arbor (BS, Biological Cybernetics, 1981-1985) and then the University of Pittsburgh School of Medicine (MD, 1990). He interned (Transitional) at Mercy Hospital of Pittsburgh (1990-1991) and did an Anesthesiology residency at Stanford (1991-1994). He was a Visiting Clinical Instructor at Stanford (1997-2001). Following residency, he worked at W.A. Foote Memorial Hospital, and was Medical Director of their Jackson Outpatient Surgery Center, Jackson, MI (1994-2004). He then was a Senior Attending Anesthesiologist at MedStar Washington Hospital Center, Washington, DC (2005-2018) where he was Director of Trauma Anesthesia and Transfusion Medicine and Medical Director of the PACUs. He was site coordinator for Georgetown University medical students and residents for obstetrics, cardiac, acute pain and trauma rotations and co-chair of the Transfusion Committee at MedStar. He then was appointed Service Chief and Medical Director of Anesthesiology, Pain Management & Perioperative Medicine at Henry Ford Jackson Hospital, Jackson, MI (2018-2023). He retired in May 2023, but returned as a part-time Senior Attending Anesthesiologist at the Henry Ford Hospitals in Detroit and Jackson (2023-Present).

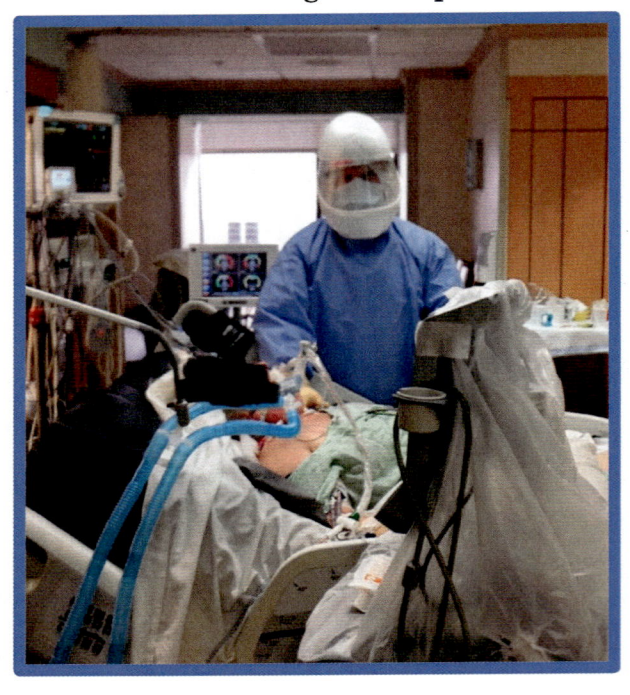

Interesting Anecdotes/Memories of Time at Stanford:
"Unforgettable memories were forged at Stanford, as I gained proficiency in my craft, and I felt privileged to experience them. My immense gratitude extends to the dedicated physicians and support staff whose contributions greatly enriched my education, though it would be impossible to adequately thank each of you. As part of my stream of consciousness, I have included a few brief recollections, in no particular order:
- *The sheer amazement of watching Tiger Woods hit golf balls at the driving range.*

- *Being cornered by Helen Bing and escorted on a personal tour of the Bing artwork in the hospital.*
- *Having the privilege of accompanying Dr. Fred Mihm to the SF Zoo to anesthetize large animals (I was fortunate to participate in the anesthesia of lion and an orangutan.*
- *Having the opportunity to fly as a member of the critical care transport and organ harvesting team. Not only did I earn some money to defray living expenses, it honed my clinical skills in unimaginable and useful ways while providing unbelievable situational experiences (seeing the SR-71's lighting up the runways at Moffitt, taking off in a helicopter with zero visibility, and sitting in the co-pilot's seat on a Lear Jet).*
- *Rescuing a fellow resident who suffered a syncopal event.*
- *The birth of our daughter Sarah Rubinstein at Stanford University Hospital during the last week of my residency. She is the light of my life!"*

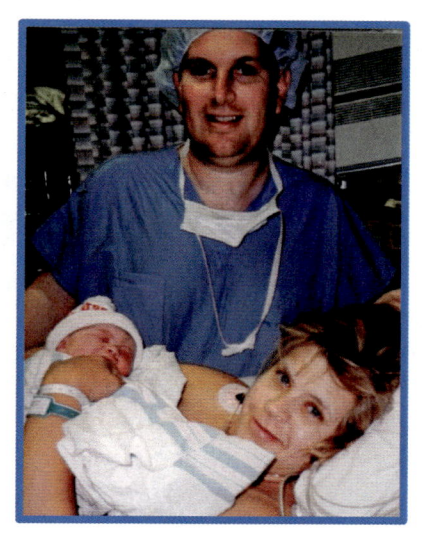

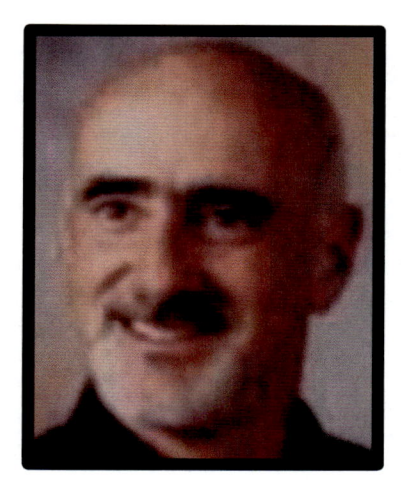

Joshua Ben Siegel was an undergraduate at UCD (Environmental Toxicology, 1977-1982) studying for a year at the Hebrew University of Jerusalem, Israel (1979-1980). He received his medical education at Tel Aviv University Sackler School of Medicine (MD, 1984-1987). He interned (Internal Medicine) at the Long Island Jewish Medical Center (1987). He then did a residency (Internal Medicine) at Stanford (1988-1990) followed by his Anesthesiology residency (1991-1993) at Stanford. He worked as an anesthesiologist and critical care physician in the San Francisco Bay Area (1994-Present). He returned to Stanford to do a Fellowship (CCM) (2012-2013).

Bryan Peter Tunink attended Claremont McKenna College (BA with honors, Biology and Psychology, 1986). He graduated from Keck School of Medicine/USC (MD, 1990) and did an internship (Internal Medicine) at SCVMC (1990-1991). He completed his Anesthesiology residency at Stanford (1991-1994).

"After leaving Stanford, I felt very well prepared to be out on my own. I thank all of the wonderful professors who taught us daily, teaching us important academic points during cases, and also the opportunities with the clinical professors who visited from the community."

He initially worked as an independent anesthesiologist at Enloe Hospital, Chico, CA (1994-1996). He moved to Texas and worked with Dallas Fort Worth (DFW) Anesthesia Associates (1996-1999). He then joined Pinnacle Anesthesia Consultants (1999-2012) as a partner, then worked with Stratus Anesthesia Associates, Southlake, TX (2012-2016). He was Chief of Anesthesiology at Forest Park Medical Center, Southlake (2015-2016).

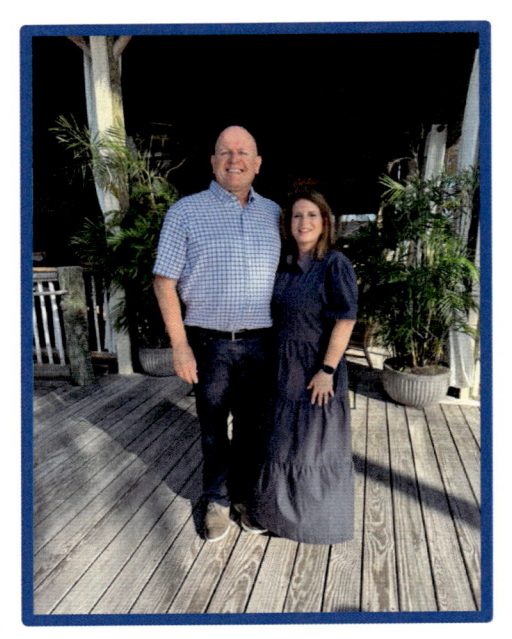

He is now with Texas Anesthesia Partners (2016-Present) and was Chief of Anesthesiology at Methodist Southlake Hospital (2016-2018).

Memories of Stanford: Jeff Clayton, Fabian Okonski, Peter Kosek, relatives, friends, my wife, my brother and I rafted on the Smith and Salmon Rivers about three months before graduating. It had rained the night and some of the week before. The river volume was higher than it had been for many years. All the boats except one flipped on our first day. But then we had a great dinner, and went right to bed, and woke up the next morning and went to the Smith River. I can remember the first day the outfitters from Ashland Oregon's Noah's Rafting told us that the height of the water under the bridge was the highest they'd seen and let us know if we decided to do it, it would be very difficult, and we'd likely be flipping the raft or thrown out of the raft part of the day. The water was very cold from snow melt. We were wearing wool socks, neoprene booties, 6 mm farmer john pants and torso wetsuits, 6 mm jacket, a wool sweater over that, splash jacket over it, and a 6 mm wetsuit hood like you would do with cold water diving. The most dangerous rapid was called Freight Train. It's called Freight Train because the rapid sounds like a freight train. Noah's guides inspected that rapid with us from the road above on the way to the boat ramp. When standing 6 inches from the person next to you and yelling, they can't hear you. We decided to go through Freight Train. We went through one raft at a time and had rescue support from other rafts below the rapid so that capsized swimmers would not go swimming through the next rapids, but could instead grab ropes that were thrown from a throw bag and hooked with carabiners into rings in the rocks below the freight train rapid. We all made it. When we returned, I'm sure more than one of us pondered that after 24 years of education this was not a good use of our time since we had given all of our effort to accomplish graduating from Stanford residency and entering the workforce, but we all made it.

- *I have a memory of Peter Kosek as my Attending during one case in the second month of cardiac anesthesia. We were doing a valve replacement on a patient with CHF, and coming off pump, we had to add amrinone in addition to the usual epi and dopamine. I think we may have had to go back on pump, before successfully coming off. We probably were also transfusing blood, but I remember thinking Peter Kosek was brilliant, as were all the cardiac attendings like Larry Siegel and Frank Sarnquist. While we were working to resuscitate the patient, he was describing the physiology, cardiac anatomy, pharmacology, and surgical interventions as if he was flawlessly reading from a textbook.*
- *Our third year was the worst year for Stanford grads finding work. Bill Clinton set up the Task Force on National Health Care Reform, headed by Hillary Clinton, to come up with a comprehensive plan to provide universal healthcare. Most of us could only obtain temporary work because Kaiser and it seemed every anesthesia group slowed developing existing projects, held future projects, and stopped offering partnership tracks. I lived in Santa Clara and wanted to stay there if possible. I was very scared and worked every break and every lunch calling hospitals in California and Oregon for opportunities to interview. I called an anesthesiologist, that graduated from Loma Linda, whom I had met in the operating room during a heart transplant harvesting. He asked me about what we were doing, and I called his boss in March the month my first daughter was born. Thankfully, I worked in California and was very excited doing neuro, cardiac, trauma, and OB anesthesia using*

the knowledge I had gained at Stanford. Then in 1996, with my wife being from Texas, I sent a CV and called the group I ended up joining in Grapevine, Texas, and was there for 16 years. The hiring environment was still very bad in 1996 as anesthesia groups did not know what the 'new national healthcare' would be. The group in Grapevine called me after they saw that I'd come from Stanford, and this is where I give a big Thank You to Jay Brodsky and John Brock-Utne whose reference letters were crucial in obtaining that employment. It turns out after interviewing with them in February 1996, two of the group members had known James Bell from the UT Southwestern Dallas program. Thank you so much Jim for offering your reference for me. It was crucial to obtaining their approval, and we successfully moved to Texas, where my second daughter was born. I remember calling Jim and thanking him; He was in Austin, excelling with their largest anesthesia group.

- *When I came out for this interview, Russell Allen was working at Baylor hospital in Dallas with another anesthesia group that ended up merging later with the group I joined, and we had a nice lunch in Deep Ellum before he had to get back to work.*
- *I realize that sometimes how anesthesia docs perform in the community is not as well done as it is at Stanford. When I would attend medical chart review meetings during my first year out, I could see the deficiencies compared to what Stanford professors and residents would have done during the same circumstances, and once or twice wrote how the circumstances could/should have been handled on chart reviews. One time, I was told, in no uncertain terms by the person who had the deficiencies that he 'did not appreciate me bringing the 'Stanford Way' to their chart review. And from that point on, I did not uphold future chart reviews to the Stanford gold standard.*
- *Dr. Phil Larson and Dr. Richard Jaffe showed us how to fiberoptically intubate using lidocaine aerosolization and sedation. I've used this technique many times, and have assisted my partners, teaching them or intubating for them. I am very grateful for that instruction.*

Joseph S. Dunn was born in Newton, KS. He received his undergraduate training at UCSD (BS Chemical Engineering, 1980-1984). He attended UCI (MD, 1988). He interned at Harborview/UCLA (1989). He started his residency (Anesthesiology) at UCLA (1989-1991) and completed his CA3 year (7/1/91-6/30/92) and a Fellowship (Pain Management) (1992-1993) at Stanford. He was a Clinical Instructor (Anesthesiology) at Stanford (1993-1994) and then Assistant Clinical Professor and Director of the Pain Fellowship at UCSD (1994-1997). He worked with Northwest Anesthesia in Oregon (1998). He then joined Peter Kosek at Pain Consultants of Oregon, Eugene, OR (1998-2014). He left that group for the NeuroSpine Institute in Eugene (2015-2016). He is currently a partner in Pain Specialists of Oregon (2016-Present). He was a President of the Pain Society of Oregon. Joe is board certified in Palliative Care and Hospice (2003-2010). He has no current plans for retirement.

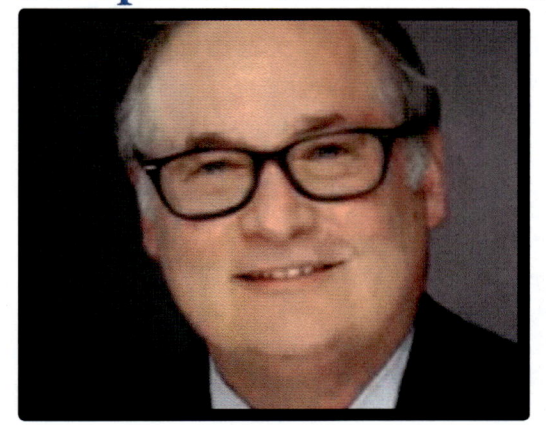

"Yuan Chi Lin used to tell me when an expert pain management consult needed --- just call 1-800 Joe Dunn."

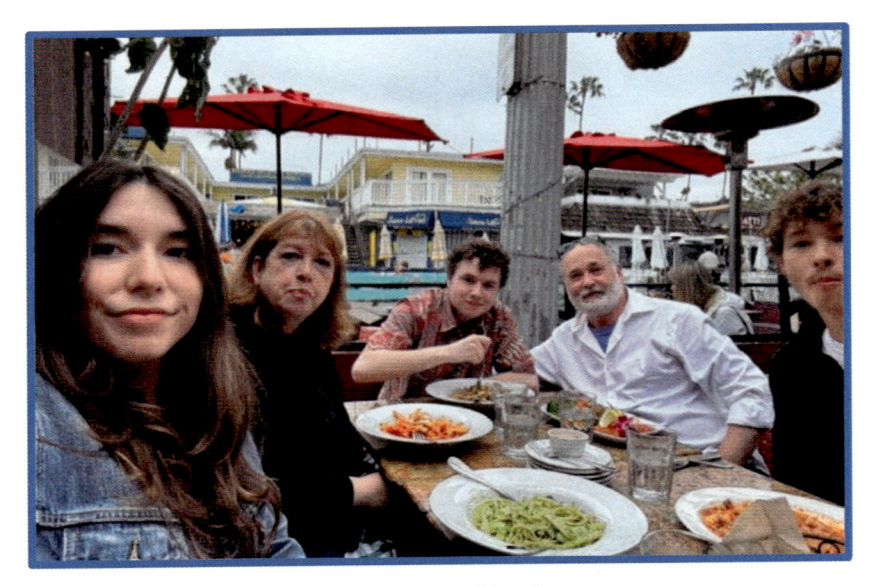

Joe Dunn and family

Doris Mary Donoghue was a UCSF medical school graduate (MD, 1989). She interned (Internal Medicine) at CPMC (1989-1990). She completed her CA1 and CA2 years of Anesthesiology training at Stanford (1/1/91-12/31/92). She changed career paths, resigned from the program, and did a residency in Psychiatry at Stanford (1993-1997). She practices psychiatry in Aptos, CA.

Thomas T. Nguyen graduated from UCLA (MD, 1990) and interned (Internal Medicine) at Kaiser - San Francisco (1990-1991). He began an Anesthesiology residency at Stanford but did not practice at a satisfactory level and only completed his CA1 year (7/1/91-7/15/92). He then completed a 3-year Anesthesiology residency at the University of Rochester, NY (1993-1996) and returned to California where he practiced in Huntington Beach and Fountain Valley, CA.

Helen Bao Tam attended (MD, 1990) and interned (Transitional) at the Medical College of Wisconsin (1990-1991). She completed several years of an Anesthesiology residency at Stanford (1991-1994) but resigned before completing the program. She has worked as an emergency medicine physician in Pleasanton, CA.

Hendrikus "Harry" J. M. Lemmens received his medical degree from Rijksuniversiteit, Utrecht, Netherlands (1981) and thereafter was a resident (Anesthesiology) at University Hospital (1986) Netherlands. After training he joined the Department of Anesthesiology at University Hospital, Leiden. In 1991 he came to the PA-VAH as a Fellow (Pharmacology) working with Don Stanski, Steve Shafer, Barry Dyck, and Talmadge Egan. He was appointed to the Stanford faculty working at Stanford Hospital. He and rose through the ranks to Professor. He is currently Chief of the Multispecialty Division (MSD) at Stanford Hospital. His research includes the pharmacology of drugs in anesthesiology.

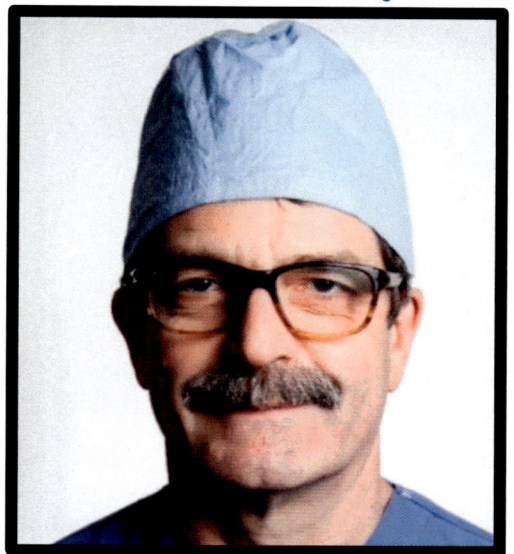

CHAPTER 12
1992

On February 1st, 1992, President George H. W. Bush and Russian President Boris Yeltsin met at Camp David and formerly declared the end of the Cold War. Two months later in April, the death of Grand Duke Vladimir Kirillovich of Russia resulted in a dispute between Prince Nicholas Romanov and Vladimir's daughter Maria for leadership of the Russian Imperial Family. Also, that April the acquittal of four police officers in the Rodney King beating criminal trial triggered massive rioting in Los Angeles resulting in 63 deaths and over $1 billion damages. The Maastricht treaty was signed by 12 countries in February 1992 formerly creating the European Union. The United States refused to sign the UN convention on *Climate Change and Biological Diversity* in Rio De Janeiro. At the Democrat Party's National Convention, Governor Bill Clinton accepted the presidential nomination on behalf of the "forgotten middle class".

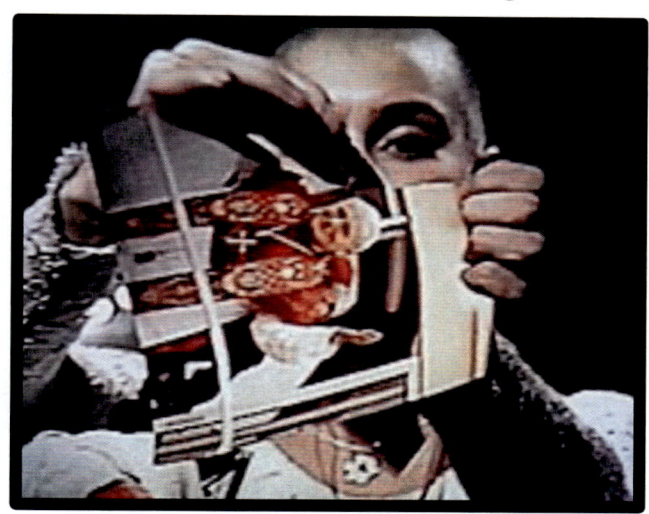

Sinead O'Connor rips a photograph of the Pope during a live SNL television broadcast.

On October 3rd during a telecast of Saturday Night Live, after performing a song protesting Church child sexual abuse Irish singer-songwriter Sinead O'Connor ripped a photograph on Pope John Paul II causing a huge controversy.

Perhaps in response, just four weeks later, finally after 350 years the Pope issued a long-awaited apology and lifted the 1633 edict of the Inquisition against Galileo Galilei. In some-what related news, the first confirmed detection of exoplanets was reported that year, and Mexico re-established diplomatic relations with Vatican City ending a break that lasted over 130 years.

The first nicotine patch was introduced to help stop smoking, and the FDA urged stopping the use of silicone gel breast implants. Stanford Medical School launched its first Family

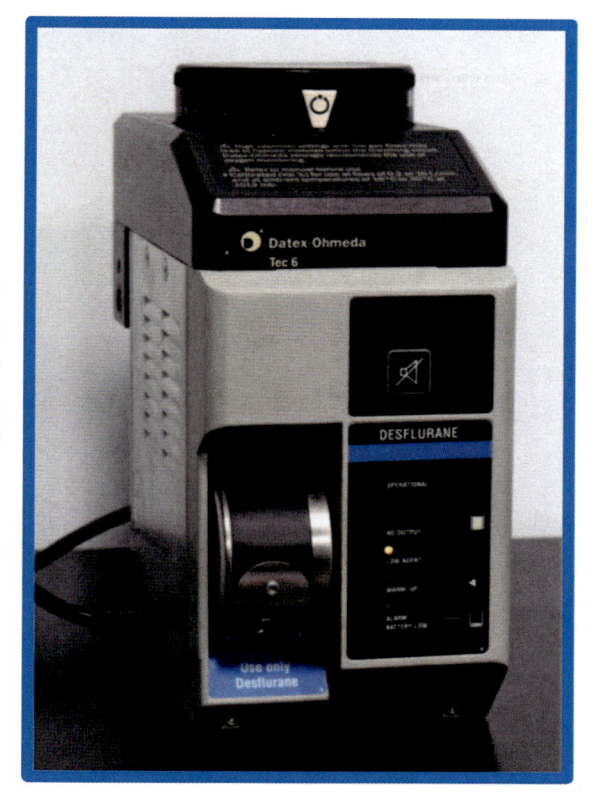

Desflurane vaporizers (like the one pictured above) were later removed from operating rooms due to the agent's greenhouse effects on global warming.

Medicine clerkship in 1992. The inhalational anesthetic desflurane was released for clinical use and dexmedetomidine was introduced as a sedative by Stanford anesthesiologist Mervyn Maze and his team. Stanford University did not see a value for dexmedetomidine and sold the patent rights for the use of the drug to the Finnish company Farmos for a pittance.

The resident group that started in 1992 were recruited during Barrie Fairley's time as Chair prior to Donald Stanski assuming that position later that year.

Russell Hughes Allen was born in Dallas. He was an undergraduate at Texas A&M University (BS, Biochemistry, 1986). He then attended University of Texas Southwestern Medical Center, Dallas (MD, 1990) and did an internship (Internal Medicine) at Pacific Presbyterian Medical Center (1990-1991). He did a year of residency (Internal Medicine) at CPMC (1991-1992) prior to starting his Anesthesiology residency at Stanford (1992-1995). He began his career at Baylor University Medical Center, Dallas (1995-2004) then moved to the University of Colorado Hospital Authority/Memorial Hospital System, in Colorado Springs, CO (2004-Present). He slowed down to half-time work in January 2024 and plans to retire in "a couple of years". Russell enjoys snow and water skiing, hiking, backcountry survival skills, traveling and spending time with his family.

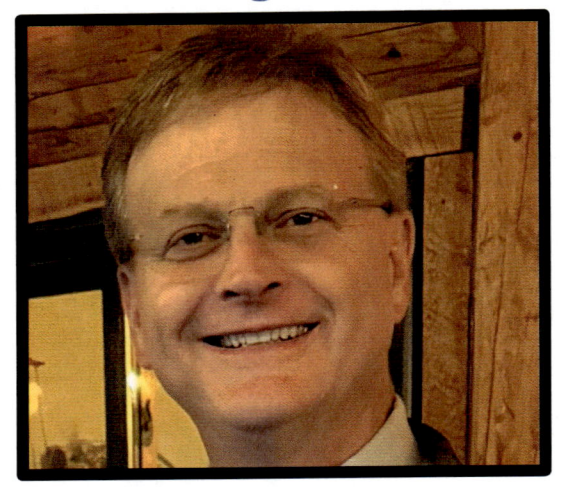

Interesting Anecdotes/Memories of Time at Stanford:
- *Drs. Jaffe and Samuels racing to Medical Records to get their favorite donuts before the residents ate them.*
- *Dr. Brock-Utne diving under the drapes to place a dorsalis pedis arterial line (I destroyed both radial arteries) and then popping up exclaiming "I got it" with his usual smiling face!*

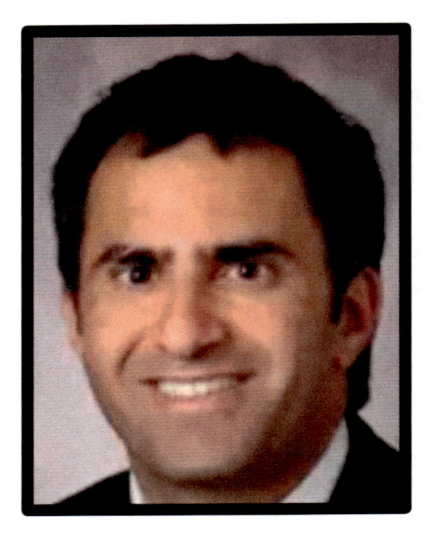

Kayvan Ariani was born in Detroit, MI. He did his undergraduate work at Stanford (BA, Human Biology, 1986). He did research in Department of Psychiatry and Behavioral Sciences at the Stanford School of Medicine. He then attended Stanford Medical School (MD, 1991) and interned (Internal Medicine) at SCVMC (1991-1992). He completed his Anesthesiology residency (1992-1995) and a Fellowship (Pain Medicine) (1995-1996) at Stanford. He initially worked at the JLR Medical Group in Orlando, FL, as an attending anesthesiologist and pain management physician (1996-2013). In 2013, JLR merged with two groups from Texas to form United States Anesthesia Partners. (USAP). He continued as a pain management physician there (2014-2019). After 5 years with USAP he helped form a smaller, strictly pain management group called Center for Pain Management (2019-present) and has been President since 2020.

His main outside interest has been music, specifically playing guitar. He has played in bands since junior high school and has continued while in medical school, playing in a band that was very active on the Stanford campus.

"I now own about 35 guitars with some being vintage pieces. About 10 years ago, I took on learning chicken pickin' guitar in the style of players like James Burton, Marty Stuart, and Vince Gill and became proficient at this style. It took a lot of practice and also involved a visit to a nail salon every 2 weeks to harden the nails on my picking hand ... until COVID ended the nail salon visits!"

He also stays active with workouts, cycling, and playing tennis.

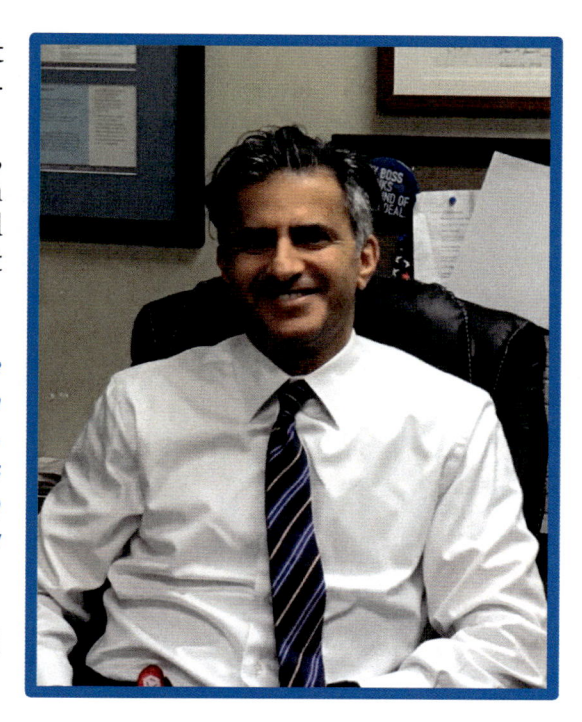

- *My interest in anesthesiology stemmed from my interest in pharmacology and physiology during my Stanford undergrad and medical school years. In those years, I did research at the Stanford Department of Psychiatry on adrenergic receptor binding and molecular biology in the old medical school research building. On the same floor, just down the hall, was the Department of Anesthesiology and I remember frequently seeing members of the department, like Dr. Fairley and Dr. Pearl, walking past the lab I worked at to their offices down the hall. It started me thinking about anesthesiology as a way to directly apply pharmacology and physiology to clinical practice. I thought of it as a possible niche for me. During medical school, I did a basic science research clerkship in Dr. Mervyn Maze's lab at the Palo Alto VAH, working on receptor binding. I believe at that time he had just started studying dexmedetomidine clinically in the ICU and I remember him telling me about the potential of this drug in clinical practice.*
- *I worked with Dr. Steve Howard at the PA-VAH and we always talked about music and tried to pick a good CD to play during cases. We were particularly fond of The Rolling Stones "Exile on Main Street". Dr. Howard was studying the effects of sleep deprivation on physician function and recruited me to the study as a subject. As part of this study, he had me wear an EEG for the entire night while on call in the ICU and providing patient care. It was a bizarre look and the next morning Dr. Feeley, who was the ICU attending, took one look at me with this contraption on my head and was mortified. He called Steve who had to immediately come over and remove the device (which he wasn't happy about).*
- *It was always pleasant and interesting to work with Dr. Brock-Utne. In addition to the "lovely party" atmosphere, he had a knack for taking any thought or question during a case and turning it into a research project. We worked on a couple of those projects together which was gratifying.*
- *Dr. Hackel was a pleasure to work with and seemed to always impart to me a kernel of his well-earned wisdom during our days together in the OR. One day we had about 5 difficult cases in a row in the pediatric room. The room was stiflingly hot, and everybody was getting a bit cranky as the day wore on. The nurses were complaining to us about something rather insignificant and Dr. Hackel was very diplomatic in his response. At one point, I looked at him and said, "Wow, how do*

you handle all this?" He just looked at me and said, "Look ... that's just a little tweak ..." as he gestured with his hand in a screwdriver motion. "You just have to let it all roll off your back ... just let it roll right off of you...". Great advice that has served me well over the years.

- *There are a lot of anecdotes, too many to write about. I am thankful for the emphasis on excellent and academically sound pre-op, intra-op, and post-op care. The standards were high, and we were coached up. The Pre-Op assessment clinic created by Dr. Stephen Fischer was ahead of its time and a great learning environment. I owe quite a bit of thanks to my Attendings during my Pain Fellowship, Dr. William Brose, Dr. Ray Gaeta, and Dr. William Longton. Early in my Fellowship, I remember a Saturday morning on call with Dr. Brose. After rounds, he spent an hour talking to me about concepts in pain management one-on-one. I remember feeling impressed and grateful that someone would spend an hour of their time on a Saturday morning teaching in that way.*

- *During my final year of residency, I went on an Interplast trip to Honduras. I was the most junior member of the anesthesia team. But I performed at a high level and the surgical and anesthesia team were impressed with me. The anesthesia leader of that trip wrote a glowing letter about me back to Dr. Stanski, who shared the letter with me. This was less of a testament to me personally as it was a testament to the type of education that was imparted to us by the faculty in the Stanford anesthesia department. Lovely party indeed."*

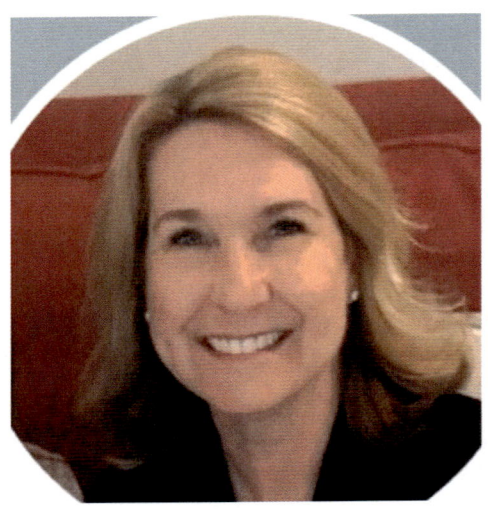

Susan Kay Browne attended Goucher College (BA, Biology, 1983-1987) and then the University of Maryland School of Medicine (MD, 1991). She did an internship (Transitional) at SCVMC (1991-1992), and her y residency at Stanford (1992-1995). She has worked as an anesthesiologist in Las Vegas since 1995. She was a member of Anesthesiology Consultants Inc (1995-2005) and then Clark County Anesthesia Consultants (2005-2016). She is currently with Desert Anesthesiologist, Las Vegas (2017-Present). She was Chief of Anesthesia at Summerlin Hospital and Medical Center (2007-2015) and is Medical Director of the Las Vegas Surgery Center/HCA Surgical Ventures (2015-Present). She enjoys traveling, cooking, hiking and spending time with her husband and daughter.

Interesting Anecdotes/Memories of Time at Stanford:
- *Best memories - Any time spent with Dr. Gail Boltz in a pediatric or peds cardiac room!*
- *ICU Rounds with Mike Rosenthal*
- *Pediatric Cardiac Outreach Trip to Russia!*
- *Most valuable skill learned - Awake fiberoptic intubation from Dr. Phil Larson.*

Charles Anthony Boudreaux was born in New Orleans. He graduated from Xavier University, New Orleans (BS Chemistry, 1987). He was a medical student at UCSF (MD, 1991). His internship (Internal Medicine) was at the UCLA-San Fernando Valley Program (1991-1992 and was an Anesthesiology resident (1992-1995). After completing his training, he worked in Albuquerque, NM (1995-2003). He has been an anesthesiologist with Central Anesthesia Services Exchange (CASE) Medical Group of Sacramento (2003-Present).

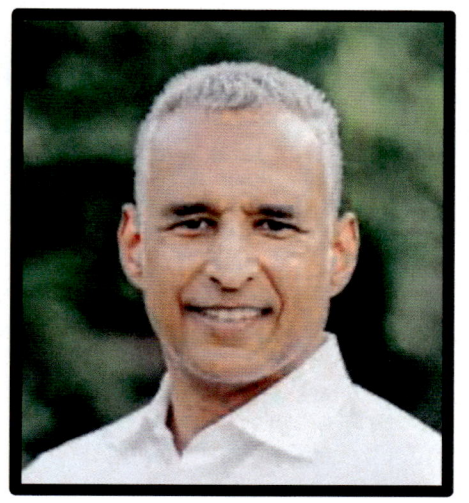

"I had great training at Stanford from a kind, generous and outstanding groups of anesthesiologists. I've spent my career doing primarily cardiac anesthesia. First 8 years in Albuquerque at St Joseph Hospital (now Lovelace) and The Heart Hospital of New Mexico, and the last 20 plus years here in Sacramento working mainly at Sutter Medical Center."

"Thanks to the guidance of Dr. Larson in 1992 -when I want to show real independence in the OR I tuck my covered ETT under my left upper arm during intubation, easy to retrieve from there, so that I don't need any assistance from the circulating nurse. Using this technique I have impressed many circulating nurses over the last 30 years."

"I'm still putting in the largest double-lumen ETT that fits easily as I was instructed by Jay Brodsky over 30 years ago. It has served me (and my partners) well throughout my career."

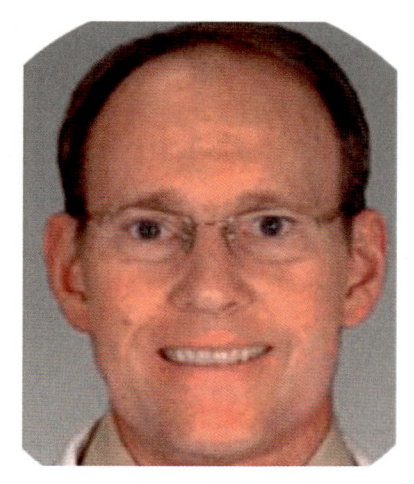

Jeffrey Paul Clayton was born in Sacramento. He graduated from UCSB (Pharmacology, 1986) and then the Medical College of Wisconsin (MD, 1990). He did an internship (Transitional) at Scripps Mercy Hospital (1990-1991). Following internship, he worked a "town" doctor at the Mopan Clinic in Benque Viejo, Belize, for 6-months in 1991. He completed his Anesthesiology residency at Stanford (1/1/92-12/31/94). He started practice with the Central Anesthesia Services Exchange (CASE) Medical Group in Sacramento in March 1995, and has worked there since (1995-Present). He plans to retire in 2025.

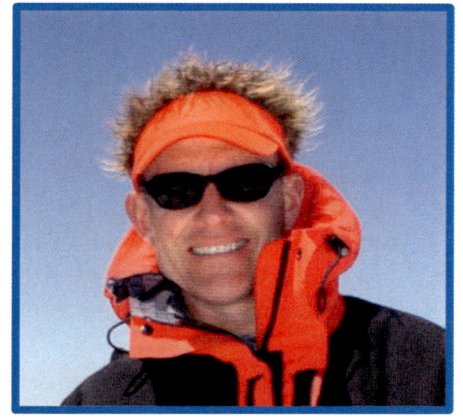

Dr. Clayton at top of Mt. Shasta (2010)

"I joined CASE Medical Group in 1995 when the anesthesia jobs market was at its nadir. It is a great group and I LOVE my job. Sutter Health is a good hospital system. I particularly love being near the Sierras and all the recreational opportunities that Northern California has to offer. I have always felt bad that I did not take John Brock-Utne's offer of doing a Cardiac Fellowship at Groote Schuur Hospital, especially since I have lots of family in South Africa. I am happily married to Ann Trowbridge from San Francisco who is an energy attorney here in Sacramento. We have one son, Aran who is an engineer major at Cal Poly San Luis Obispo. He is going to meet me in Norway in July 2024 and together we will cycle 400 miles from Trondheim to Oslo. Norway is the holy grail of cycling. My son is an oarsman and a very good cyclist ("see you dad, meet you at the top")."

Jeff has been Recruiting Coordinator for his group for the past 27 years. There are 110 members of the physician-only practice with Sutter Hospitals from Davis up to Auburn. The two big campuses are Sutter Medical Center Sacramento (Dr. Clayton's hospital) and Sutter Roseville Medical Center. Some former Stanford Residents (all of whom Jeff hired) are Drs. Nate Simon, Rohith Piyaratna, Ioana Brisc, Doug Crocket, Maninder Atwal, Charles Boudreaux, Bob Sanborn, Josh Melvin, and others.

"We can always use more Stanford residents! So, if you know of any residents with interests or ties to Northern California, we remain the best private practice going - truly independent and thriving, NOT investor owned!"

Jeff had stage 4 squamous cell cancer of the floor of his mouth that was operated successfully at Stanford in 2013. He has been back at work full time for the past 10 years.

"Dr. Mike Kaplan did a great job with bilateral radical neck dissection, floor of mouth resection and reconstruction, 13.5 hours, in February 2013. That was followed by chemoradiation at Sutter in Sacramento. Vlad Nekhendzy, Harry Lemmens, and anesthesiology resident Dr. Jared Pearson took care of me. Norm Risk extubated me the next day in ICU."

"I do have some favorite sayings from residency that still echo in my ear while I'm working and make me smile:

- *"A tube is never a problem, only a solution" —— Dr. Frank Sarnquist*
- *"In the OR, babies are either pink or blue, and the goal is to keep them pink" —— Dr. John Brock-Utne*
- *"Babies cry, that's what they do" —— Dr. Harry Lemmens*
- *"If you do nothing else for your patient, just put oxygen in their trachea and move it back and forth" —— Dr. Steve Shafer (Something that Dr. Conrad Murray failed to do)*
- *"The DMA is closely followed by the MOT" —— Dr. David Gaba*
  (DMA = daily miracle of anesthesia (the return of spontaneous respirations), MOT = the moment of truth (extubation!)
- *"You can make another record, but you can't make another patient" —— Dr. Yuan-Chi Lin*
- *"Did you give him some glycol?" —— Dr. Buechel*
- *"Scope - tube - tape - airway - introducer - suction" —— Dr. Frank Sarnquist*
- *"For break, lunch and dinner for the next 7 days, calculate the triggering pressure of the oxygen ratio monitor control valve on the Drager Narcomed 2B" —— Dr. Richard Jaffe*
- *"Never waken a sleeping monkey" —— Dr. Bhati (We never figured out what that means)*

- *"Wow, twins! It's like having puppies, except you can sell puppies" —— Dr. Joe Dunn*
- *"Three things you gotta learn in anesthesia: 1) keep a good airway, 2) they stand, you sit, and 3) if someone comes to give you a break they should only see your back." —— Dr. Peter Kosek*
- *"Bones heal, pain is temporary, chicks dig scars and glory lasts forever" —— Dr. Fabian Okonski*
- *"Your patient will survive a bad surgeon, but he won't survive a bad anesthesiologist" —— Dr. Bob Sanborn*
- *"This may look like the O.B. ward, but it's not, this is Da Nang and the VC are out there waiting. There are snipers in the trees, you can hear the choppers now … and Sergeant Brodsky will be calling your name …" Dr. Clint Warne*

There are other notable quotes, for sure and many of my Stanford colleagues will be able to recall more. It was an amazing time in my life, and I own my life (quite literally) to Stanford and my Stanford residency education.

Douglas Eugene Crockett

was born in Taipei, Taiwan. He was an undergraduate at UCD (Zoology, 1986), and received his medical degree from the University of Pittsburgh School of Medicine (MD, 1991). He did an internship (Internal Medicine) at Mercy Hospital/UPMC (1991-1992). He then did his Anesthesiology residency at Stanford (1992-1995) followed by a Fellowship (Pediatric Anesthesiology) at Children's Hospital of Philadelphia (1996-1997). He worked as a staff anesthesiologist at Lucile Packard Children's Hospital (1997-1998). Dr. Crockett has worked with the Central Anesthesia Service Exchange (CASE) in Sacramento with CASE Medical Group (1998-Present).

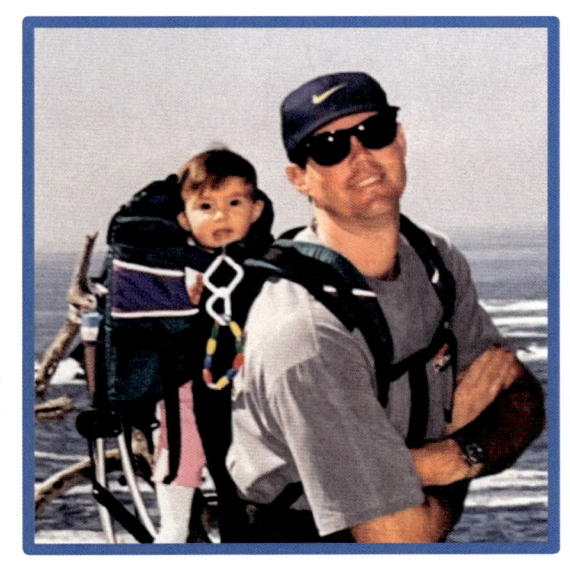

With my daughter who was born at Stanford when I was on staff. She is now a 4th year medical student UCSF

Michael Patrick Keating

a graduate of Columbia University College of Physicians & Surgeons (MD, 1991) and the Stanford Anesthesiology residency (1992-1995) and works in California.

Steven Paul Laitin attended Tufts University School of Medicine (MD, 1991) and then interned (Internal Medicine) at St. Mary's Medical Center (1991-1992). Following Anesthesiology residency (1992-1995) he did a Fellowship (Pain Medicine) at UCSD (1995-1996).

Richard Cary Mantin

was an undergraduate at Yale (BA, Physics, 1987). He then attended Stanford (MD, 1991) and interned (Internal Medicine) at Kaiser - Santa Clara (1991-1992). He was a Stanford resident (1992-1995). Following residency he did a Fellowship (Cardiothoracic Anesthesia) at Emory University (1995-1996). He has been in private practice with US Anesthesia Partners Nevada, Las Vegas, specializing in cardiothoracic anesthesia (1996-Present). He enjoys bicycle riding putting in 8-10K miles each year.

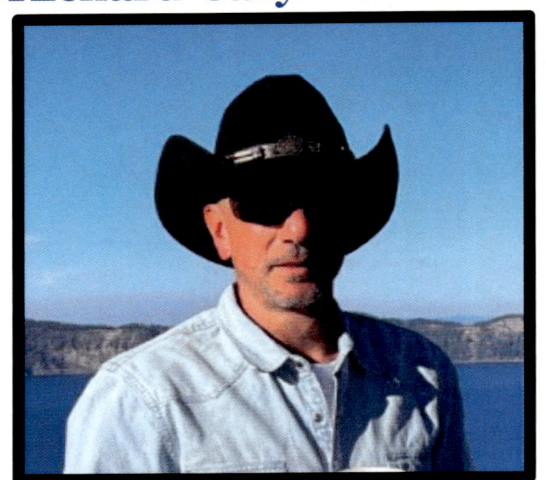

"On my first clinical rotation as a medical student my future wife, Sheila, who was a Pediatric Intensive Care RN in the "old" Stanford Hospital. When we first met, Sheila told him that one of the main jobs of a Peds ICU RN was to protect the patients from the medical students and residents!" Sheila and I have been married since 1992 and had twin boys in 1997."

Memories from Stanford:
- *"When I first entered medical school, my plans were to become an orthopedic surgeon. During clinical rotations I enjoyed Ortho, but also had the chance to take an anesthesia rotation at Kaiser Santa Clara. With my physics background, I was immediately drawn to Anesthesia – recognizing that it was applied physics, engineering, and pharmacology – all in real time. My decision was finalized after taking an ICU Rotation at Stanford. Mike Rosenthal became my mentor, along with Tom Feeley. These were the guys that could take care of the sickest of the sickest at a tertiary care facility – Wow!"*
- *During anesthesia residency at Stanford, I remember taking a one-month Thoracic Anesthesia Rotation with Jay Brodsky. At that time, Jay had an ongoing "debate" with Jon Benumof regarding the necessity of using a fiberoptic scope to place a double lumen endotracheal tube. Jay's position was that the*

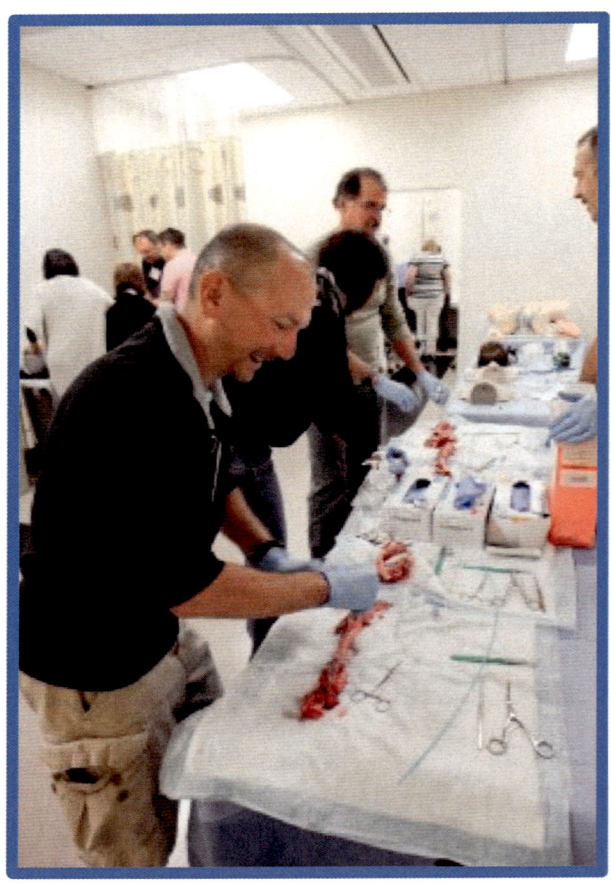

tube could be easily placed blindly and confirmed by auscultation. When I started the rotation, Jay was running a study on the success rate for blindly placing a left sided double lumen ETT. I had never placed a DL ETT before and was there to learn. Jay taught me how to place a DL ETT. With Jay standing there at the bedside, instructing me, I proceeded to place the next 8 left-sided DL ETT's into the RIGHT main stem bronchus – completely wrecking his study. In my 29 years of practicing Cardio-Thoracic Anesthesia, I continue to use Jay's technique (and then confirm with FOB after positioning) – and have placed maybe 1-2 into the right-main stem in 29 years."

- *"One night I was on call in house carrying the code beeper for Stanford Hospital. A code was called on the medical ward for an unfortunate 82-year-old man with advanced metastatic prostate cancer. When I arrived, there were multiple Medicine interns and residents in the room, but not much resuscitation going on. I asked who was in charge of the patient, and a Medicine intern raised his hand. I asked if he really wanted to code this patient and he said "Yes". They had been talking to the family about code status, but no decision had been made. I proceeded to intubate the patient, push EPI and run the code. At some point, the Medicine resident left, and came back to tell me that he had spoken with the family, and the patient was a "No Code" now. I told him it was a little bit too late; the patient had already been resuscitated. In all fairness, code status and discussions were not yet a routine part of care back then like they are today …"*

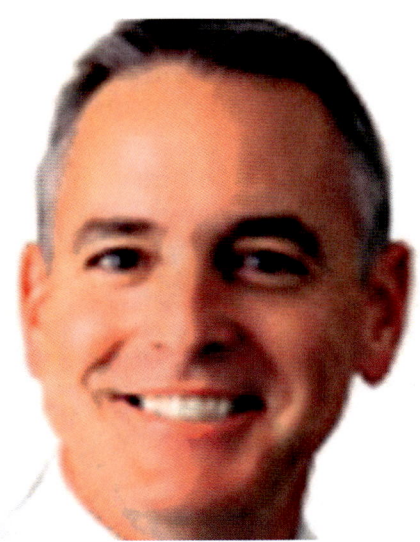

John Edward Massey was born in San Jose. As an undergraduate he attended Santa Clara University (BS, Biology, 1985). He graduated from the Stanford (MD, 1991) and interned (Internal Medicine) at SCVMC (1991-1992). He was an Anesthesiology resident (1992-1995) and Fellow (Pain Management) (1995-1996) at Stanford. He remained on the faculty as an Assistant Clinical Professor (1997-1998). Dr. Massey was a co-founder of the Bay Area Pain and Wellness Center (2005) in Los Gatos, CA. He later sold it to private equity and retired. John has also been an Adjunct Clinical Assistant Professor (Anesthesiology) at Stanford.

"The Stanford OR was pretty uptight and academic … which was appropriate and good but stressful. Some crazy cases. SCVMC was laid back but very busy … it was not uncommon to do 11 C-sections in one call day. The PA-VAH was mellow … Overall, I found the training life changing."

"I remember … make sure the air is going in and out and blood is going round and round."

"Dr. Brodsky was the most likely attending to chew my ass and let me know when he thought I could do better. Crusty on the outside but turned out to be one of my real mentors during training. Very caring about detail and execution. Once he trusted you, he was pretty funny … great sense of humor."

"Brodsky and other senior attendings could always be found in front of the "big white board" in the OR … the schedule. The bulk of the work in the rooms was done by the senior residents, with attendings popping in and out to check our work. If you were a good reliable resident (meaning … they could leave you alone in a room, you were very likely to get nabbed for an add-on case at the end of the day. My

way around being pulled back into a late case was to go to the Pain Clinic on the 4th floor of the Grant Building in the medical school. Drs. Brose and Gaeta would give me a patient to see in the clinic. If Jay Brodsky called trying to find me for a late case, they would tell him that I was already busy with other work ... I always got out early .... True story."

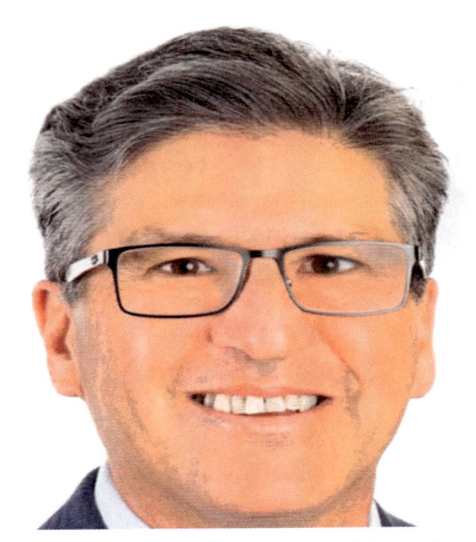

Ricardo "Rick" Barraza Ronquillo

was born in Mexico and raised in Sacramento, CA. He attended Stanford (BS, 1985) and graduated from the Stanford School of Medicine (MD, 1991). He interned (Internal Medicine) and then was an Anesthesiology resident (1991-1995). He was Chief Resident his CA3 year. Following that, he was a Fellow (CCM) at Stanford (1995-1996). He was a Clinical Instructor (Anesthesiology) during his Fellowship year.

"Stanford Cardinal through and through!"

He moved to San Jose in 1996 and joined Group Anesthesia Services, along with other Stanford alums that included Fabian Okonski, Chris Vasil, Mark Singleton, Mark Jamieson, and Ann Marie Mallat. The anesthesia practice is now named G2 Anesthesia. He has been at the same location, Good Samaritan Hospital, San Jose, and surrounding facilities for 28 years. Rick is an avid golfer and cyclist. He recently started tandem cycling with his wife and Cal alum, Stephanie.

"I have enjoyed international travel for the love of the game of golf (Scotland of course, Canada, Mexico, Argentina, Ireland, England and Spain). I'm a member at San Jose Country Club (Men's Club Champion 2017 and Men's Senior Club Champion 2019)."

Memories of Stanford & Influential faculty:

"The first two years of residency were a blur, but my third year was very memorable in that I was Chief Resident. One of many responsibilities was making a call schedule for all residents and the call schedule for the Transport Service. The Transport Service exciting and gratifying. My most memorable transport was a 350 lb. intubated stroke patient in the Life Flight helicopter from Hollister to Stanford; truly a harrowing experience. I wasn't sure the helicopter could take off although the pilot was reassuring, and we made it just fine although there was very little wiggle room in the patient bay. He needed to be hand-ventilated the entire way because the portable

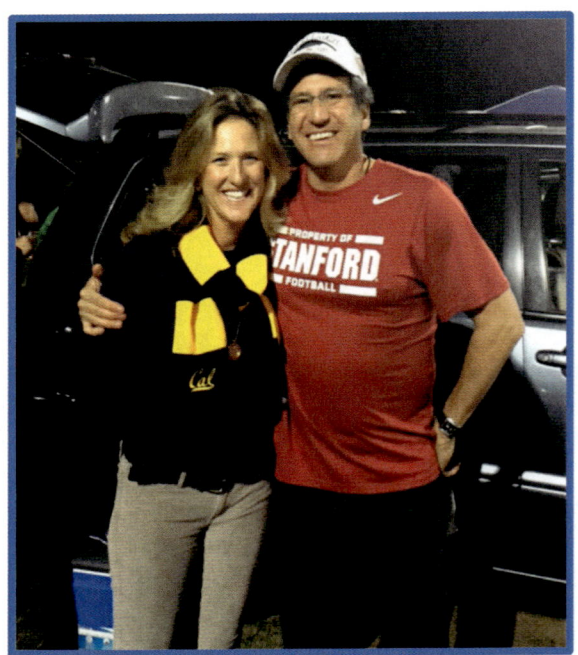

Stanford fan Rick with CAL fan Stephanie at Big Game

ventilator could not deliver adequate tidal volumes. Also, the many overnight organ harvests were made especially difficult since you had to return to your assigned day and Jay showed little mercy when requesting an early day."

"I also truly enjoyed and learned many lasting valuable lessons from Mike Rosenthal, Ron Pearl, Mike Feeley, Fred Mihm, and Norm Rizk, while a CCM Fellow. I had invaluable experiences of doing many thoracic cases with Drs Mark and Cannon under the tutelage of Jay Brodsky and then being the Attending for all thoracic cases when Jay went on sabbatical. There were many great, practical, and sometimes very nuanced lessons taught by Dr. Richard Jaffe, while doing extremely long Gary Steinberg neurosurgical cases. In fact, the most memorable was a young lady who had an 8-hour awake craniotomy who about 6 hours into it asked if she could call her husband to tell him she was doing ok. The look on her face and the joy in her voice is something I'll never forget

"In all, I look back at my 5 years in the department as extremely tiring, stressful, and immensely valuable. The program prepared me for a lasting and successful career. I have nothing but great memories of those years."

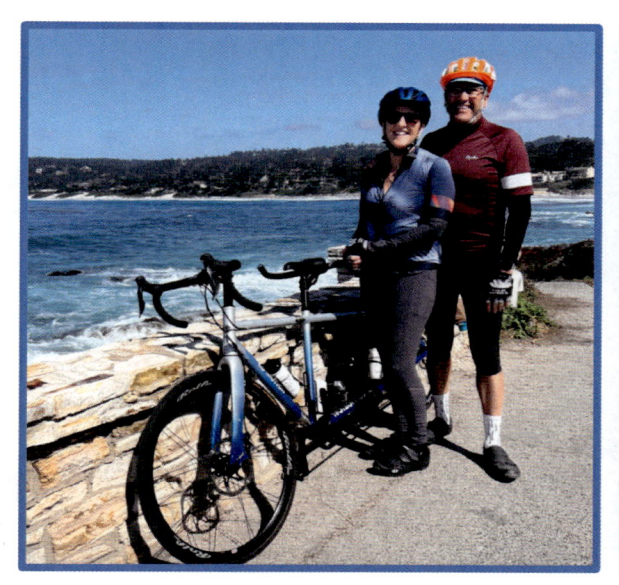

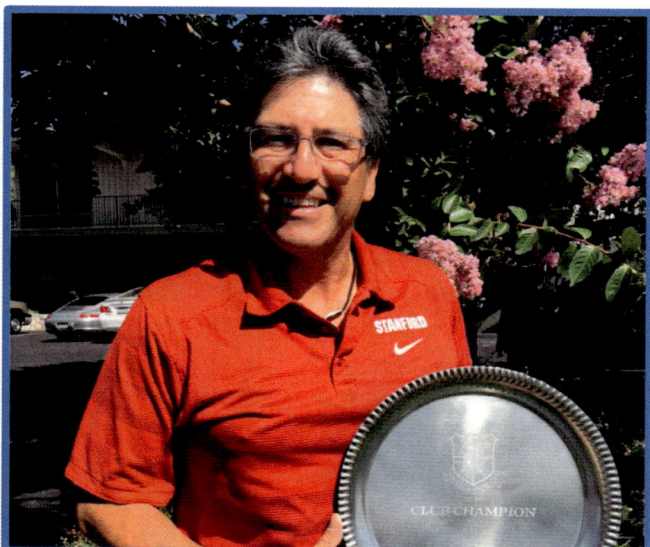

Dean Stanton Walker graduated from UCSD (MD, 1991) and interned (Transitional) at Cambridge Health Alliance (1991-1992). He completed his Anesthesiology residency (1992-1995) followed by a Fellowship (Obstetrical Anesthesia) at Stanford. He works in Portland, OR.

James M. Bell was born in Austin, TX. He was an undergraduate at University of Texas, Auston (BS, 1986) and a medical student at the University of Texas, Medical Branch (MD, 1990). He interned at Methodist Hospital, Dallas (1991-1992) and then began his Anesthesiology residency at the University of Texas Southwestern (1991-1992). He transferred to Stanford for his CA2 and CA3 years (7/1/92-6/30/94). He practiced with Southwest Anesthesia, Houston (1994-1995), then with the Austin Anesthesia Group (1995-2005). He works with Capital Anesthesiology Association (now USAP), Austin (1995-Present). He practices at Ascension Seton Medical Center and University Medical Center at Brackenridge, both in Austin, TX.

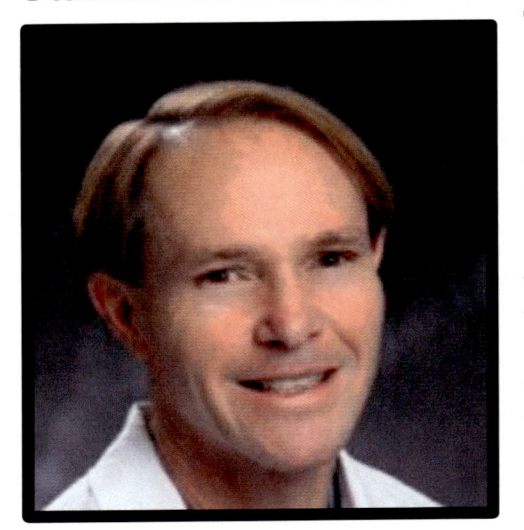

Memories of Stanford:
- *Aud Pullens was like a Godmother to me and all the residents.*
- *Phil Larson was incredibly calm, despite our patient's systolic BP of 30.*
- *Richard Jaffe's enthusiasm to teach.*
- *Stanley Samuels friendliness and team spirit.*
- *The collegial relationship between Anesthesia and Cardiovascular Surgery.*
- *The down-to-earth approachability of Dr. Norman Shumway.*
- *Dr. Craig Miller's surgical skill, relaxing manner and cowboy boots.*
- *Mike Rosenthal's real-life teaching of the Frank Starling curve on ICU rounds.*
- *Al Hackel's blinding white OR shoes.*
- *The unexpected "pheo" case I did in the patient who had a negative workup for pheo.*
- *Coming very close to losing the airway on one of the biggest shipping magnates in Asia on the first day of my CA3 year, with my staff having just finished his CA3 year. This was a patient who had extensive radiation to the head and neck. We were assured by Dr. Fee, the ENT surgeon, that the patient's airway was "fine". Post-op, after ordering a CXR in the PACU, my attending was unceremoniously chewed-out by Dr. Fee for ordering an unnecessary test and costing our patient unnecessary expense.* **(Ed note: we all have similar memories of Willard Fee)**

Helmuth Thorlakur Billy was a graduate of UC-Berkeley (Molecular Biology) and UCD (MD, 1990). He resigned from the Anesthesiology residency after just 6 months (1/1/92-6/30/92) leaving to train in Surgery. He is a bariatric surgeon working in Ventura and Santa Barbara.

CHAPTER 13

CLINICAL and RESEARCH FACULTY and ADMINISTRATIVE STAFF (1983-1992)

During the ten years covered by this book (1983-1992) the Department of Anesthesiology at Stanford continued to grow. With the expansion of Stanford University Medical Center and the opening of the new Lucile Packard Children's Hospital there was an increased need for clinical anesthesia services, especially for pediatric anesthesiologists. The majority of the faculty appointments during this 10-year period were former Stanford trained anesthesiology residents and clinical Fellows.

A partial list of Assistant Professors hired from 1983 until mid-1992 (before Donald Stanski became Chair) include Anne Fischell (1984), Ray Engstrom (1986), Dave Fitzgerald (1986), Darrel Tanelian (1988), Bill Brose (1989), Kristi Peterson (1991), Price Stover (1991), Chris Vasil (1991), Greg Botz (1991), and Ellen Finch (1992). Many left Stanford within a year or two. Other faculty initially hired as Assistant Professors remained at Stanford long enough to be promoted before leaving. That group includes Ray Gaeta (Associate Professor 1995-2011) and Emily Ratner (Clinical Professor 2001-2014). Several Assistant Professors remained at Stanford and after long careers retired from the Department as an Emeriti Professor (Stephen Fischer, Rona Giffard, Ed Riley, Steve Shafer). At the present time (2024) several former residents (Larry Siegel, Alex Macario, Ronald Pearl) have reached the full Professor level and remain active in the Department. Sadly, while still on the active faculty, Professor (Anesthesiology and Neurosurgery) Richard Jaffe passed away in June 2023.

A group of attendings were recruited to the faculty from the outside, mainly to support our rapidly expanding pediatric anesthesia, particularly pediatric cardiac surgery, needs. Almost all stayed for a short period of time before departing.

CLINICAL FACULTY

Bruce Allen Bollen graduated from the Keck School of Medicine/USC (1982) and was an intern and resident (Anesthesiology) at the University of Iowa Hospitals and Clinics (1982-1986). He also did a Fellowship (Cardiovascular Research) at the University of Iowa. He joined the cardiac anesthesia team at Stanford. After her left he practiced in Iowa, Missoula MT, and California.

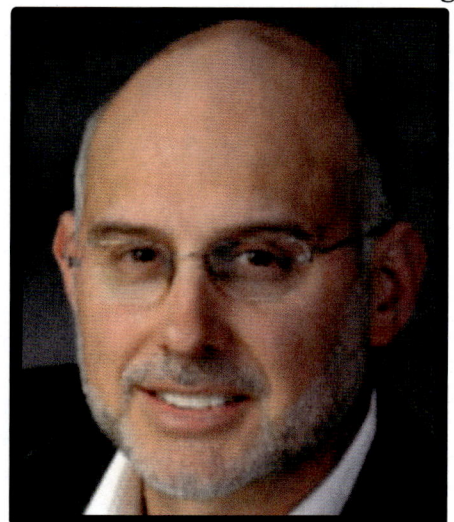

"When I arrived at Stanford the cardiac group had suddenly vanished with most people leaving for private practice (certainly not expected by me). Alan Ream was the sole remaining "senior" member of the group. Dr. Fairley then assembled Robert McKlveen (from Brigham, and recruited initially for OB anesthesia), John Urbanowicz (a former Stanford resident returning from Fellowship with Mike Cahalan at UCSF), and me.

Larry Siegel (from U Penn) had arrived for LVAD Fellowship with Allen Ream but transitioned to Cardiac Team after working with Ron Pearl. Ellen Finch (another former Stanford resident) returned to join staff just prior to Norm Shumway hiring Vaughn Starnes. Vaughn had returned from Great Ormond London Hospital where he had done a Pediatric Cardiac Surgery Fellowship. He would take advantage of pediatric cardiac surgery referrals to Stanford which had changed dramatically with retirement of UCSF peds cardiac surgeons. Vaughn was an incredibly gifted surgeon and quickly increased the pediatric volume. Bob McKlveen and John Urbanowicz and I left about the same time, Ellen Finch also left a bit later. Ray Engstrom and Dave Fitzgerald who were our first CA3 residents working with Ellen and John solely doing Starnes cases stayed on to provide anesthesia for pediatric cardiac cases. I recall Mike Champeau, current ASA President, was on the staff as a pediatric anesthesiologist."

Lawrence Howard Feld

attended Rutgers University (BA, 1976) and graduated from SUNY - Downstate Medical Center (MD, 1980). He then completed his internship and residency (Pediatrics) at CPMC (1980-1983) and his Anesthesiology residency at McGaw Medical Center/Northwestern University (1983-1985). He did a Fellowship (Pediatric Anesthesiology) at Children's Hospital of Boston (1985-1986). He joined the faculty at Stanford (1986-1990), then left to work at CPMC at the St. Luke's Campus in San Francisco (1990-Present). He is currently Medical Director of Surgery/Interventional at CPMC. Dr. Feld lives in Sonoma where he grows pinot noir grapes and enjoys playing the guitar.

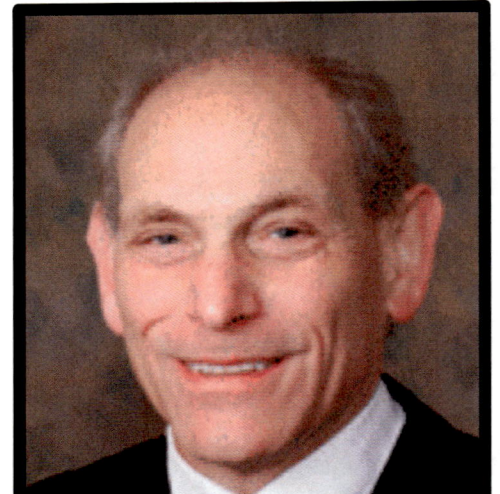

"I was a part of a team spearheading pediatric anesthesiology at Stanford – a new subspecialty and was a founding member of BAYPAC along with Al Hackel."

Gordon Rowat Haddow

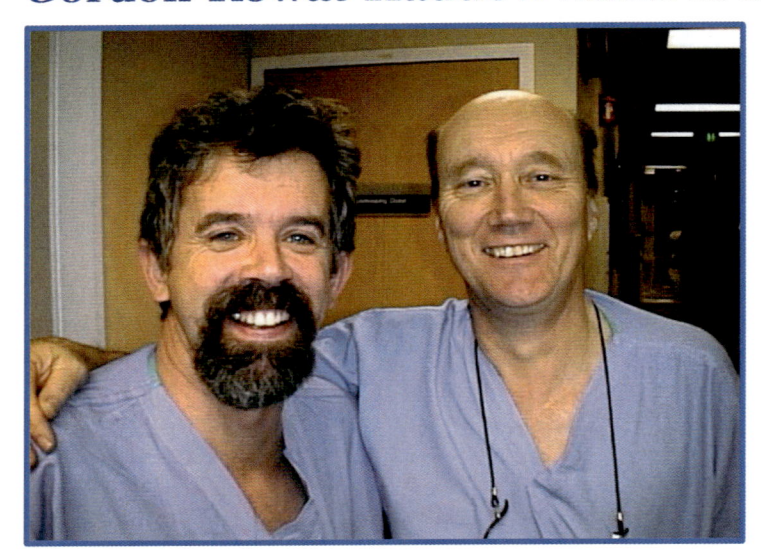

received his medical training at the University of Cape Town Faculty of Medicine (1979). He interned at Edendale Hospital and did a residency in Anaesthesia at the University of Natal, Durban (1983-1987) working with John Brock-Utne. He also did Cardiothoracic Anesthesia at the University of Natal (1987-1988). He came to Stanford in 1988 as Assistant Professor (Anesthesiology) and was later promoted to Associate Professor. He was Chief of Cardiac Anesthesia and the Chief of Liver Transplantation while at Stanford. After he left in 2000 and has worked in several local Kaiser hospitals in the SF Bay area. He was Chief of Cardiac Anesthesia at the Kaiser-Santa Clara (2008-2020). He was also an Adjunct Clinical Associate Professor training Stanford Cardiothoracic Fellows at his Kaiser locations. Gordon Haddow retired January 2022. He lives in the SF Bay area and enjoys photography, hiking and traveling.

John Brock-Utne ... "Gordon Haddow and I worked together in South Africa at in the time when halothane was the inhalational agent of choice. During cases using this agent arrythmias were often seen. Gordon was taking over a halothane general anesthetic from one of his colleagues during his time in Zululand. He noticed the EKG showed an arrhythmia. His colleagues also saw it and said, "Don't worry, ... when you see an arrythmia do two things - turn off the EKG and turn down the halothane. Works like a charm every time."

Yuan-Chi Lin was born in Taiwan. He attended medical school at Kaohsiung Medical University, Taiwan (1981). He then received an MPH degree from the Harvard School of Public Health (1984). He interned at Nationwide Children's Hospital, Columbus, OH (1985) and did a residency (Pediatrics) at Ohio State University, Columbus, OH (1985-1987). This was followed by an Anesthesiology residency at the Hospital of the University of Pennsylvania (1987-1989). Following his residency he completed a Fellowship at Boston Children's Hospital/Harvard Medical School (Pediatric Anesthesia, 1990) and another Fellowship at Stanford (Pain Medicine, 1991). He was recruited at Stanford as an Assistant Professor (Anesthesiology and Pediatrics) (1991-1996) and promoted to Associate Professor in 1997 (1997-2000). At Stanford he was Director of Medical Students Course in Anesthesia Medicine (1993-1998), Director of non-anesthesia Trainees for Anesthesia Experience (1993-1998), Founder and Director of Pediatric Pain Medicine (1992-2000), Founder and Director of the Pediatric Anesthesia Fellowship (1993-2000) and Founder and Director of the Medical Acupuncture Service (1994-2000).

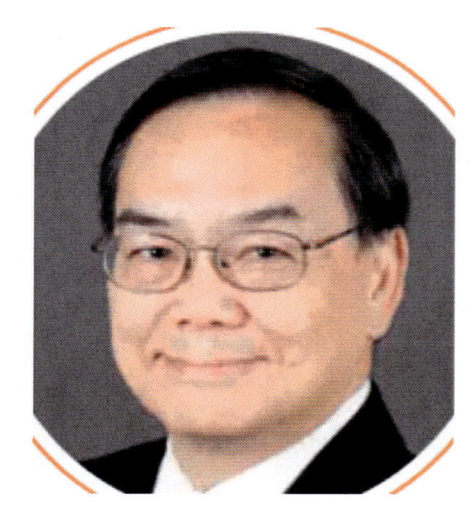

In 2001 he left Stanford for Boston and was appointed an Associate Professor (Anaesthesia and Pediatrics) at Harvard Medical School. He was Founder and Director of Medical Acupuncture Services at Boston Children's Hospital and Senior Associate in Perioperative Anesthesia and Pain Medicine, Department of Anesthesiology, Critical Care and Pain Medicine, Boston Children's Hospital/Harvard Medical School.

Dr. Lin is President of the Society of Pediatric Pain Medicine and President of the American Board of Medical Acupuncture.

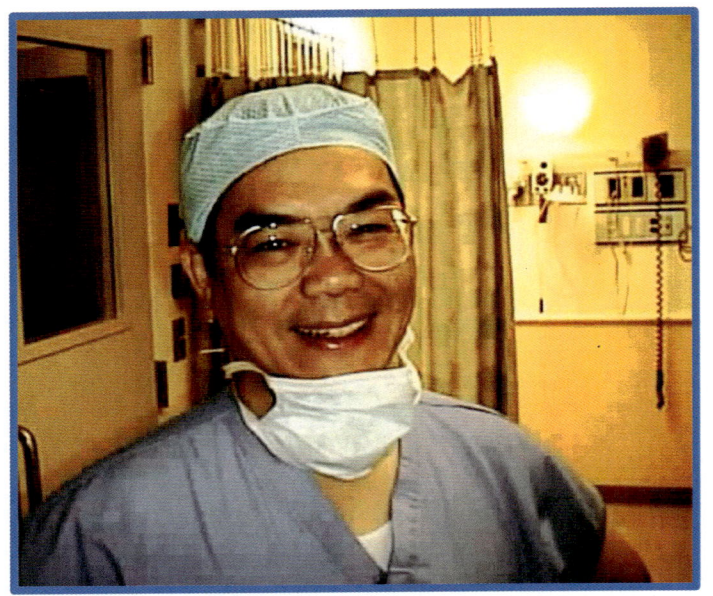

"Promoting the wellbeing in the medical community is one of my goals. I have been elected and served as the President of the Medical Staff at Boston Children's Hospital. The Massachusetts Medical Board requires physicians to have three credit hours in Pain Management and two hours of end-of-life care CME units. I have created a course for physicians to fulfill this requirement. For the past eight years, the conference has been very well received. To educate physicians in acupuncture as a complementary medical therapy, I have founded the New England Society of Medical Acupuncture. I have established the Acupuncture Workshop at the ASA Annual Meeting. This is one of the longest running workshops at the ASA. I am President of the American Board of Medical Acupuncture which is the only Board certification organization for physician acupuncturists. I also serve as President of the Society for Pediatric Pain Medicine (SPPM) which is the leading medical organization for pediatric pain medicine."

Dr. Lin has received numerous honors and awards during his career including teaching awards at Ohio State, at the University of Pennsylvania, and at Stanford. At Stanford he was the recipient of the Ellis Cohen Award and the medical school's High-Five Award in recognition of his outstanding contributions in medical school education. At Harvard he received the Outstanding Tutor Teaching Award for excellence in tutoring four times. At Boston Children's Hospital he was the recipients of the Staff Organization Recognition Award as a physician who has made a significant effort in improving the lives of other physicians at Boston Children's Hospital.

"During my decade-long tenure at Stanford, I cultivated countless cherished memories. Notably, under the chairmanship of Dr. H. Barrie Fairley, Lucile Packard Children's Hospital (LPCH) at Stanford opened its doors in April 1991, marking a significant milestone in Stanford's history. Initially, LPCH lacked its own operating room, so we relied on Stanford's main OR team. At night, we had to wait for adult cases to finish before using the emergency Pediatric OR. I distinctly remember providing anesthesia care at OR number 6 for pediatric surgeries, as one of the two attending pediatric anesthesiologists. Often, I found myself fielding most night calls, patiently anticipating the start of pediatric emergency cases. There were occasions when I remained within the hospital premises for several consecutive nights, fueled by the commitment to successfully complete pediatric cases.

When I was a junior faculty member at Stanford, many clinicians believed that neonates, infants, and children experienced less pain than adults. I am grateful to Dr. William G. Brose for training me in Pain Medicine. Under his guidance, I established the pediatric pain management service at LPCH. For almost three years, I took weekend pediatric pain calls solo until Dr. Elliot Krane joined in 1994. Dr. Julie Good also completed a month-long rotation in pediatric pain medicine, demonstrating a keen interest in pursuing it as a career. I drafted the first curriculum for a Stanford pediatric pain medicine Fellowship, which incorporated training in acupuncture medicine as part of the Fellowship."

Not until I became a pediatric pain practitioner did I realize that for children, we cannot rely solely on pain medications or regional anesthesia nerve blocks for pain management. I explored and studied acupuncture medicine, drawing upon my upbringing in Taiwan and my knowledge of Chinese, which helped me understand the ancient texts of Traditional Chinese Medicine. With the support of Drs. Donald Stanski and Elliot Krane, I established the Medical Acupuncture Service as part of pediatric pain management at LPCH. Additionally, I had the pleasure of working with Dr. David Spiegel to open the acupuncture service at the Stanford Center for Integrative Medicine. With the assistance of Dean Eugene Bauer, Stanford School of Medicine granted me permission to offer a course in acupuncture medicine, marking one of the first times acupuncture medicine was taught in a major medical school in the country. Dr. Brenda Golianu continues this tradition by offering courses in acupuncture medicine at Stanford.

I maintained a spreadsheet listing the major topics in pediatric anesthesia along with the names of all anesthesia residents. For each resident, I documented the topics discussed during our OR sessions. I ensured that fresh topics and handouts were prepared for trainees every time we worked together. Many anesthesia residents expressed interest in pediatric anesthesia, and I often guided them towards pediatric anesthesia Fellowships in Boston until we established our own pediatric anesthesia Fellowship program. I vividly remember writing and submitting the first ACGME application for a Stanford pediatric anesthesia Fellowship program.

Stanford's inclusion of anesthesia as a required rotation for all medical students is commendable. I proposed to our chairman, Dr. Donald Stanski, a revised learning experience for medical students and trainees in other disciplines during their anesthesia rotation. With the assistance of Drs. Pamela Fish and David Gaba, we were among the first institutions to introduce medical simulation training for medical students. I arranged for medical students to work directly with an assigned anesthesia resident for a week at a time, enhancing their educational experience. Additionally, I initiated the Resident Teaching Awards, which are still presented during the graduation dinner. The anesthesia medical student rotation received High-Five Award from Stanford University recognizing outstanding contribution in medical school education.

I believe in the importance of valuing our work, prioritizing family, and consistently delivering the highest quality care to our patients. Educating and mentoring future generations of anesthesiologists and pain specialists was deeply fulfilling. My time at Stanford was incredibly rewarding and enriching."

Lawrence Litt attended Columbia College (BA magna cum laude, Physics, 1963). He had a Fellowship at Harvard University (1964) and then received a PhD (Philosophy in Physics) from the Harvard University Graduate School of Arts and Sciences (1971). His work at Harvard was based on elementary particle experiments at the Cambridge Electron Accelerator.

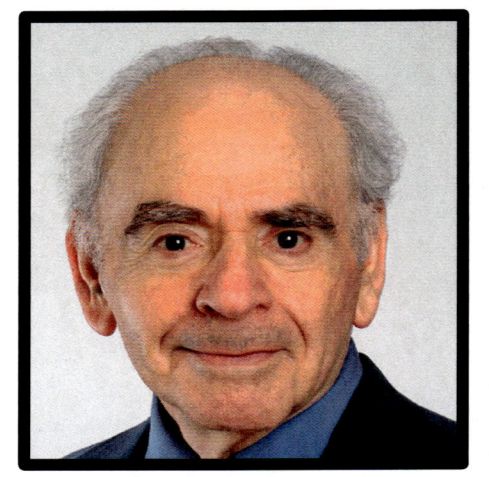

A summer neuroscience course at Cold Spring Harbor Laboratory initiated thoughts about having a medical career. The switch to medicine was delayed by a postdoctoral physics research position at Rockefeller University (1971-1974). He worked at the Centre Européenne pour la Recherche Nucléaire (CERN), Geneva, Switzerland (1971-1973), and at Brookhaven, and Fermilab laboratories.

He was appointed an Assistant Professor (Physics) at Michigan State University (1974-1977) before attending medical school. He was awarded his medical degree at the University of Miami Miller School of Medicine (MD, 1979). He interned at University of Miami Affiliated Hospitals. He then completed an Anesthesiology residency at UCSF (1980-1982). In July 1982 Litt was appointed an Assistant Professor (Anesthesiology) at Stanford (1982-1983). It was during his short time at Stanford that this renowned physicist and physician co-authored one of his most important papers.

"At Stanford my officemate Jay Brodsky and I had composed a facetious "Letter to the Editor" of The New England Journal of Medicine [NEJM] entitled, "Nurse Surgeons: A New Role for Nurses. In my first week back at UCSF I was walking down the hall when Professor Paul Ebert happened to be coming towards me on the way to his office. He was the most powerful person in the hospital, Chief of UCSF's Department of Surgery, Chief of the Division of Cardiothoracic Surgery, influential on every department or committee. I was surprised when he stopped me and asked me to accompany him back to his office. He sat me down at a table in front of a stack

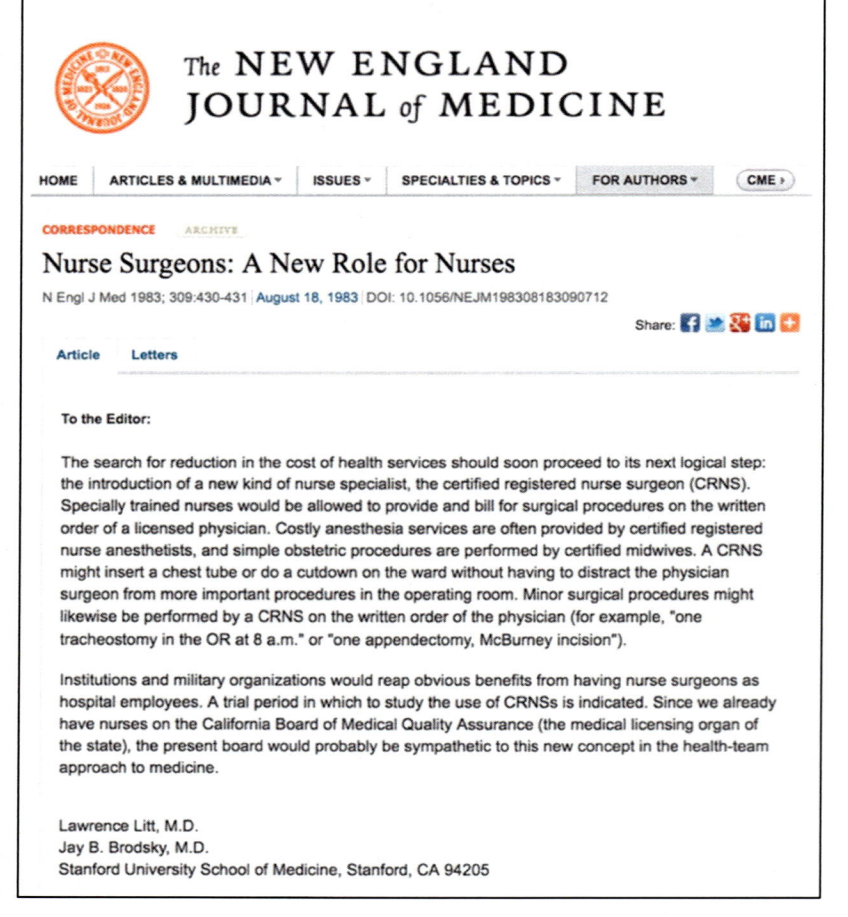

210

of papers and said, "I've been saving for you these letters that I received." There were approximately 20 serious letters from ICU nurses across the country, all requesting that UCSF be the first medical center to establish a Nurse Surgeons program to which they could apply. I spent a couple of hours reading many passionate descriptions about each writer's strong work ethic, their love for nursing and surgery, and for having a crucial role in helping people. The jolt from the letters affected all of my thoughts, making me better appreciate the humanity in everyone in the hospital: all patients, physicians, nurses, health professionals, supportive staff, and visitors. Such was the epiphany I experienced while sitting in Dr. Ebert's empty office that when I left the office, having been a former UCSF anesthesia resident and a Stanford faculty member suddenly seemed way back in an ancient past. I felt that I was starting a new life."

Dr. Litt returned to UCSF as an Assistant Professor (Anesthesiology, 1983-1988) and an Assistant Professor (Radiology, 1985-1988). He was promoted to Associate Professor (Anesthesiology and Radiology, 1988). He retired from UCSF in 2022 as Emeritus Professor (Anesthesiology and Radiology).

His anesthesia-related laboratory research began in 1988 and was subsequently supported by 28 years of NIH RO1 grant funding with Dr. Litt as principal investigator. He performed magnetic-resonance studies of brain hypoxia and ischemia. His preclinical studies of adult and neonatal brain metabolism provided insight to anesthesia protection and rescue in brain hypoxia and ischemia. He was a member of NIH Neurology A Study Section for 7 years, and a member of NIH Surgery, Anesthesiology, and Trauma Study Section for 5 years.

Clinically at UCSF he specialized in anesthesia for neurological surgery working at the Moffitt Hospital. He was a member of the Society for Neuroscience in Anesthesiology and Critical Care. He is a Fellow of the American Physical Society, the American College of Physicians, and the UK Royal Society of Medicine. He authored numerous peer-reviewed publications in major professional journals. He is in Marquis Who's Who of top educators, a list that is selected based on the current reference value of the member's publications.

John Richard Loftus

was born in Denver. He received his undergraduate education at Colorado State University (BS, Pre-Medical Studies, 1977). He then graduated from the George Washington University School of Medicine (MD, 1983). He interned (Internal Medicine) (1983-1984), followed by an Anesthesiology residency (1984-1986) at George Washington University. He then did a Fellowship (Obstetrical Anesthesia) at Stanford (1988-1989) during which time he was a Clinical Instructor (1988-1989). He was on the Voluntary Clinical faculty (1989-1996). He worked at Kaiser - South San Francisco (1986-1994)) then Kaiser - Oakland (1994-2018). He was Chair, Board of Directors, TPMG Mid-Atlantic region (2014-2018). He retired on July 1, 2018. He lists his outside interests as hiking, travel, gardening and duplicate bridge.

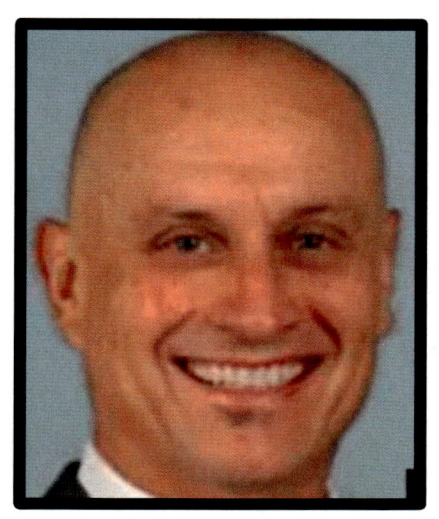

"The most important memory I have of my time at Stanford is centered on the amazing mentorship and inspiration I received as a Fellow under Dr. Sheila Cohen. Sheila was a remarkable teacher both clinically

and in terms of patient centered research. Both of these areas of my Fellowship in Obstetrical Anesthesia were intellectually stimulating and invaluable to me throughout my career. In addition to these incredible educational aspects of working with Sheila, she is one of the warmest and fun people I ever worked beside. Through all of the challenging patients and clinical research, we had a lot of fun together. She always will have my unwavering respect and admiration."

Robert E. McKlveen graduated from Northwestern University School of Medicine (MD, 1982), interned (Internal Medicine) at Tufts Medical Center (1982-1983), and was a resident (Anesthesiology) at Brigham and Women's Hospital, Boston (1983-1986). He was an Instructor (Anesthesiology) at Harvard (1986-1987) while doing a Fellowship (Obstetrical Anesthesia). He arrived at Stanford as an Acting Assistant Professor (Anesthesiology, 1987-1989). He was initially interested in OB Anesthesia, but then joined the Cardiac Anesthesia team. After leaving Stanford he moved to Minneapolis, MN, and entered private practice at Abbott Northwestern Hospital (1989-2019). After a clinical career focused on both high-risk obstetric care and cardiothoracic anesthesia, he retired in 2019.

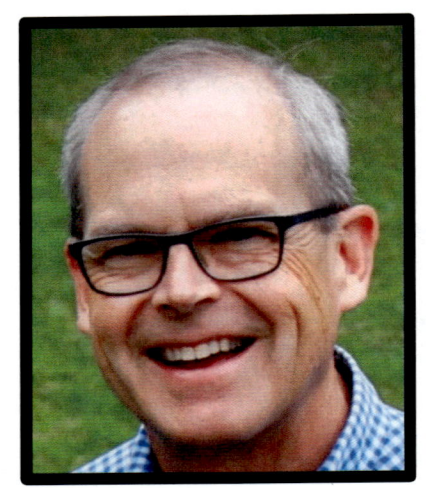

He has worked as a volunteer and leader on medical missions with Guatemala Surgery/Common Hope for 3 weeks each year for almost 30 years. This group provides surgical care at Hermano Pedro Hospital in Antigua, Guatemala. Although now clinically retired, he still participates and functions on trips as translator and team leader. He also works with a Twin Cities nonprofit as a qualified neutral facilitative mediator for community and family conflict, and on the board of a youth wilderness camp. In his spare time, he enjoys nordic skiing, biking, sailing, and hiking.

"My move from Boston to Palo Alto was motivated by my desire to be closer to Ellen, who was living in San Francisco. We had been dating VERY long-distance for about 18 months, and now we have been married for over 36 years. While we both loved the Bay Area and Stanford, and I found teaching at Stanford to be extremely fulfilling, I wanted to do more direct patient care and less lab and writing work. Plus, we had our roots in the Midwest, so we headed to Minneapolis. My practice here offered me the opportunity to use my skills in anesthesia for high-risk OB as well as cardiac anesthesia, and we've enjoyed raising our family here. Still, we miss the weather, the Stanford Hills, and wonderful colleagues of Stanford."

"As I was preparing for my oral Boards, Jay Brodsky helped me out by giving me a practice exam. Jay asked me a question to which I didn't really know the answer, so I dug myself a bit of a hole trying to answer it. His follow up

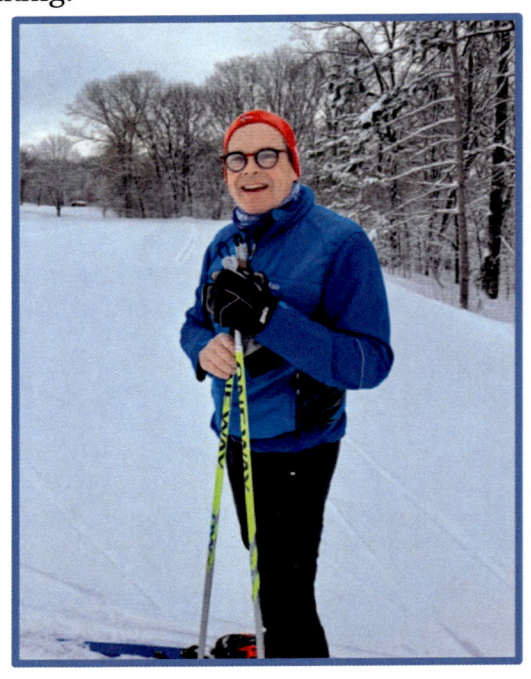

questions led me to dig that hole deeper and deeper, until I was so far down that there was no ladder long enough to climb back out. Finally, Jay said, "Bob, it's OK to say, 'I don't know.' No one knows everything. You just can't say it too often." That was excellent advice that serves me well to this day."

"Around the holidays, residents had a tradition of putting on a skit roasting the faculty. But in 1988, knowing that I had taken a position in private practice in Minnesota beginning in early 1989, they instead created a video called 'Heart Rooms of Darkness' fashioned after Conrad's 'Heart of Darkness'. But instead of featuring Kurtz who has "gone native" up the Congo River, it featured McKlveen (me) who had "gone native" and disappeared into the North Woods of Minnesota, and the residents are on a mad search for him. It was lots of fun, and featured vignettes of residents impersonating various faculty and highlighting their quirks. And it closed with a grainy photo of a balding, obese man flanked by two alluring young ladies, standing on a dock somewhere in the North Woods. McKlveen found!"

Robert Joseph Moynihan was an undergraduate at the University of Massachusetts Amherst (1974-1979). He then attended University of Massachusetts Medical School (MD, 1983) and completed residencies in both Pediatrics (1983-1985) and Anesthesiology (1986-1988) at the MGH. From there he completed Fellowship Training at Children's Hospital of Philadelphia in Pediatric Anesthesiology, Pediatric Critical Care and Pediatric Cardiac Anesthesiology (1988-1989) before coming to Stanford (1990-1992). Dr. Moynihan has been with Sutter Health in Sacramento (1993-Present). He was the founder and Medical Director of Pediatric Anesthesiology at Sutter Medical creating the first in the region all Fellowship Trained Department thus establishing a community standard. Dr Moynihan has also been very active for the 29 hospitals in the Sutter Health System with wide electric health record (EHR) implementation as Pediatrics & Anesthesiology SME (Subject Matter Expert), Epic OpTime Anesthesia EHR - Anesthesia Work Group member, Lead Physician for Sutter Health Sacramento Sierra Region.

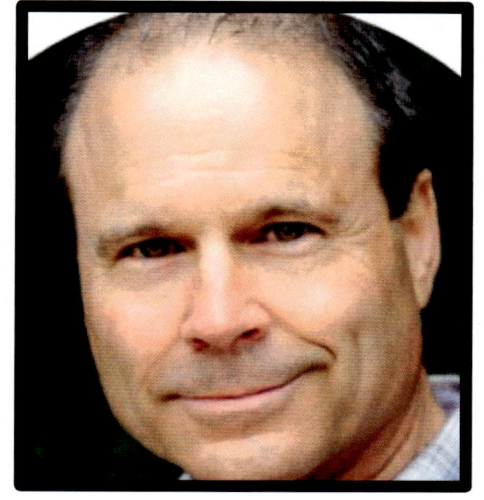

He obtained Teacher Certification for the Alexander Technique from the Pacific Institute for the Alexander Technique (2003-2006).

The Alexander Technique is a way of learning to move mindfully through life. The Alexander process shines a light on inefficient habits of movement and patterns of accumulated tension, which interferes with our innate ability to move easily and according to how we are designed. It's a simple yet powerful approach that offers the opportunity to take charge of one's own learning and healing process, because it's not a series of passive treatments but an active exploration that changes the way one thinks and responds in activity. It produces a skill set that can be applied in every situation. Lessons leave one feeling lighter, freer, and more grounded.

He also studied at the David Geffen School of Medicine/UCLA in Medical Acupuncture (2004-2005) and the Helms Medical Institute (Chinese Scalp Acupuncture, 2007). He also trained in Functional Medicine by the Institute for Functional Medicine (2012-2020). From 2016-2018 he received a certificate (Residential Rental and Property

Management) from the California Apartment Association, and in 2018 was enrolled in the Emerging Leaders Program for the US Small Business Administration earning an MBA thus empowering his role as Executive Director, Mobile Medical Team International, Inc.(MMTI).

Since 2007 MMTI has provided at-risk and disaster response focused health care services, technologies, systems and educational programs using innovative, sustainable and scalable methodologies while simultaneously incorporating and melding with local customs and cultures. MMTI's programs are in more than 65 countries, spanning five continents and expertise ranging the US Government, DARPA, World Bank, WHO, UN, US Department of State, CDC, Foundation CEOs, and Field Specialists in North America, Europe, Africa, Asia and South America.

Dr Moynihan also serves as Executive Advisor and Venture Partner with Global Health Impact Network Inc.

Global Health Impact Fund, LLC. is a quantum opportunity for clinical healthcare angel investors to participate alongside trusted VC's and institutional investors and act as clinical advisors/consultants during the due diligence phase and post investment. The Network is a unique strategic healthcare community/network of like-minded healthcare professionals who share a common vision to actively participate in molding and directing the current healthcare digital revolution.

In 2017 he was honored by a resolution of the Sacramento Board of Supervisors, County of Sacramento, for his 13 years of service as a member and Board Chairman of the Sacramento County Maternal, Child and Adolescent Health Advisory Board.

Interesting Anecdotes/Memories of Time at Stanford:
- *Building of the Packard Children's Hospital*
- *Building of the Pediatric Cardiac Surgical Service (Starnes years)*
- *Initiating the Pediatric Pain Service (Dr Yuan Chi Lin)*
- *Opus One Cabernet at "Red Barn Restaurant" for Dr. Lin's Recruitment dinner and Dr Hackel's $ concerns!*
- *Commuting by bike to Stanford along the Alameda De Las Pulgas*
- *Transition from the old anesthesia offices (Old but openable windows looking out into green courtyard, long commute to OR's) to the new (very close to OR's but modern sterile without windows) after Children's Hospital opened.*

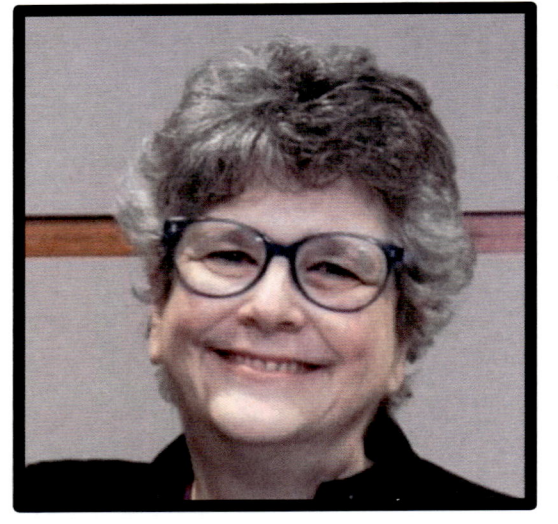

Audrey C. Shafer graduated from Harvard University (AB, Biochemistry). At Harvard she was an active athlete on the women's swim and water polo teams. She received her MD from Stanford and then trained in Anesthesiology (1984-1986) and completed a Fellowship (Clinical Pharmacology) (1986-1987) at the University of Pennsylvania. She was appointed an Assistant Professor at the PA-VAH in 1989 and worked there until her retirement as Professor of Anesthesiology, Perioperative and

Pain Medicine, Emeritum. Dr. Shafer has been on the faculty of the Stanford Center for Biomedical Ethics (2003-Present) and was founding co-director of Biomedical Ethics & Medical Humanities Scholarly Concentration (2003-2021), and founder of the Stanford Medicine and the Muse Program: Medical Humanities and the Arts (2003-Present). She was the inaugural recipient of the Leadership and Service Award, Health Humanities Consortium (2022). She also received the Henry J. Kaiser Foundation Award for Outstanding & Innovative Contributions to Medical Education, Stanford University School of Medicine (2007) and the Ellis N. Cohen MD Achievement Award (2018).

Dr. Shafer is an acclaimed novelist and poet.

The Department of Anesthesiology had a long tradition, beginning in the early 1960s, when John Bunker would invite clinical and research anesthesiologists from around the world to come to Stanford to work and study. In many cases these visitors would assume a significant portion of clinical activities in the operating rooms at Stanford Hospital and at the PA-VAH. This allowed Bunker's full-time faculty additional time for their research. These "Acting" staff appointments were often junior faculty wanting to experience a year or two of additional work experiences or training in the United States. Most, but not all, returned to their home country after leaving Stanford and proudly added a *'Been to America'* notation on their curriculum vitae. During Phil Larson's tenure as Chair many anesthesiologists coming for an initial one-year appointment stayed on for a full-time career at Stanford. (See Table)

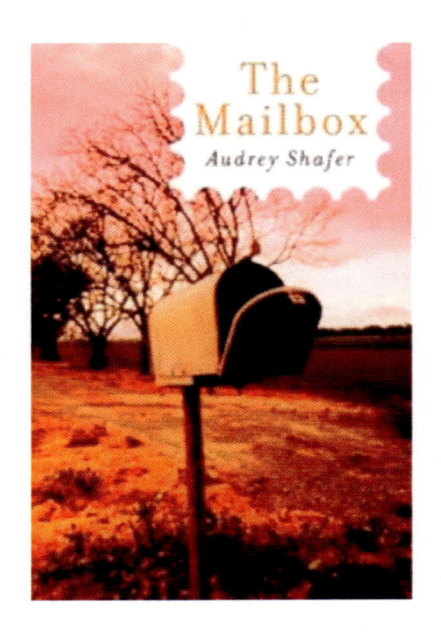

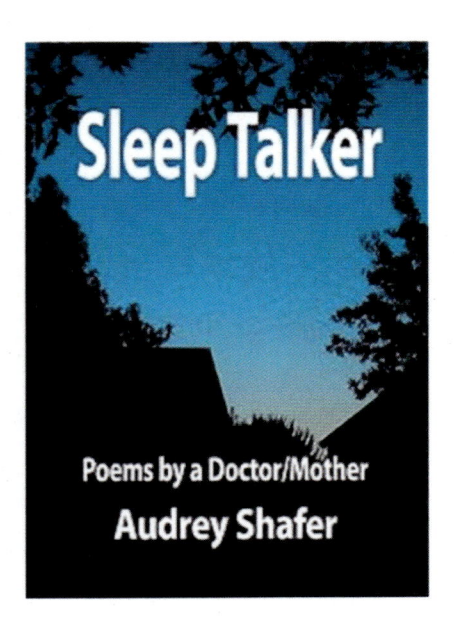

VISITING CLINICAL FACULTY

Diana Gillian Beeby (McGregor)

was born in London. She graduated from the University of London, Charing Cross and Westminster Medical School (1971). She was a registrar in the Department of Anaesthetics, Norfolk and Norwich Hospital, Norwich, UK and Addenbrooks Hospital, Cambridge. She did advanced training in cardiac and neuroanesthesia, and pediatrics and pain at Papworth and Addenbrooks Hospital, at Great Ormond Street Children's Hospital, London, and Norwich Hospitals. She came to Stanford as an Acting Assistant Professor (Anesthesiology) (1982-1984). After 2 years she returned to the UK as a consultant at Newcastle Hospital (1984-1987). She then worked as a anesthesiologist at the Mayo Clinic (1987-2005) before returning to Stanford in 2005 She remained associated with Stanford as a Clinical Associate Professor (Anesthesiology) (2005-2012). She married Stanford cardiac surgeon Chris McGregor. Dr. Diana McGregor was Chair of the ASA Task Force on Waste Anesthetic Gases and the ASA Occupational Health Committee. She retired November 2012.

"In the early days, breakfast with colleagues was the highlight my day with such interesting discussions."

Acting (Visiting) Instructor or Assistant Professor

1960-1972 (Bunker)

David J. Bowen	Wales
James Defares	Belgium
Stanley Feldman	England
Valeer Derijcke	Belgium
Berwyn Thomas	Wales
Thomas Shakespeare	Australia
Malcolm Tyrrell	England
Gordon Taylor	England
Arno Hollman	Finland
Michael Cousins	Australia
Colin Brown	Australia
Michael Skivington	England
Jeanette Thirwell	Australia
J. Alastair Lack	England
David Crankshaw	Australia
Frederick Camu	Belgium

1973-1982 (Larson)

Sheila Cohen	England
Stanley Samuels	England
Alex Thurlow	England
Ian Carson	Ireland
Jeffrey Baden	Australia
John Brock-Utne	South Africa

(Partial List)

Barry Cristopher Sellick

graduated medical school from St Thomas's Hospital, London (1975). Following various jobs in the south of England he took a post in Cape Town, South Africa, working at the Groote Schuur Hospital. He returned to the UK and worked in Nottingham and at St. Georges Hospitals. He spent a year as an Acting Assistant Professor (Anesthesiology) at Stanford (1984-1985). He says his first child is proud to say, "Born in the USA". He is currently a Consultant Anaesthetist in the Intensive Care Unit at Ashford and St. Peter's Hospitals, UK.

James Justin Margary

was a Senior Registrar in the Department of Anaesthetics at St George's Hospital, London in 1986. In 1986-1988 he was on the Stanford faculty as an Acting Assistant Professor (Anesthesiology) working mainly at the

PA-VAH. He was Lead for Obstetric Anaesthesia in the Anaesthetic Department at St. Peter's Hospital, Surrey, UK.

Charles F. Minto was born on the Falkland Islands. He studied at the University of Auckland, New Zealand obtaining a degree in Human Biology (BHB, 1982) and Medicine and Surgery (MBChB, 1985). After working for six months as a Medical Officer (Resident) in Anesthesiology in Hong Kong (1987), he completed his training in Anesthesiology at Waikato Hospital, Hamilton, NZ, and Christchurch Hospital, Christchurch, NZ. He was awarded the inaugural BWT Ritchie Scholarship to support a two-year research Fellowship (Anesthesiology and Clinical Pharmacology) at Stanford with Don Stanski and Steve Shafer. He arrived at Stanford in 1992. He worked initially with Talmage Egan on the pharmacokinetics and pharmacodynamics of remifentanil. During his time at the PA-VAH he also had a faculty role supervising residents and doing clinical anesthesia. He was appointed to the voluntary Clinical Faculty at Stanford where he worked as a pediatric anesthesiologist at Lucile Packard Children's Hospital and did neuroanesthesia at Stanford Hospital. After completing his Fellowship, he was appointed a staff anesthesiologist in the department.

After three years he moved to Australia to complete a Ph.D. at Sydney University and to work as a clinical academic at Royal North Shore Hospital. He currently works in private practice with a focus on neuroanesthesia and neuromonitoring at North Shore Private, Westmead Private and Sydney Adventist Hospitals. He and Professor Thomas Schnider, former PA-VAH Pharmacology Fellow and recently retired Chair of Anaesthesia, Kantonsspital St. Gallen, Switzerland, are the co-founders of The Open TCI Initiative, a website began in January 2008 to encourage open discussions on TIVA and TCI. They held their first meeting, chaired by Steve Shafer (then at Columbia University), in Cape Town, South Africa (March 2008). Minto was elected the second Chair at the Second World Congress of TIVA-TCI in Berlin (2009). Minto continues to collaborate and publish research studies with Schnider, and with Talmage Egan.

"My Stanford Years were some of my best experiences as a doctor and I am very proud to be part the story."

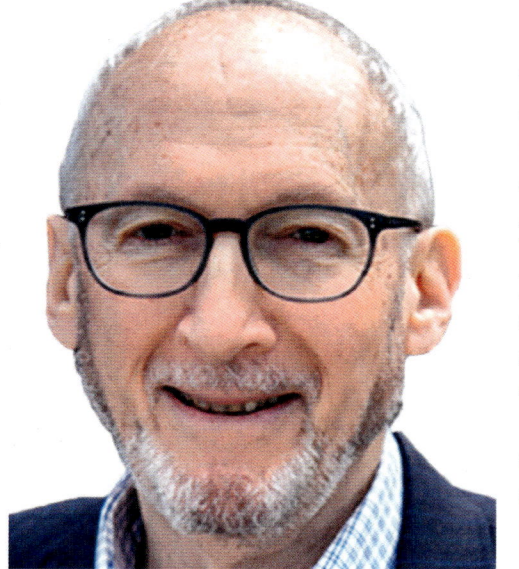

John Zelcer arrived from Australia and was appointed an Acting Assistant Professor (Anesthesiology) at Stanford (1985). He has worked as an anaesthetist at several hospitals in Melbourne Australia including the University of Melbourne, St. Vincent's Hospital, and the Royal Women's Hospital. His clinical practice interests focused on obstetrical, urology, pediatric, and head and neck cancer anesthesia. He is currently an adjunct Professor on the faculty for LaTrobe University, Melbourne.

Dr. Zelcer was an early and passionate proponent of digital medicine and remains deeply engaged in developing information technology solutions to help enhance the quality and impact of clinical care, with a current emphasis on artificial intelligence and machine learning for clinical decision support.

Digital Medicine: Software-driven connected technologies have created a fundamental shift in health data and information flows. Digital medicine describes the use of these technologies as tools for measurement and intervention in human health. Digital medicine products are driven by hardware and software that support the practice of medicine broadly, including treatment, recovery, disease prevention, and health promotion for individuals and across populations. Digital medicine products can be used independently or in concert with pharmaceuticals, biologics, devices, or other products to optimize patient care and health outcomes. Digital medicine empowers patients and healthcare providers with intelligent and accessible tools to address a wide range of conditions through high-quality, safe, and effective measurements and data-driven interventions. As a discipline, digital medicine encapsulates both broad professional expertise and responsibilities concerning the use of these digital tools. Digital medicine focuses on evidence-generation to support the use of these technologies.

His career has spanned clinical and academic medicine, management consulting and business leadership roles in Australia and the United States. His early research focus was on safe anaesthesia practice and the beneficial role of information technology, continuing now in digital health strategy and application. He has held strategy management consulting and senior executive management roles for over 35 years. His business roles included board chairmanships and directorships, and senior executive roles in strategic planning and business development. He was a board director of Eastern Health in Victoria, for nine years, and involved with the Health Informatics Society of Australia, Epworth Healthcare, the Victorian Clinical Genetics Service and Jewish Care Victoria. He has provided extensive management consulting and professional advice to government and diverse healthcare sector organizations since 1979, including: Organization governance, leadership, and management; Healthcare strategic planning and healthcare management; Clinical governance and risk mitigation in healthcare delivery; Clinical information management strategies, business cases, governance and safety; Facilitation and advice on corporate strategic planning and operations. He has also provided master level, evidence-based executive coaching, and mentoring support to senior leaders at board, executive and senior management levels spanning more than 20 years.

Richard Joseph Flynn received his medical degree from University College Cork, Ireland (1978). He is currently a consultant anaesthetist at Cork. He was on the faculty as an Acting Assistant Professor (Anesthesiology) at Stanford (1990-1991). We have no information on **John Walker** (1984) and **Robin Lee Davidson** (1991-1992). Both are listed in the Stanford Medical School annual bulletin as having one-year "acting" appointments in the Department of Anesthesiology.

RESEARCH FACULTY

Several Research Associates were appointed to the Department's faculty during 1983-1992.

Masahiko "Mas" Fujinaga joined the PA-VAH in the mid-1980s. Mas was a physician anesthesiologist but did not do any clinical anesthesia and only worked in the PA-VAH research labs. He was very prolific and published dozens of research papers with Dick Mazze, Jeff Baden, and other VAH faculty. He left in 1999 to join Mervyn Maze at the Imperial College in London. After 4 years there he returned to Japan and has practiced clinical anesthesia.

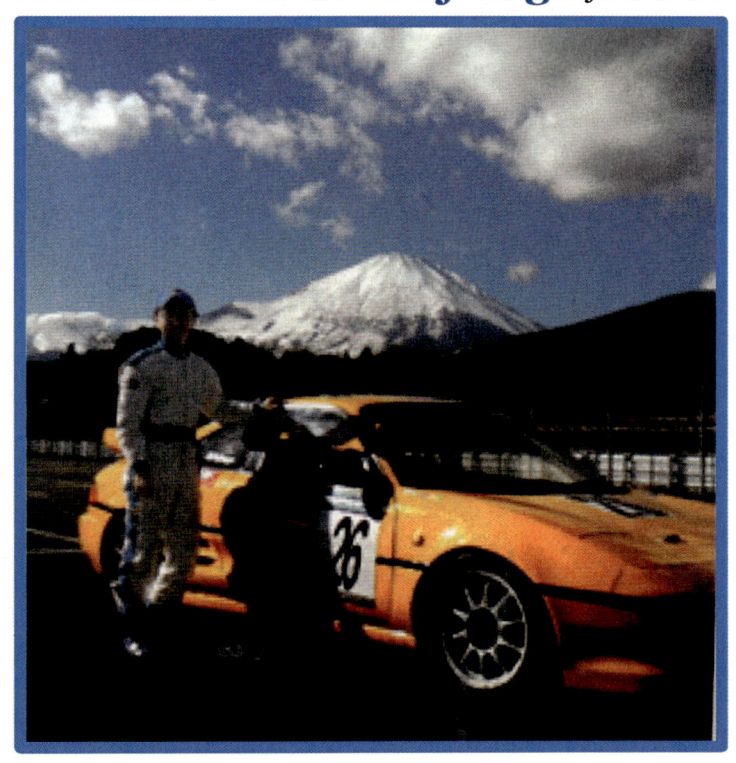

Mas Fujinaga races his Toyota MR2 at the Fuji Speedway in Japan

William F. Ebling attended Temple University and then studied SUNY - Buffalo (PhD, Pharmaceutics, 1977-1985). He was appointed Assistant Professor (Research) in the Stanford Anesthesiology Department and worked at the PA-VAH with Don Stanski (1991-1992). He was an Assistant Professor of Pharmacology at the University of Buffalo and Stanford University. He was Senior Clinical Pharmacologist at DuPont Merck Pharmaceuticals, a former Senior Consultant, Pharmaceutical Services at Pharsight (2000-2007) and President of Emergent Insights Consulting (2007-Present).

M. Bruce MacIver attended the University of Calgary, Alberta (MSc, Pharmacology 1981) and a PhD (Neuroscience, 1985). He joined the Stanford Anesthesiology Department in 1987 initially as a postdoctoral Fellow. He was appointed an Assistant Professor (Neurophysiology) at Stanford in the Department of Anesthesiology (1991-1998), then promoted to Associate Professor (1998-2010), and subsequently Professor of Neurophysiology in Anesthesia. His research was funded by numerous NIH grants for the study of the effects of anesthetic agents on CNS activity.

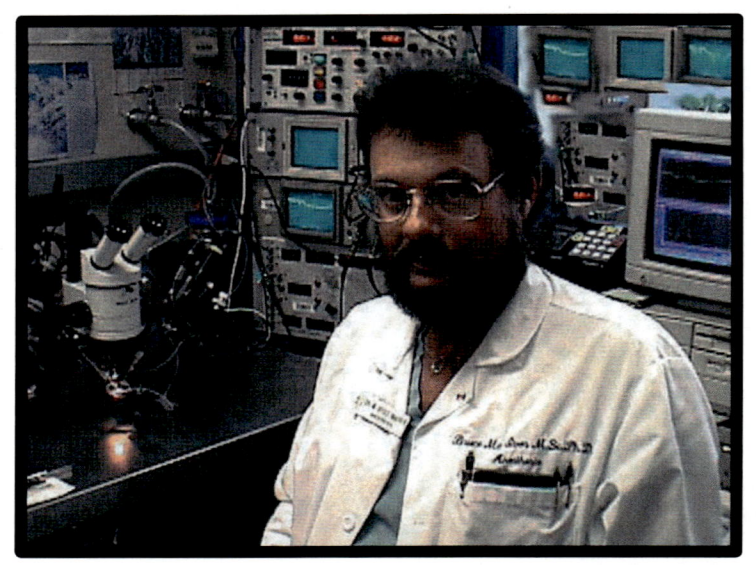

Bruce MacIver was Director and NIH Principal Investigator of the Neuropharmacology Laboratory at Stanford Medical School. He was Neuroscience Program Executive (1997-2005), on the Neuroscience Admissions Panel (2000-2005) and the Study Section - Adjunct, for the NIH (2004-2020). He served on the Stanford Medical School Faculty Senate (2008-2017). At Stanford University he was on the Committee on Graduate Studies (2008-2011) and a member of Environmental Health & Safety Committee (2006-2009). He was also a File Reviewer for the Stanford Neuroscience PhD Program (2017-Present), on the ASA's Neuroscience Subcommittee (2006-2013), an associate editor for the Journal of Neurophysiology (2020-Present), on the editorial Board of Trends in Anaesthesia and Critical Care (2020-Present), and an associate editor of Anesthesia & Analgesia (2022-Present).

Among his numerous awards and honors is the Allen V. Cox Medal, Stanford University (2004) and the Elmer Zsigmond Award, International Society for Anaesthetic Pharmacology (2017).

The Cox Medal is awarded annually to a Stanford faculty member who has established a record of excellence directing undergraduate research. The citation for Bruce MacIver's award acknowledged "his long-standing and widely acknowledged commitment to undergraduate research and lifelong mentoring that has moved students from initial exposure to cutting edge work to careers in their own biomedical laboratories. MacIver fostered independent thinking in a supportive, but intellectually rigorous research environment that encourages the development of scientific thinking as well as technical virtuosity—

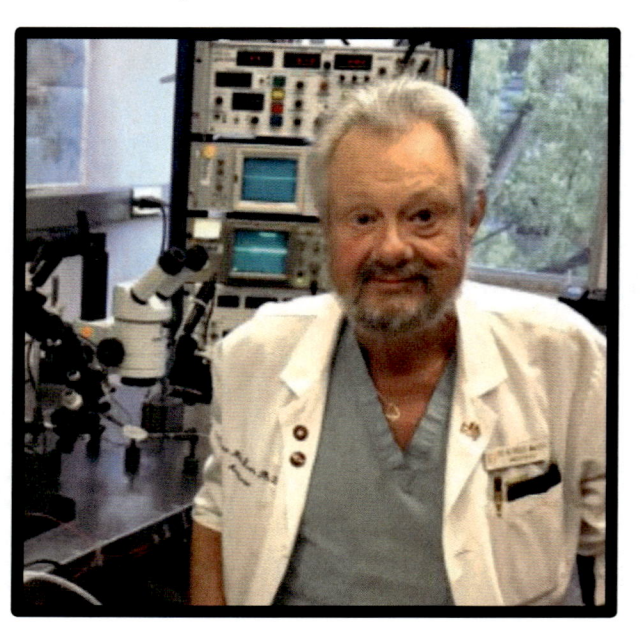

training which has garnered prestigious awards for his students".

Bruce MacIver recently retired as Emeritus Professor (Research) in the Department of Anesthesiology, Perioperative and Pain Medicine.

ADMINISTRATIVE STAFF

From its beginning in 1960, the Department of Anesthesiology has always had outstanding administrative and secretarial support. Many individuals have filled those roles, but unfortunately, we have records of very few of them. There are two that deserve special mention.

Virginia F. Tse was born in Casablanca, Morocco, to an American father in the military and a French mother. The family moved to Champagne, IL, soon after her birth. After that, there was a succession of moves to Japan, Hawaii, the Azores, Idaho, Nebraska, Southern California, and Virginia. When she was 15 the family settled in the SF Bay area. She attended Skyline Junior College in San Bruno. After graduation she worked in San Francisco before joining the staff in the Department of Anesthesia at UCSF as a secretary (1977-1978) and Administrative Assistant (1978-1985).

In 1985 Virginia joined the Stanford Department of Anesthesiology when Barrie Fairley took over as Chair. She had been Dr. Fairley's secretary and assistant at UCSF/SFGH since 1977. Her initial appointment at Stanford was Administrative Assistant (1985-1988) promoted to Management Service Officer (1998-2024). Virginia took over Adena Goodart's post. Adena had started in our department in 1965 and was Phil Larson's administrative assistant after he became Chair. After Phil stepped down, Adena left to work for Norman Shumway in the Cardiothoracic Department.

Virginia's served as department faculty affairs advisor by preparing all recommendations for faculty appointments, reappointments, and promotions. She also supervised clerical and office staff. Virginia stayed at Stanford for the remainder of her career and retired in 2024 after 39 years.

"When Dr. Fairley and I arrived in the Department, staffing consisted of approximately 30 faculty and 12 administrative staff. I remember Dr. Fairley telling me that the staff and faculty were not only coworkers, but also friends. The entire department fit in one hallway in the Grant Building."

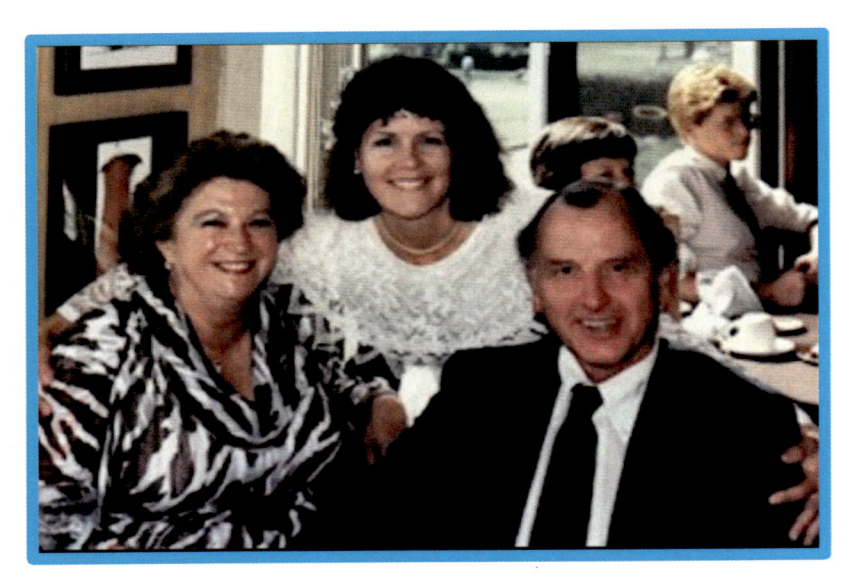

Dr. and Mrs. Fairley at Virginia's wedding reception, June 20, 1987

Audrey "Aud" Gladys Clewes Ramage (Pullens) (deceased) was

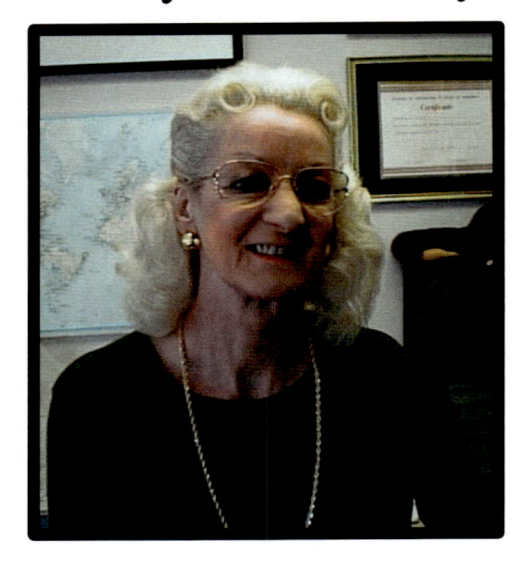

born on August 31st, 1936, in Edinburgh, Scotland, the second of four children and the only daughter of Andrew and Charlotte Ramage. She grew up in a working-class family during WW2 and graduated Tynecastle High School (1950). She then attended Skerry's College in Edinburgh. At 18 she left on the Queen Elizabeth for New York City. She was originally hired as a "children's nurse," then worked as a shop window dresser. She eventually found work as a flight attendant with KLM Royal Dutch Airlines at Idlewild Airport, NYC (now JFK Airport).

In 1959, while working for KLM Audrey met a tall blond Dutchman named Wim. It must have been "love at first sight" since they were married after knowing each other only one day! They settled in Curaçao where their first child, son Andrew was born in 1961.

Several years later the family moved to California where their second child, daughter Tineke was born in 1964. In 1973 they settled in Redwood City. Tragically, in 1976 Wim was killed in an automobile accident. Audrey never remarried.

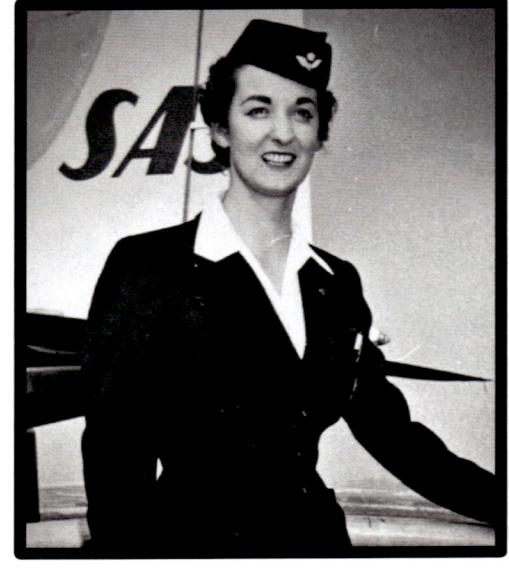

Audrey's career included working as a radio DJ, as an insurance coder, and in retail management, including as the deli manager at Roberts Market in Woodside. She eventually came to work in our Department in the early 1980s and remained there until her retirement in 2005. Audrey served as secretarial support for several faculty and as the "welcoming" person at the front desk of the main office. She passed away peacefully on 27 April 2023 at home in Redwood City, at age 86.

Jay Brodsky, "Audrey Pullens was a real character. She took great pride in keeping her office immaculate. Every surface was always dusted and polished, and everything was always in its place. We would "tease" her by moving items on her desk at night after she left work. She eventually solved this problem by gluing everything (her stapler, her mail inbox, her pen holder, everything) to their proper place on the desk. Her family says she was busy cleaning her apartment right up to her last day."

John Brock-Utne, "The first time I met Aud was in January 1989. I liked her immediately as she preferred to be called Aud, a good old Norwegian name. This got us off to a good start. Aud was known to the residents at "Mother Aud". A very appropriate name. She was always very supportive of all of them, and they loved her for it."

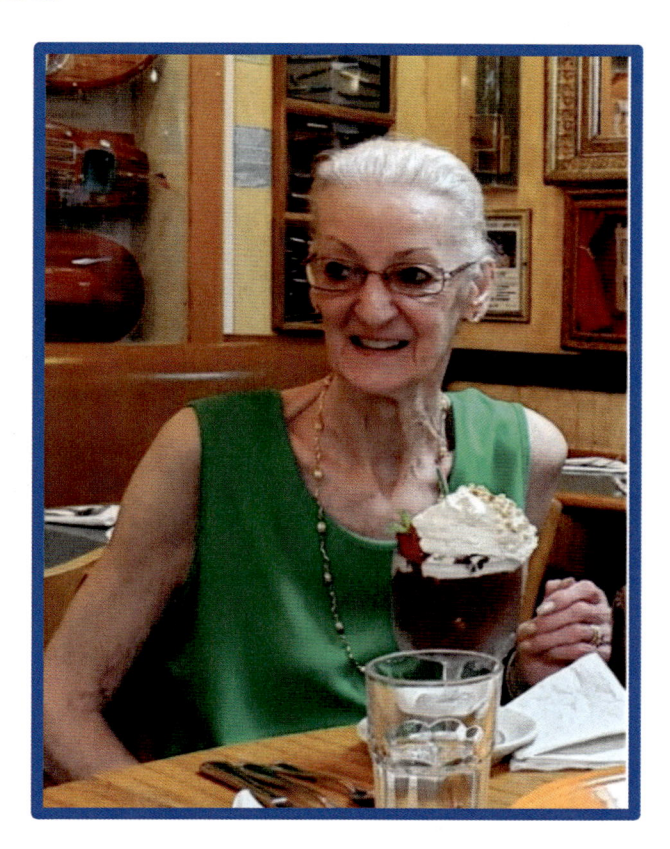

Chapter 14

TRANSITION

In 1992 when Barrie Fairley decided to step down from his leadership position the Department was in serious financial straits. Working with a large mix of uninsured patients in the same operating rooms next to the well insured patients going to PAMF and the AAMG groups meant the Department couldn't match the income of the competing with the local private practice anesthesiologists. To make matters worse, the medical school's Dean introduced a new tax directing that clinical profits from departments like Anesthesiology with few or no out-patient clinics go to other financially strained departments in order to support their poorly reimbursed clinics. The situation made it difficult to recruit new faculty and even more challenging to retain those who did come to Stanford. The majority of clinical attendings joining the faculty were recent graduates of our residency and Fellowship programs. Most stayed on for only a short period before leaving for higher paying jobs. Frank Sarnquist took over the temporary leadership of the Department until Donald Stanski moved from the PA-

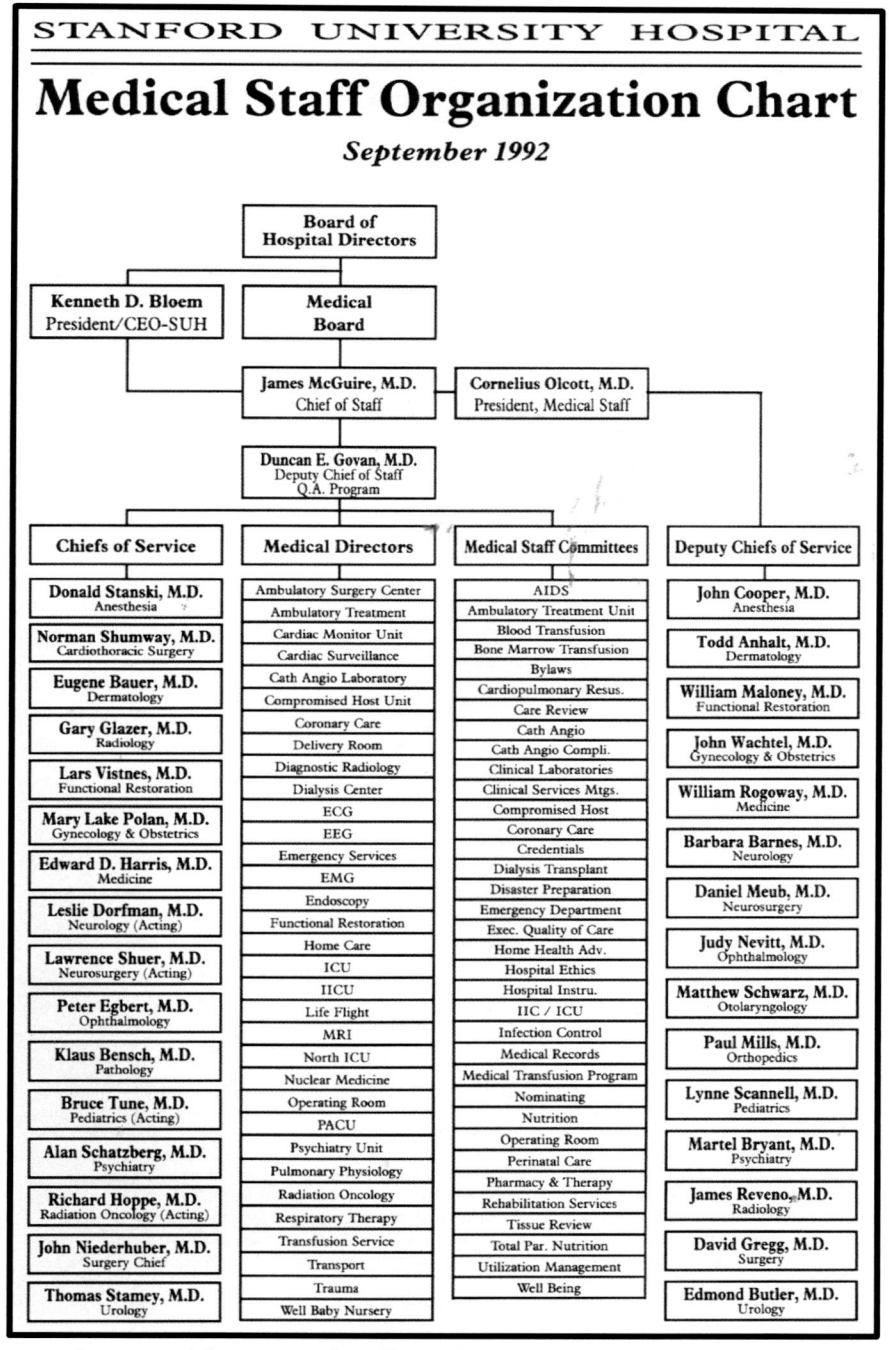

VAH to become the fourth full-time Chair of the Stanford Department of Anesthesiology. Dr. Stanski inherited the serious problems that Dr. Fairley had faced.

In September 1992 Stanford University Hospital published a Pictorial Membership Roster of the nearly 1,700 physicians then practicing there "to facilitate familiarity with fellow staff members". The list included the names and photographs of academic full-time and retired emeriti faculty, private physicians working at Stanford Hospital (AAMG and PAMF anesthesiologists), and volunteer adjunct teaching faculty based elsewhere. More than 40 of the 100 attending anesthesiologists listed (below) were anesthesiology residents or fellows at some time during the 1983-1992 period covered in this book.

ANESTHESIOLOGY

AHLERING, JOHN
ARCHER, JOHN H
ATKINSON, RHETT W
BADEN, JEFFREY M
BAER, EDWARD R
BAHL, CAROLYN
BERGER, DAVID L
BERNARD, WALTER
BERNER, GERALD
BRINKS, HEINRICH A
BRIZGYS, RAY C
BROCK-UTNE, JOHN G
BRODSKY, JAY B
BROSE, WILLIAM G
BUECHEL, D ROBERT
CHAMPEAU, MICHAEL W
CHERRY, CARTER
COHEN, ELLIS N
COHEN, SHEILA E
COOPER, JOHN R
CULLY, MICHAEL
CURTIS, PATRICIA
DAMRON, JOHN C
DANIELS, DAVID N
DAVIDSON, ROBIN LEE
DESAI, JAYSHREE
DOLAN, WILLIAM
DUEKER, CHRISTOPHER
EGAN, TALMAGE
ENGSTROM, RAY H
FAIRLEY, H BARRIE
FEELEY, THOMAS W
FELD, LAWRENCE H
FINCH, ELLEN L

FISCHELL, ANNE A
FISH, KEVIN J
FISH, PAMELA M
FISK, STEPHEN
FITZGERALD, DAVID
FORREST, W H, JR
GABA, DAVID M
GAETA, RAYMOND
GARMAN, J KENT
GASTON, THOMAS L
GIFFARD, RONA G
HACKEL, ALVIN
HADDOW, GORDON R
HALPERIN, BRUCE D
HOLGUIN, GERALD
HOMER, TERRI D
HSU, ERIC
JAFFE, RICHARD A
KREITZMAN, TED
LARSON, C PHILIP, JR
LEE, JEFFREY S
LIN, YUANG-CHI
LOFTUS, JOHN R
MASON, DONALD
MAZE, MERVYN
MAZZE, RICHARD I
MCFARLAND, DANIEL J
MELLENTHIN, MICHAEL
MERLONE, STEVEN C
MIHM, FREDERICK G
MOYNIHAN, ROBERT J
NEGUS, JEAN B
NEW, WILLIAM, JR
NOVAK, RICHARD J

PEARL, RONALD G
PETERSON, KRISTI L
PROPST, JON
RATNER, EMILY
REDPATH, JOHN H
ROSENSTOCK, LYNN L B
ROSENTHAL, MYER H
ROSNOW, JAN M
SAMUELS, STANLEY I
SARNQUIST, FRANK H
SAUNDERS, LISA
SCAVONE, JOHN A
SCHARES, THOMAS
SHAFER, AUDREY
SHAFER, STEVEN L
SIEGEL, LAWRENCE C
SINGLETON, MARK A
SORBO, SONJA
STANSKI, DONALD R
STOCKER, WILLIAM A
STRITTER, GWEN
SUGAR, ROBERT
TAYLOR, GORDON
URBANOWICZ, JOHN H
VASIL, CHRISTOPHER
WHEATON, KEVIN R
WHITCHER, CHARLES E
WINCHESTER, LYNN W
WYNER, JANET
ZWENG, JOSEPH

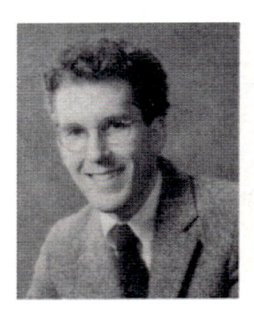

Archer, John H
Anesthesiology
Stanford Univ Med Ctr
Dept of Anesthesia
Stanford, CA 94305
723-6411
Asst Prof

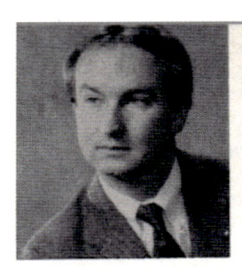

Baer, Edward R
Anesthesiology *
Critical Care Medicine *
701 Welch Rd #216
Palo Alto, CA 94304
323-0617
Clin Instr

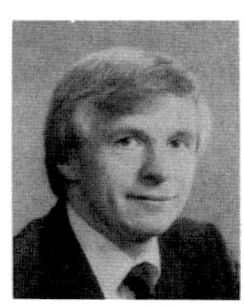

Baden, Jeffrey M
Anesthesiology *
Veterans Hospital
Palo Alto, CA   94304
858-3938
Assoc Prof

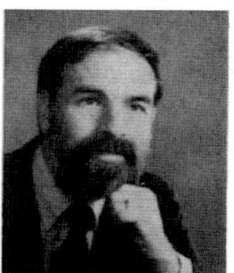

Brodsky, Jay B
Anesthesiology *
Stanford Univ Med Ctr
#S-278
Stanford, CA   94305
723-6411
Prof

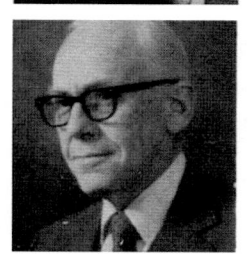

Buechel, D Robert
Anesthesiology
751 S Bascom Ave
San Jose, CA   95128
299-6341
Prof

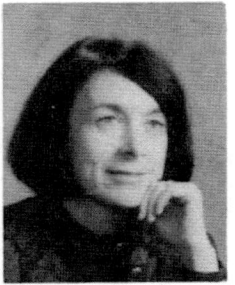

Cohen, Sheila E
Anesthesiology
Stanford Univ Med Ctr
#S-278
Stanford, CA   94305
723-6411
Prof

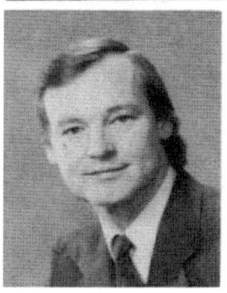

Courtesy
Engstrom, Ray H
Anesthesiology *
305 Lennon Ave
#S-236A
Walnut Creek, CA   94598
723-6411
Asst Prof

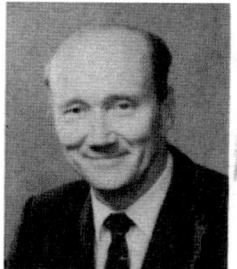

Brock-Utne, John G
Anesthesiology
Stanford Univ Med Ctr
Dept of Anesthesia #S-278
Stanford, CA   94305
723-6411
Prof

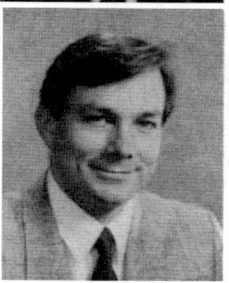

Brose, William G
Anesthesiology *
Stanford Univ Med Ctr
Dept of Anesthesia #A283
Stanford, CA   94305
723-6411
Asst Prof

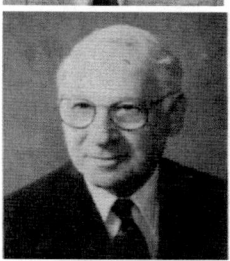

Cohen, Ellis N
Anesthesiology *
Stanford Univ Med Ctr
Stanford, CA   94305
857-0681
Prof Emer

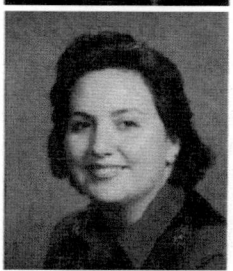

Davidson, Robin Lee
Anesthesioiogy *
Stanford Med Ctr
#H-3583
Stanford, CA   94305
723-6411
Clin Asst Prof

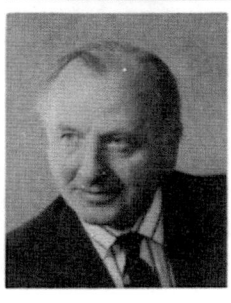

Fairley, H Barrie
Anesthesiology *
Stanford Med Ctr
#S-278
Stanford, CA   94305
723-5024
Prof

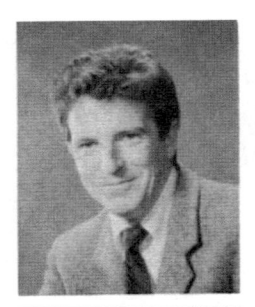

Feeley, Thomas W
Anesthesiology *
Critical Care Medicine *
Stanford Univ Med Ctr
#S-278
Stanford, CA 94305
723-6411
Prof

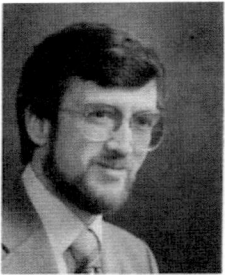

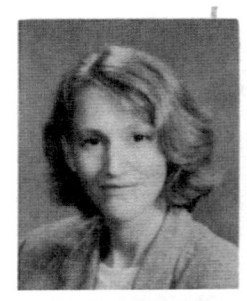

Fischell, Anne A
Anesthesiology *
Pediatrics *
Stanford Univ Med Ctr
#S-278
Stanford, CA 94305
723-6411
Asst Prof

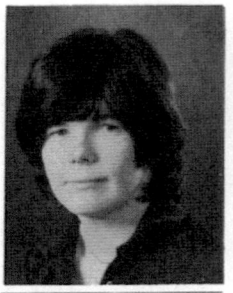

Fish, Kevin J
Anesthesiology
Stanford Univ Med Ctr
#S-278
Stanford, CA 94305
723-6411
Assoc Prof

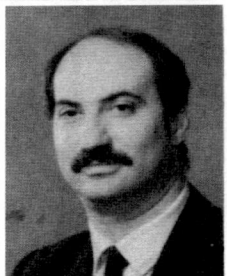

Fish, Pamela M
Anesthesiology
VAH 112-A
Palo Alto, CA 94306
323-0617
Clin Asst Prof

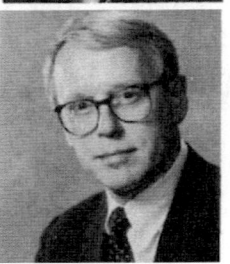

Gaba, David M
Anesthesiology *
Palo Alto VA Med Ctr
#S-278C
Palo Alto, CA 94304
723-6411
Asst Prof

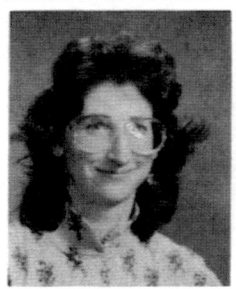

Garman, J Kent
Anesthesiology
27742 Stirrup Way
Los Altos Hills, CA
(408) 949-3470
Clin Prof

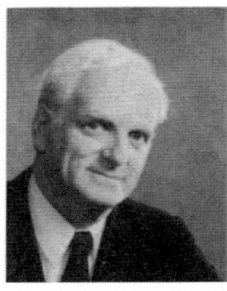

Giffard, Rona G
Anesthesiology *
Stanford Univ Med Ctr
#S-278
Stanford, CA 94305
723-6411
Asst Prof

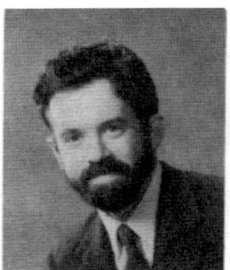

Hackel, Alvin
Anesthesiology *
Pediatrics *
Stanford Med Ctr
Dept of Anesthesia
Stanford, CA 94305
723-6307
Prof

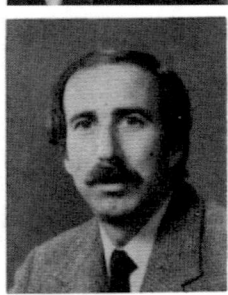

Haddow, Gordon R
Anesthesiology
Dept of Anesthesia *
Stanford Med Sch
Stanford, CA 94305
723-6415
Asst Prof

Halperin, Bruce D
Anesthesiology *
Critical Care Medicine
701 Welch Rd #216
Palo Alto, CA 94304
323-0617
Asst Clin Prof

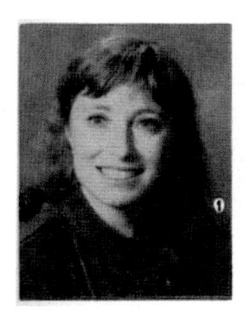

Homer, Terri D
Anesthesiology *
701 Welch Rd #216
Palo Alto, CA   94304
323-0617
Vol Clin Faculty

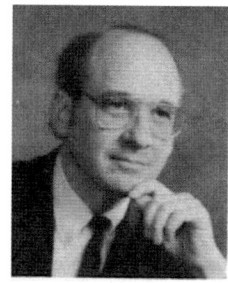

Jaffe, Richard A
Anesthesiology *
Stanford Univ Med Ctr
Dept of Anesthesia
Stanford, CA   94305
723-6411
Asst Prof

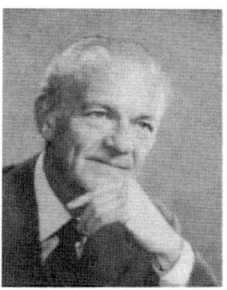

Larson, C Philip, Jr
Anesthesiology *
Stanford Univ Med Ctr
Dept of Anesthesia
Stanford, CA   94305
723-5439
Prof

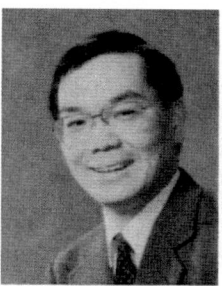

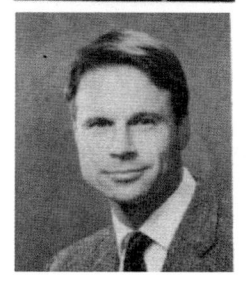

Lin, Yuan-Chi
Anesthesiology
Pediatrics *
Stanford Univ Med Ctr
Dept of Anesthesia
Stanford, CA   94305
723-6415
Asst Prof

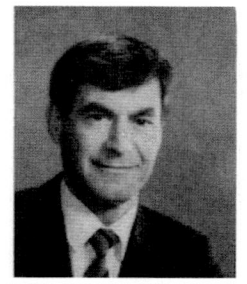

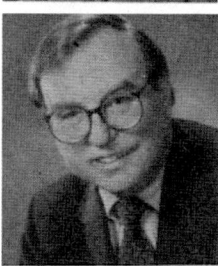

Maze, Mervyn
Anesthesiology *
Gastroenterology *
Stanford Univ Med Ctr
Dept Anesthesia #M-5117
Stanford, CA   94305
858-3938
Assoc Prof

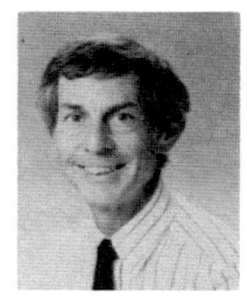

Mazze, Richard I
Anesthesiology
3801 Miranda Ave
Palo Alto, CA   94304
493-5000
Prof

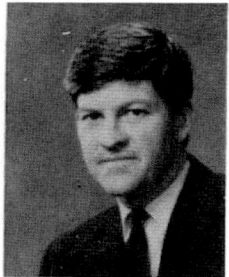

Merlone, Steven C
Anesthesiology *
300 Homer Ave
Palo Alto, CA   94301
321-4121
Clin Prof

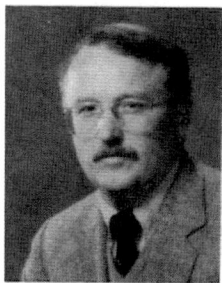

Mihm, Frederick G
Anesthesiology *
Critical Care Medicine *
Stanford Univ Med Ctr
Dept of Anesthesia #H-3585
Stanford, CA   94305
723-6415
Assoc Prof

Moynihan, Robert J
Anesthesiology
Pediatrics
Stanford Univ Med Ctr
Dept of Anesthesia
Stanford, CA   94305
723-7562
Asst Prof

New, William, Jr
Anesthesiology *
124 University Ave
Palo Alto, CA   94301
328-4000
Clin Assoc Prof

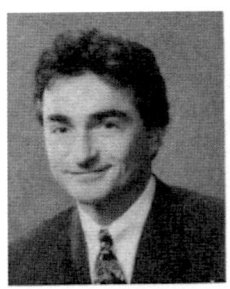

Novak, Richard J
Anesthesiology *
Internal Medicine *
701 Welch Rd #216
Palo Alto, CA   94304
323-0617
Clin Instr

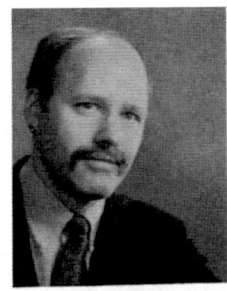

Pearl, Ronald G
Anesthesiology *
Internal Medicine *
Stanford Univ Med Ctr
Dept of Anesthesia
Stanford, CA   94305
725-5875
Asst Prof

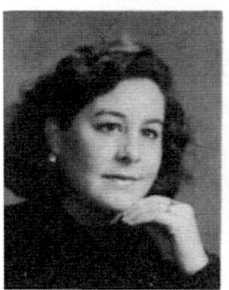

Peterson, Kristi L
Anesthesiology *
Stanford Univ Med Ctr
Anesthesia Dept
Stanford, CA   94305
858-3938
Clin Asst Prof

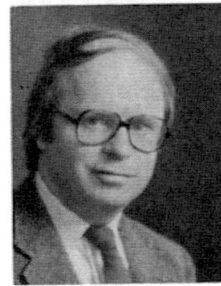

Redpath, John H
Anesthesiology
300 Homer Ave
Palo Alto, CA   94301
321-4121
Clin Assoc Prof

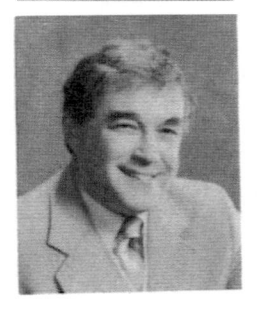

Rosenthal, Myer H
Anesthesiology *
Critical Care Medicine *
Stanford Univ Med Ctr
#S-278
Stanford, CA   94305
723-7662
Prof

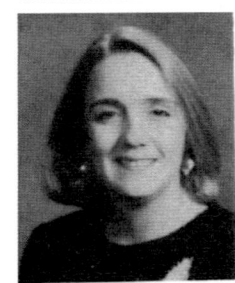

Rosnow, Jan M
Anesthesiology *
Pediatrics
900 Kiely Blvd
Santa Clara, CA   95051
(408) 236-5025
Vol Clin Faculty

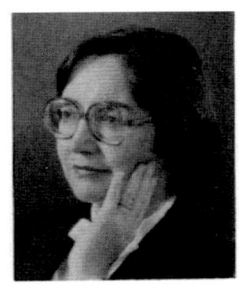

Rosenstock, Lynn L B
Anesthesiology
701 Welch Rd #216
Palo Alto, CA   94301
323-0617
Clin Asst Prof

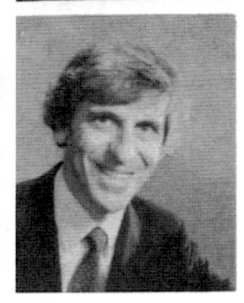

Samuels, Stanley I
Anesthesiology *
Stanford Univ Med Sch
Dept of Anesthesia
Stanford, CA   94305
723-6411
Prof

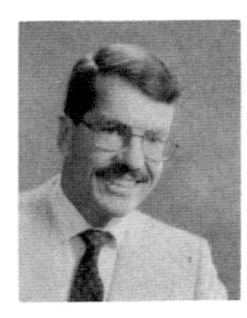

Sarnquist, Frank H
Anesthesiology *
Stanford Univ Med Ctr
Dept of Anesthsia #H-3580
Stanford, CA   94305
723-6411
Assoc Prof

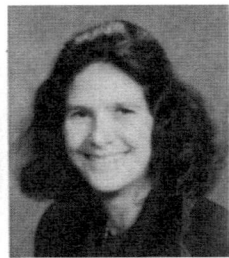

Shafer, Audrey
Anesthesiology *
Palo Alto Med Clinic
Dept of Anesthesia
Palo Alto, CA   94304
858-3938
Asst Prof

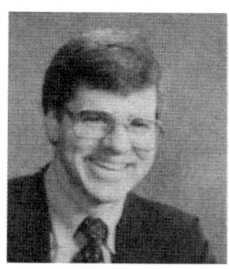

Shafer, Steven L
Anesthesiology *
Pharmacology, Clinical
3801 Miranda
Palo Alto, CA 94304
852-3419
Asst Prof

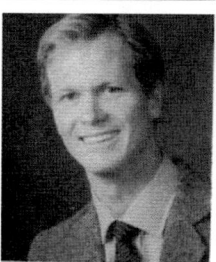

Singleton, Mark A
Anesthesiology
111 Alta Tierra Ct
Los Gatos, CA 95032
(408) 395-6838
Clin Asst Prof

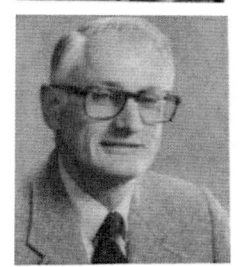

Stocker, William A
Anesthesiology *
701 Welch Rd
Palo Alto, CA 94306
323-0617
Clin Faculty

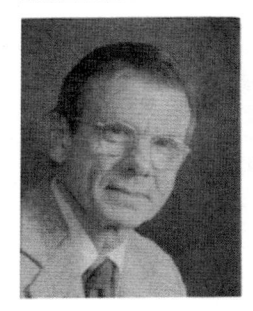

Whitcher, Charles E
Anesthesiology
Stanford Univ Med Ctr
#S-278
Stanford, CA 94305
723-6411
Prof

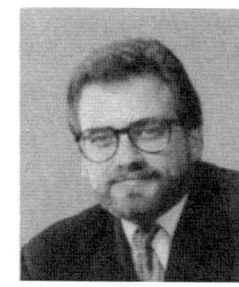

Siegel, Lawrence C
Anesthesiology *
Stanford Univ Med Ctr
Dept of Anesthesia
Stanford, CA 94305
723-6411
Asst Prof

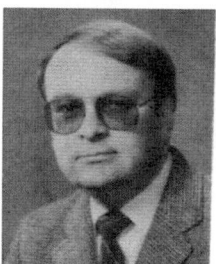

Stanski, Donald R
Anesthesiology *
3801 Miranda Ave
Palo Alto, CA 94304
723-5910
Prof

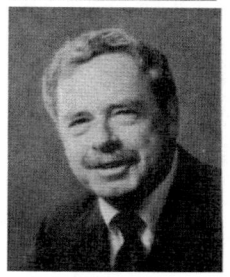

Wheaton, Kevin R
Anesthesiology *
300 Homer
Palo Alto, CA 94321
321-4121
Clin Prof

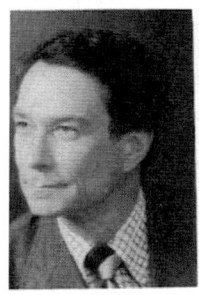

Winchester, Lynn W
Anesthesiology
300 Homer Ave
Palo Alto, CA 94301
321-4121
Clin Prof

[NO PHOTOGRAPH]

Carolyn Bahl	Courtesy Teaching
Walter Bernard	Courtesy Teaching
Michael Champeau	Clinical Assistant Professor
John Cooper	Clinical Instructor
Michael Cully	Courtesy Teaching
Patricia Curtis	Clinical Instructor
Larry Feld	Clinical Assistant Professor
David Fitzgerald	Active
William Forrest	Professor
Thomas Gaston	Clinical Instructor
Gerald Holguin	Clinical Instructor
John Loftus	Clinical Instructor
Michael Mellenthin	Courtesy Teaching
Lisa Saunders	Clinical Instructor
Thomas Schares	Clinical Instructor
Sonja Sorbo	Clinical Assistant Professor
Gwen Stritter	Active
Gordon Taylor	Clinical Professor
John Urbanowicz	Clinical Assistant Professor
Christopher Vasil	Assistant Professor
Janet Wyner	Clinical Associate Professor
Joseph Zweng	Active

CHAPTER 15

PHOTOGRAPHS

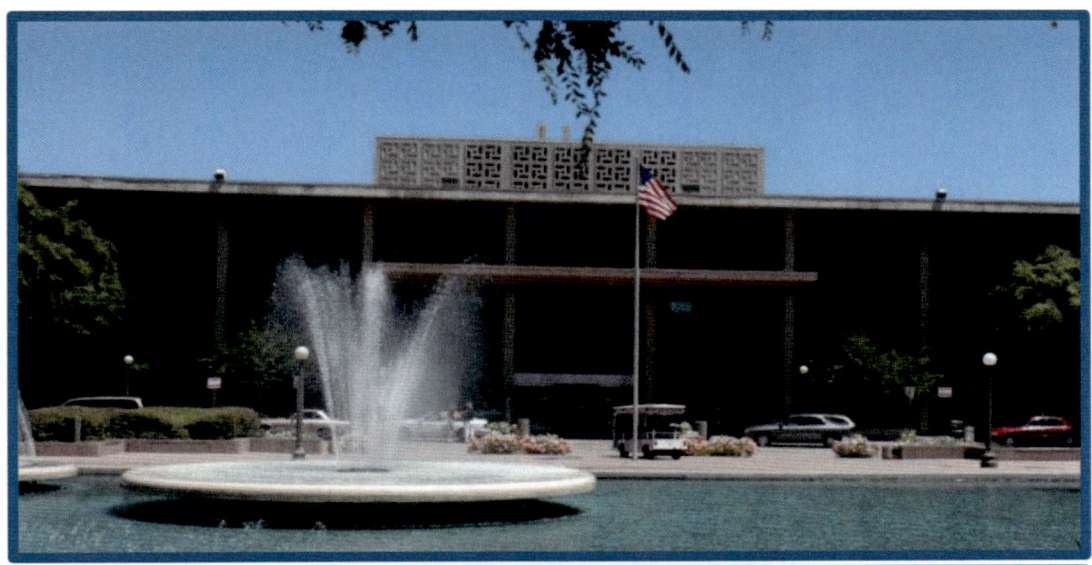

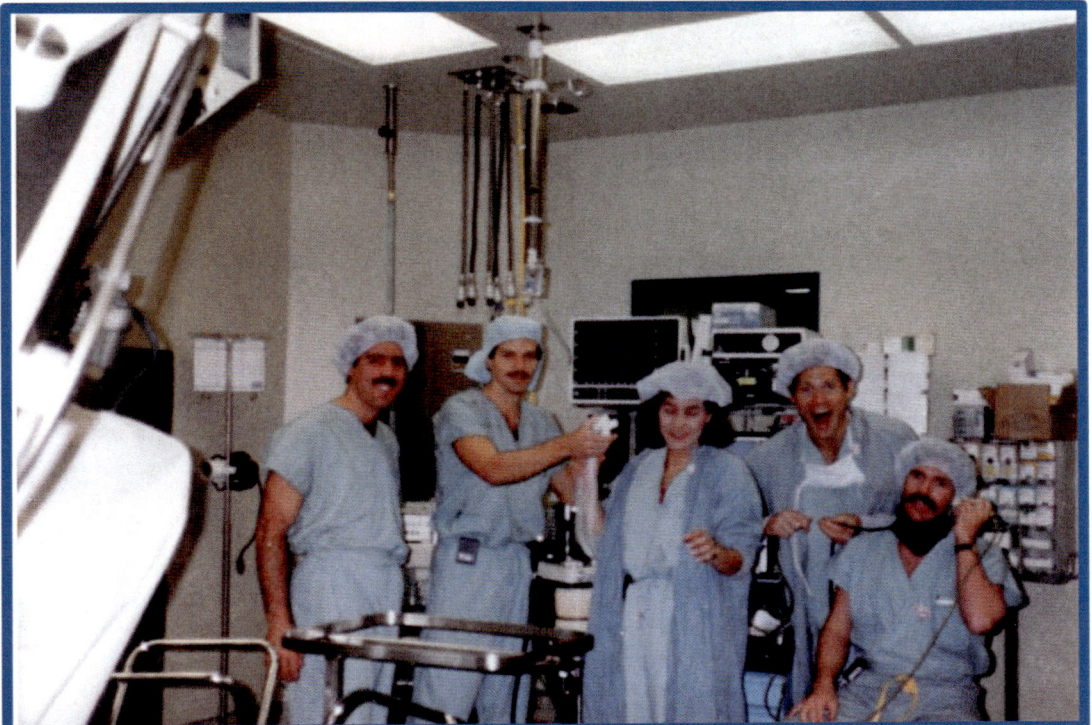

Moving into the new Operating Rooms at 500 Pasteur Dr (1989)
(L-R) Darell Tanelian, Dave Fitzgerald, Kristi Peterson, George Wakerlin, Brad Beebe

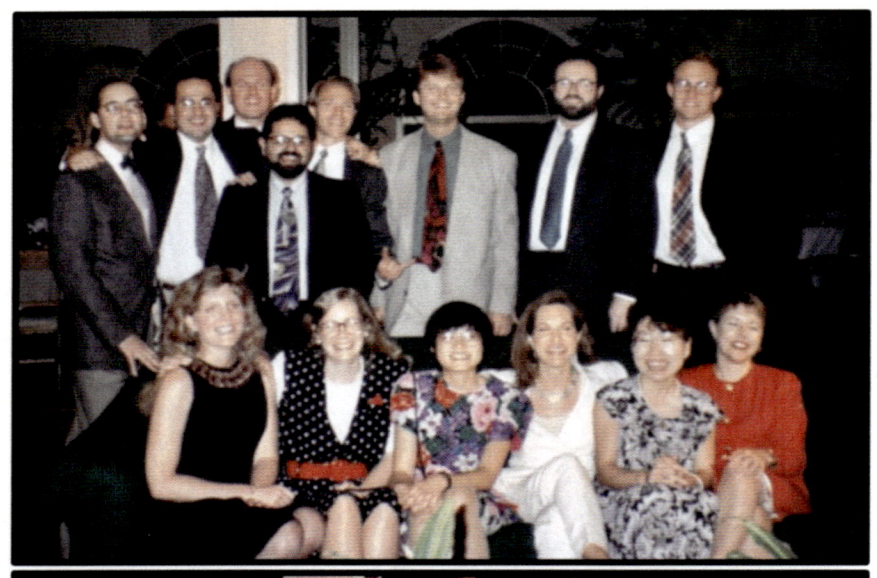

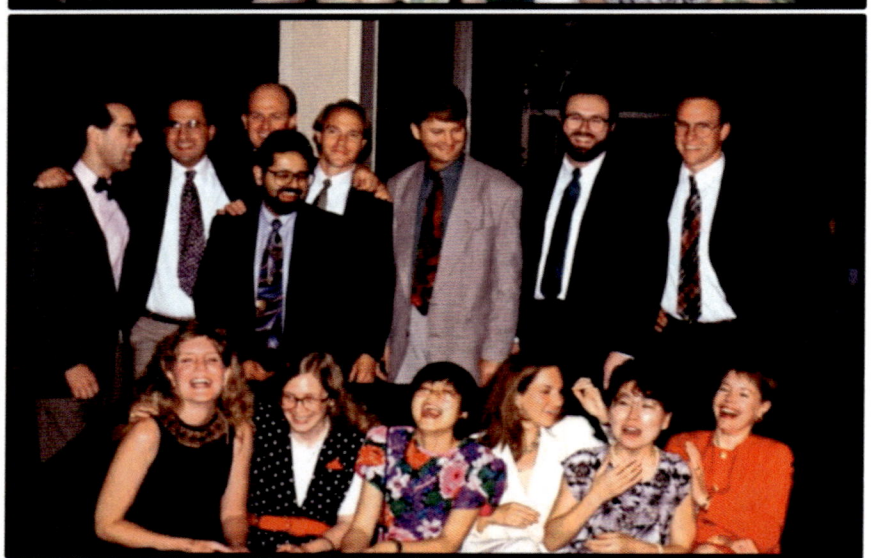

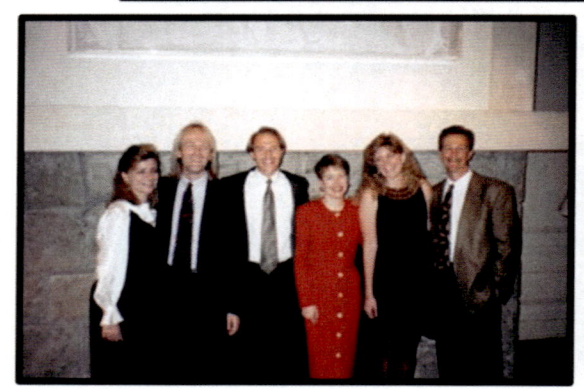

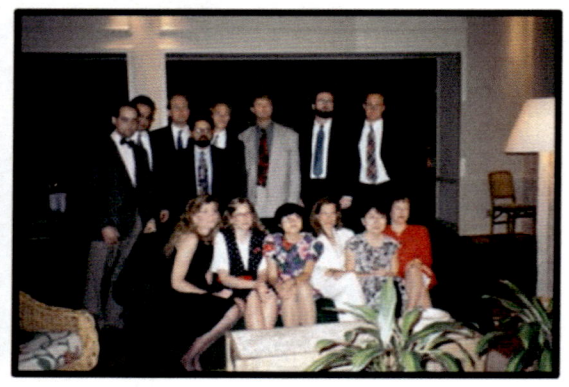

1991-1994 Resident graduation
[Missing Fabian Okonski]

235

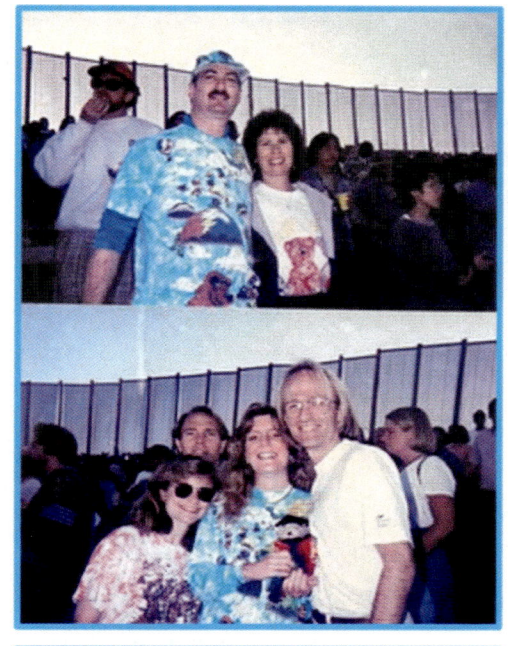

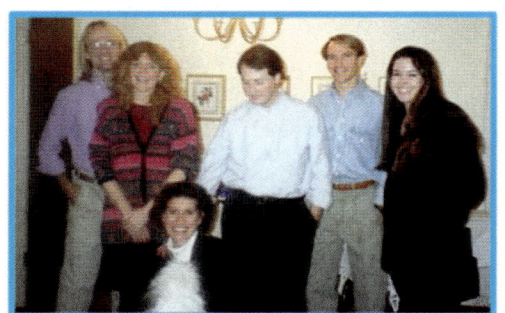

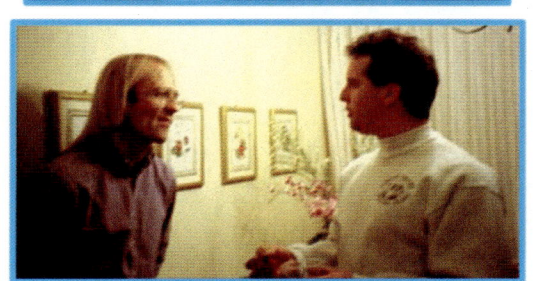

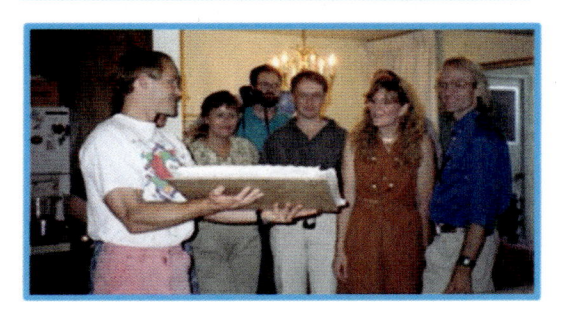

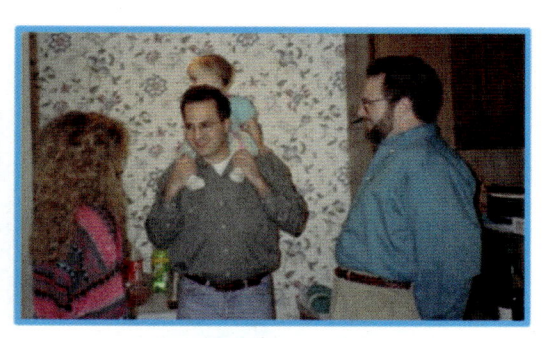

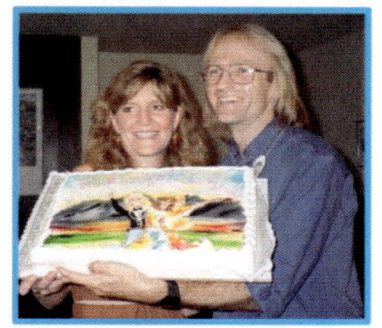

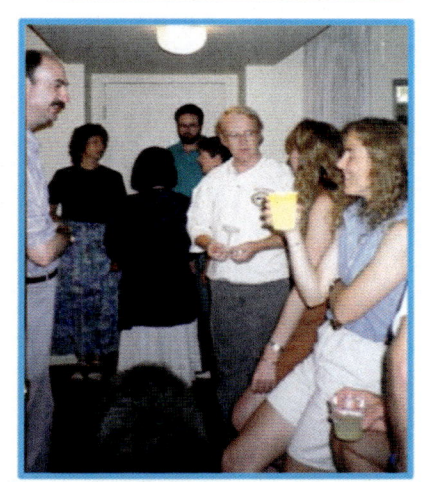

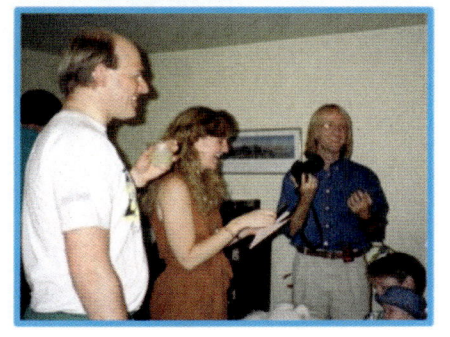

236

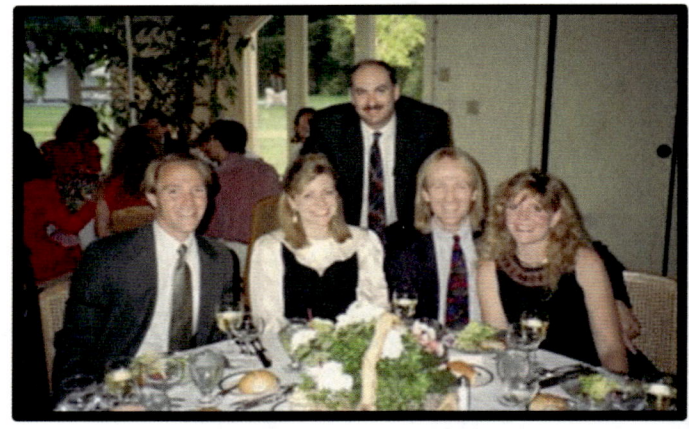

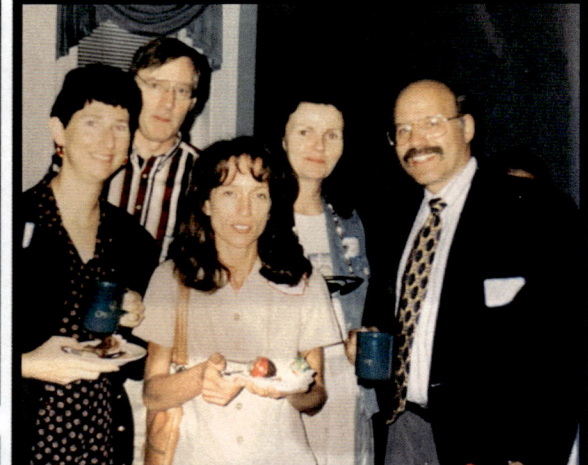

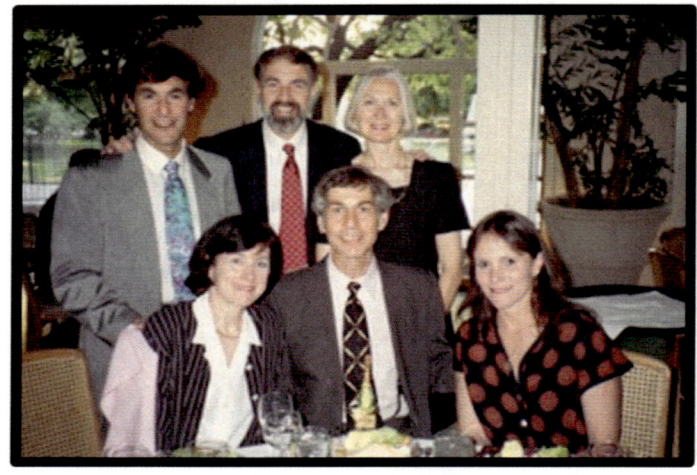

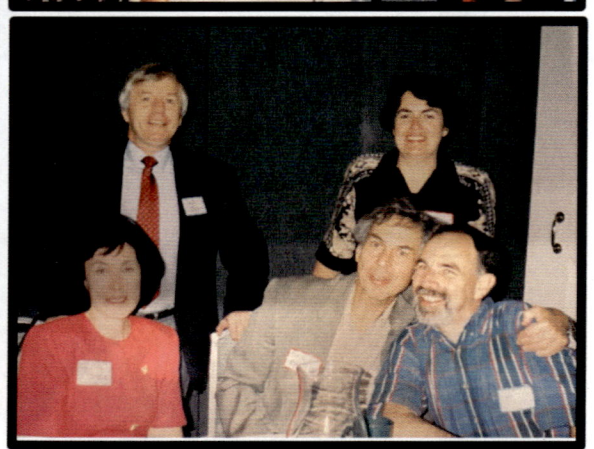

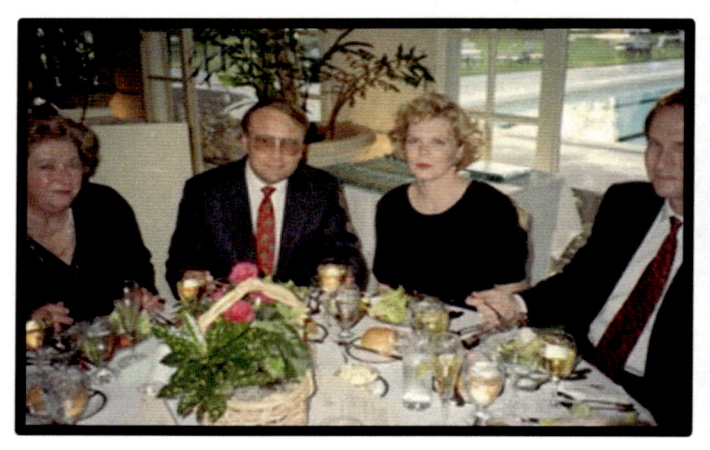

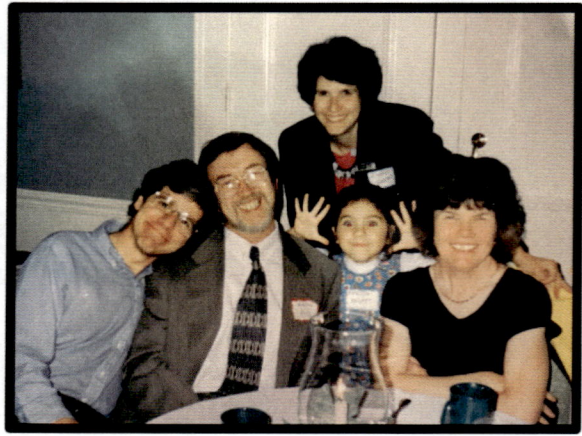

Associated Anesthesiologists Medical Group (AAMG) and guests throughout the years

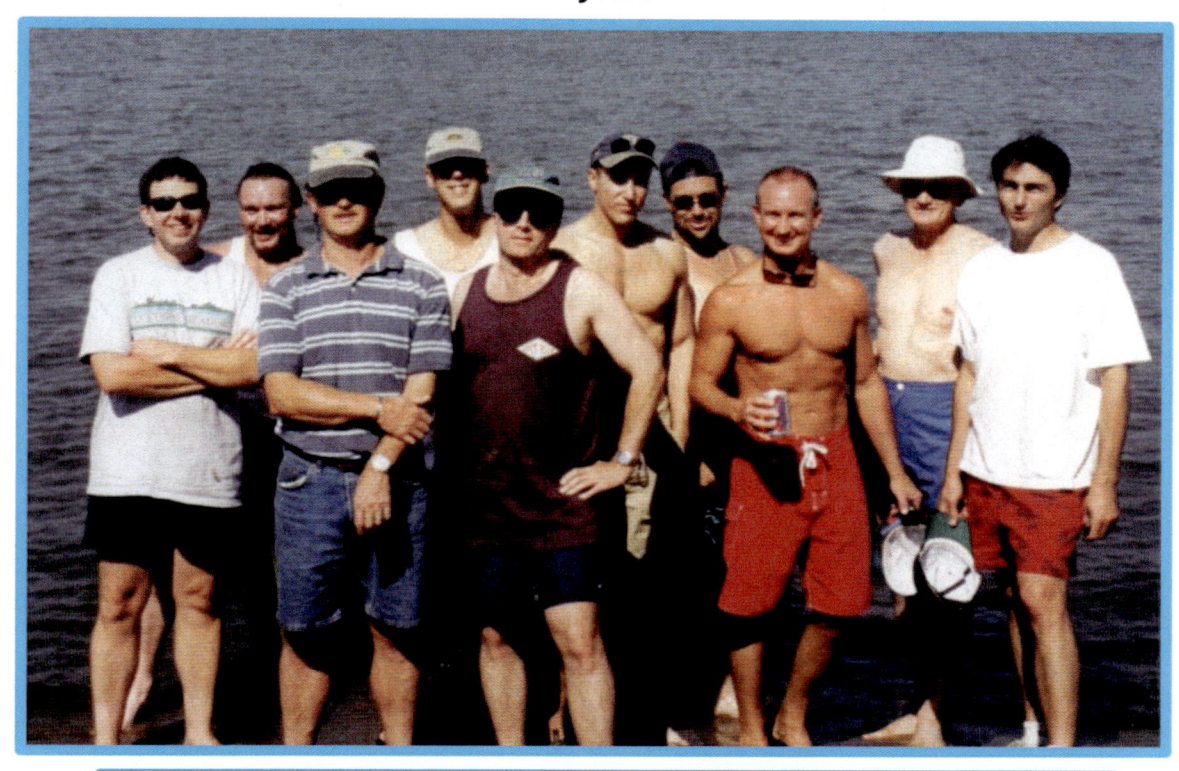

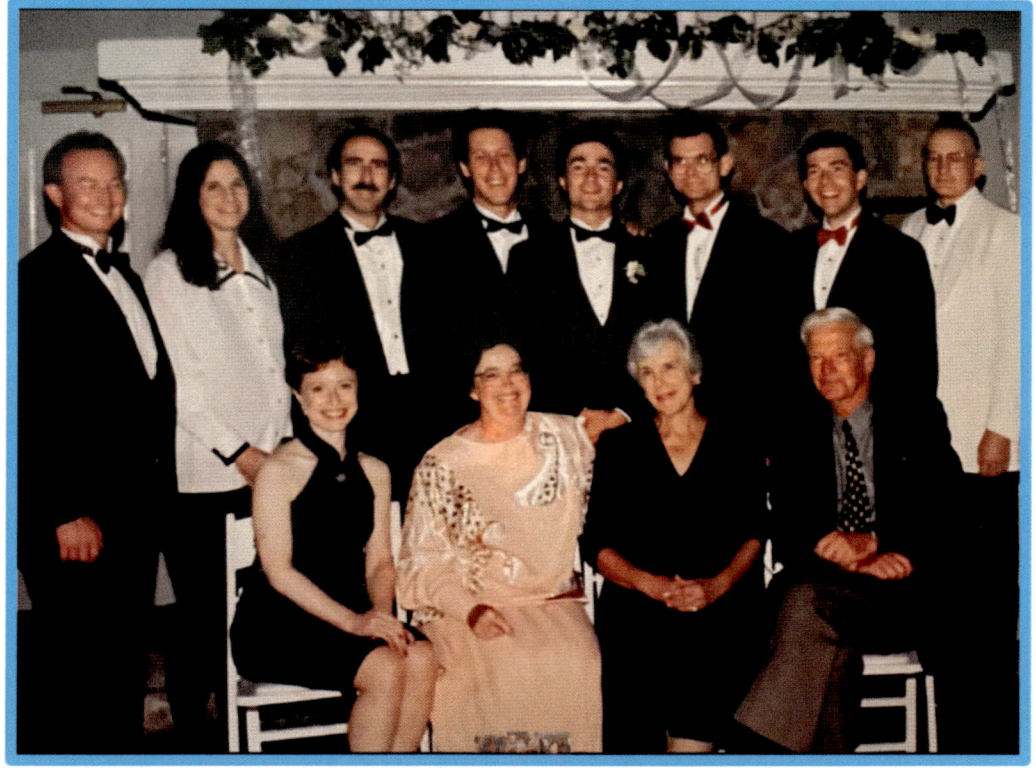

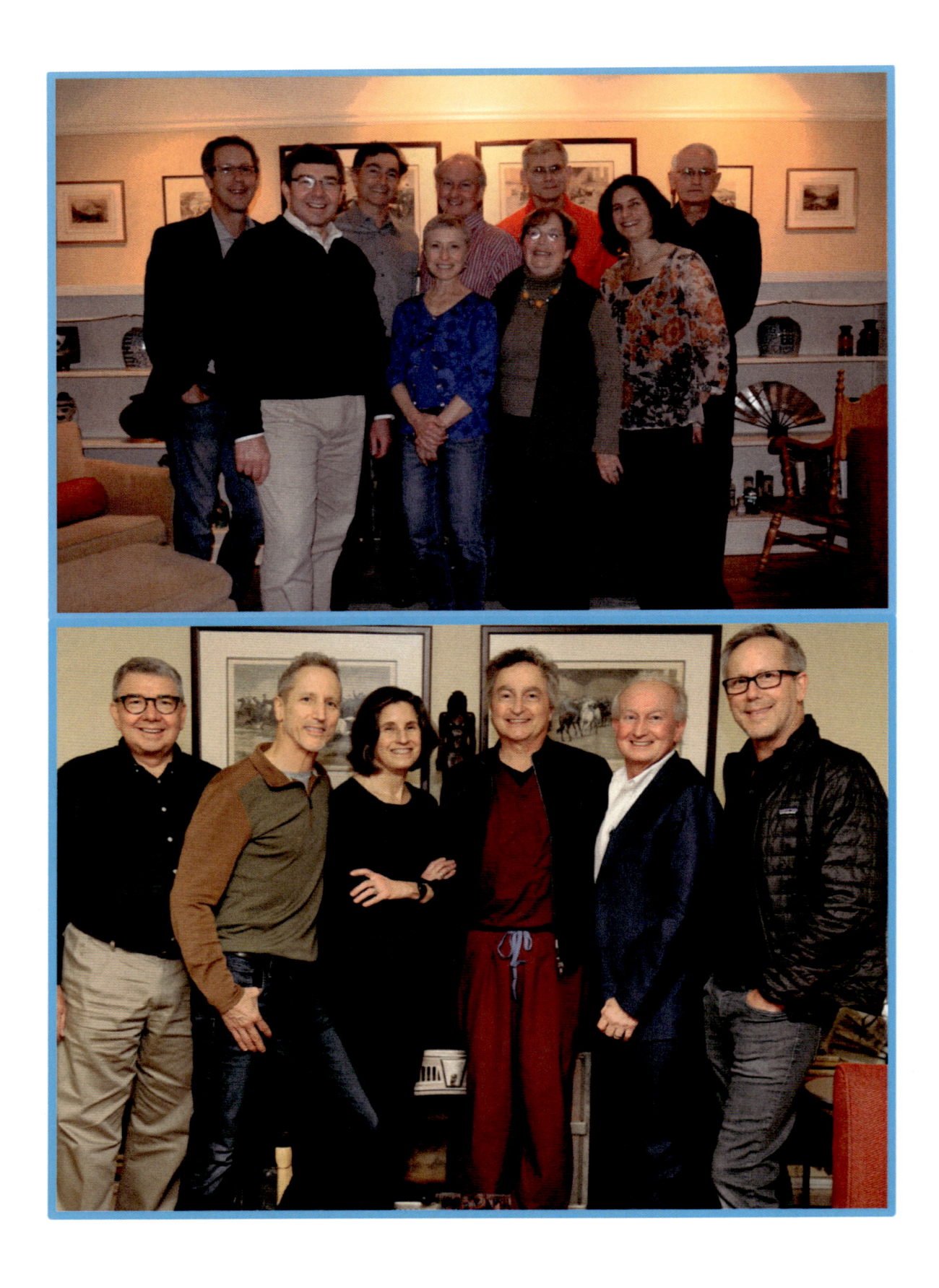

(L-R) Steve Shafer, Thomas Schnider, Charles Minto, and Talmage Egan at a conference honoring Dr. Schnider's retirement (Salzburg, Austria, August 2023)

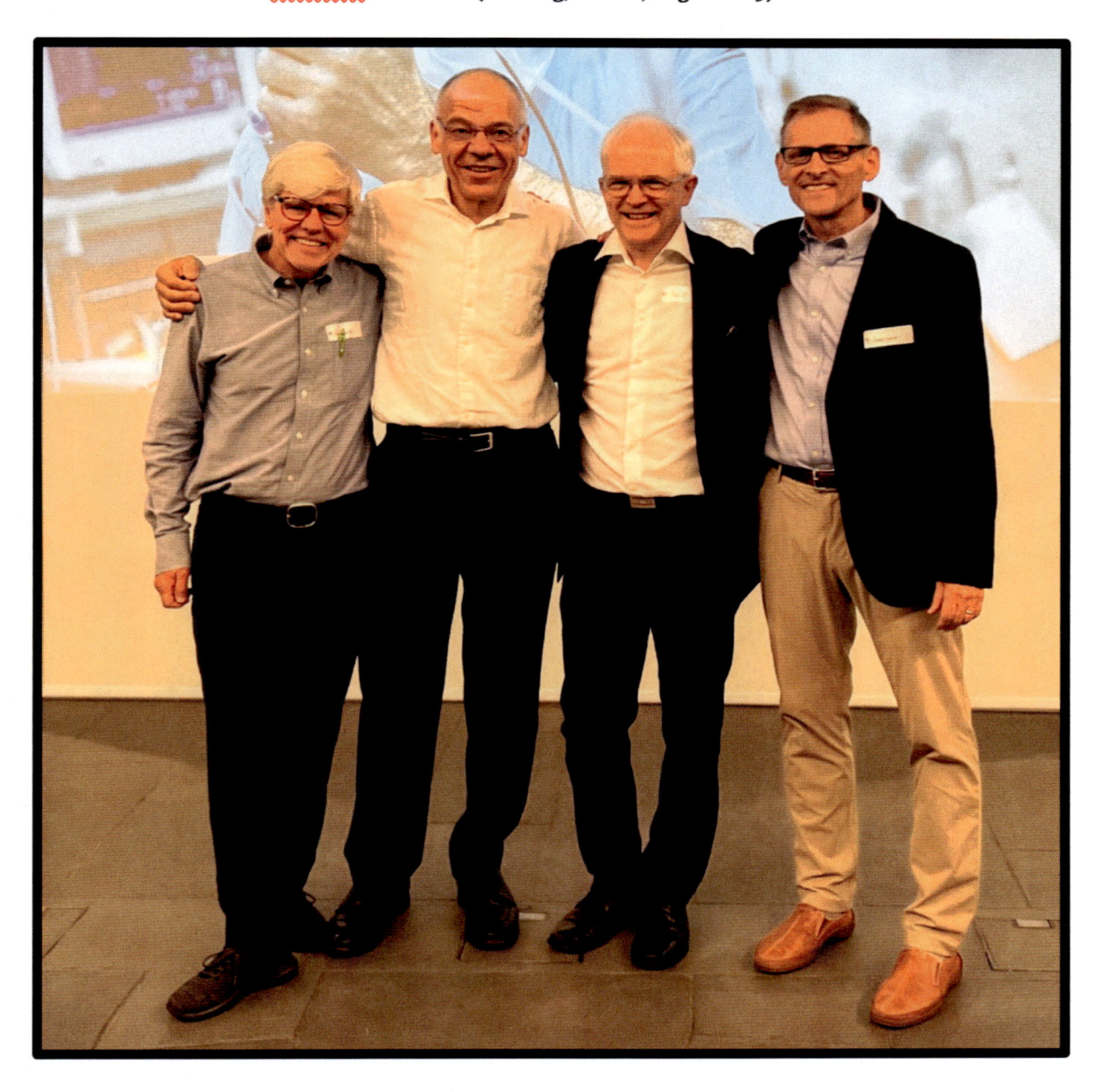

2016

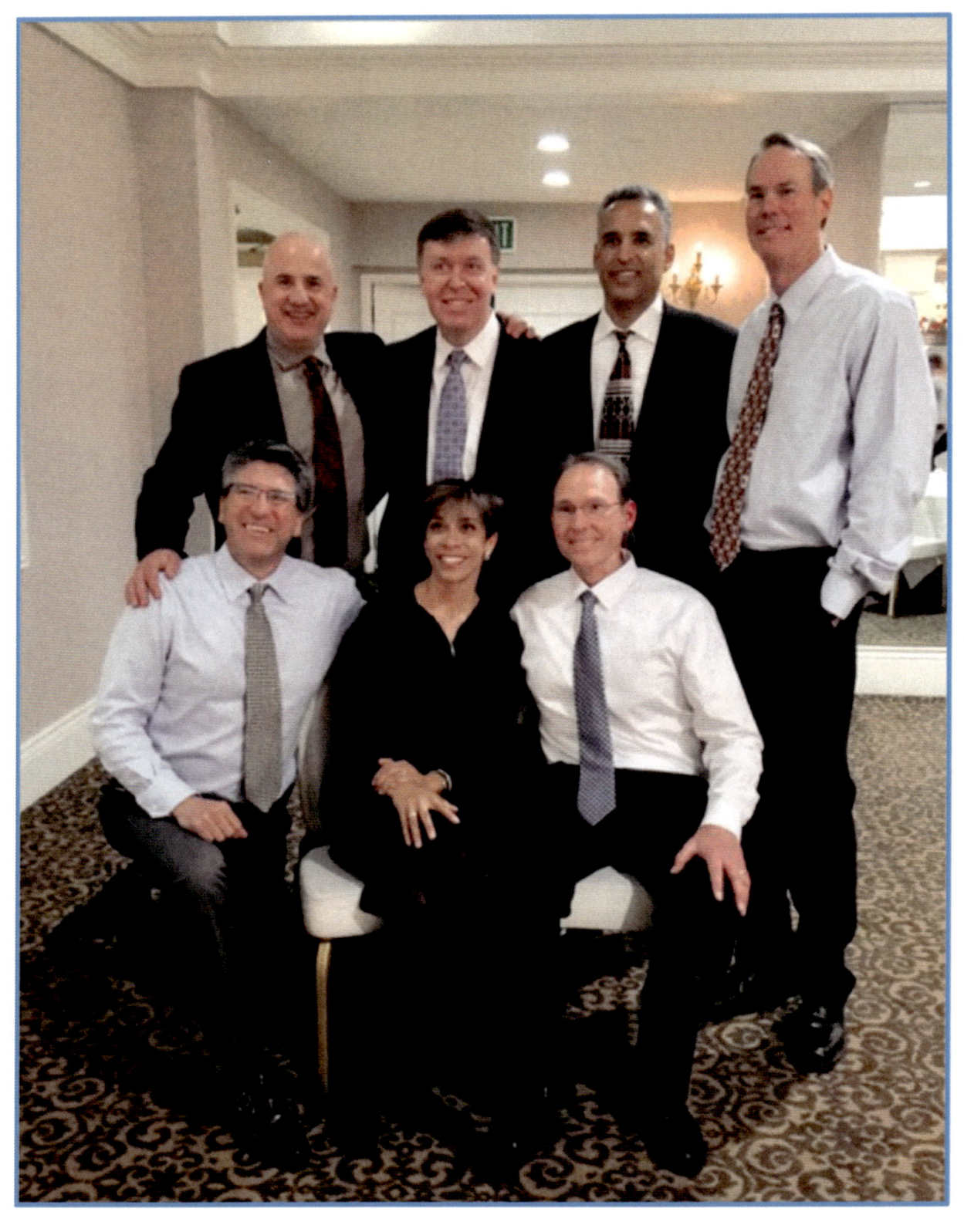

241

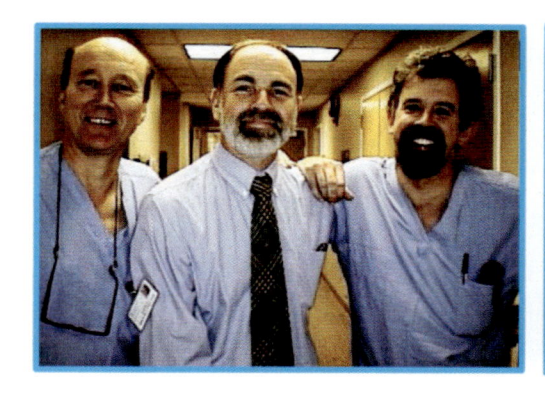

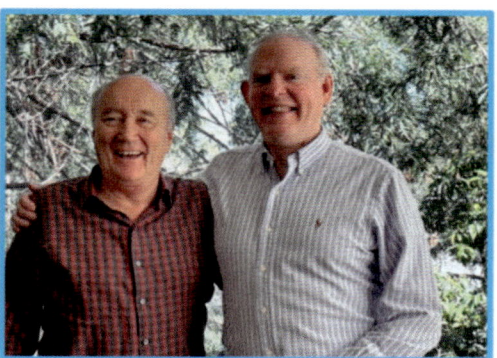

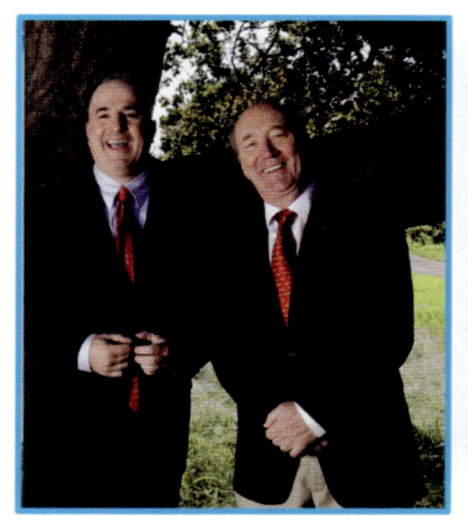

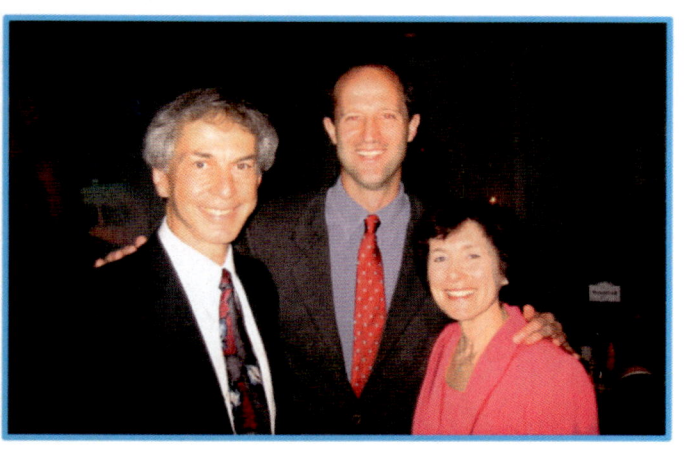

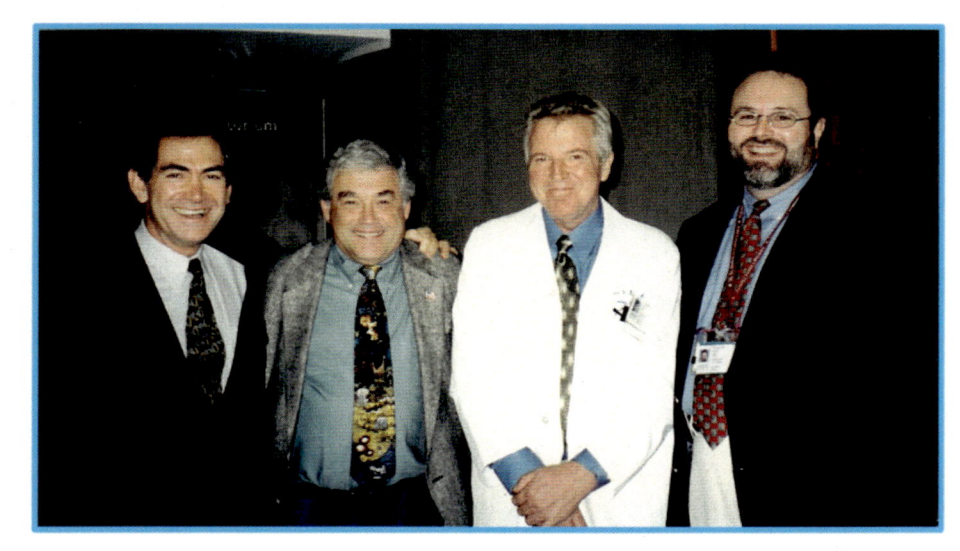

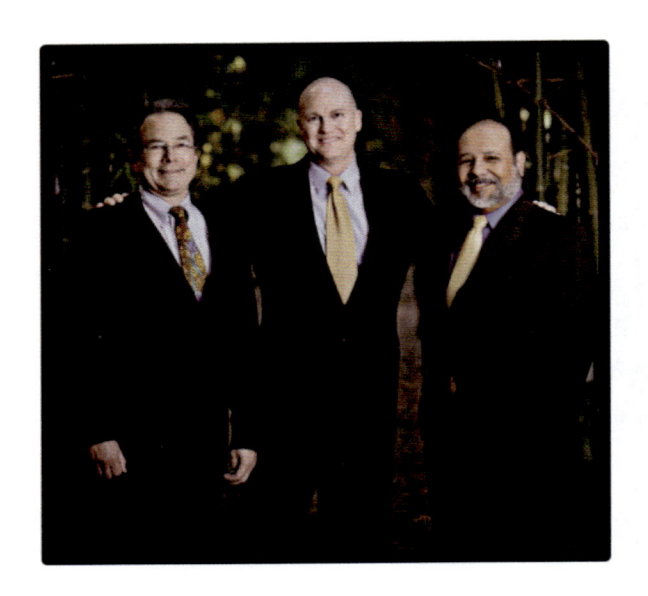

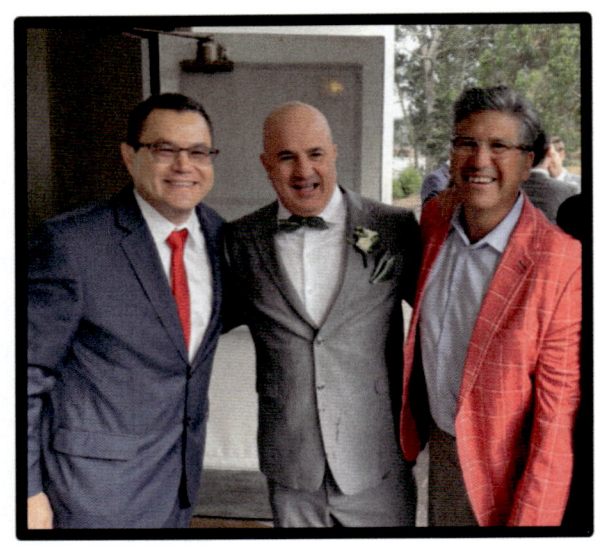

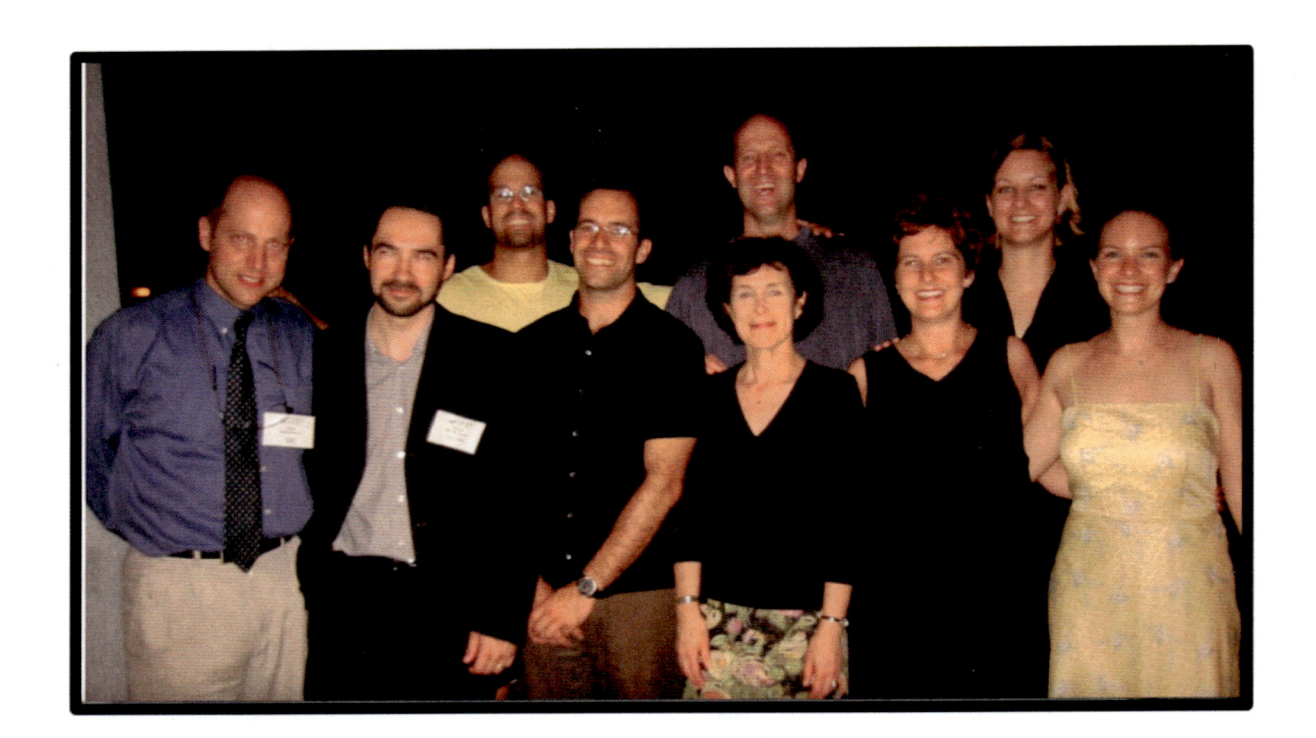

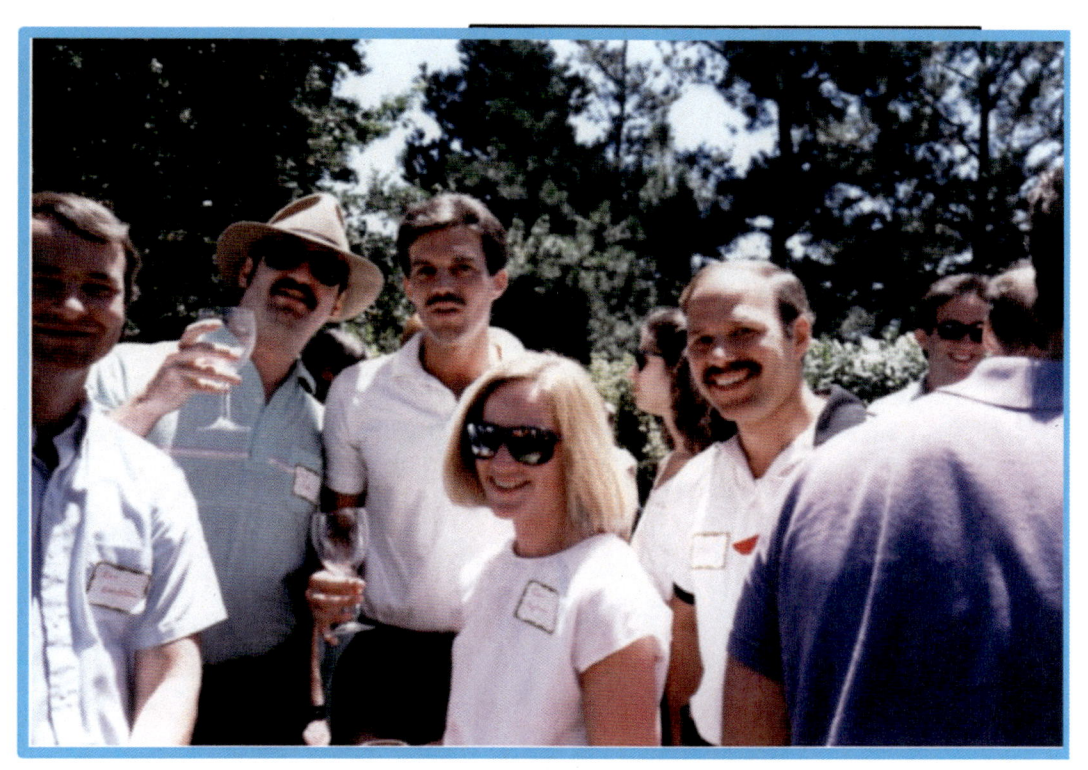

(L-R) Ray Engstrom, Dave Gaba, Dave Fitzgerald, Chris Engstrom (Ray's wife), Ron Pearl, with Lisa Saunders and Ted Kreitzman in background (1990)

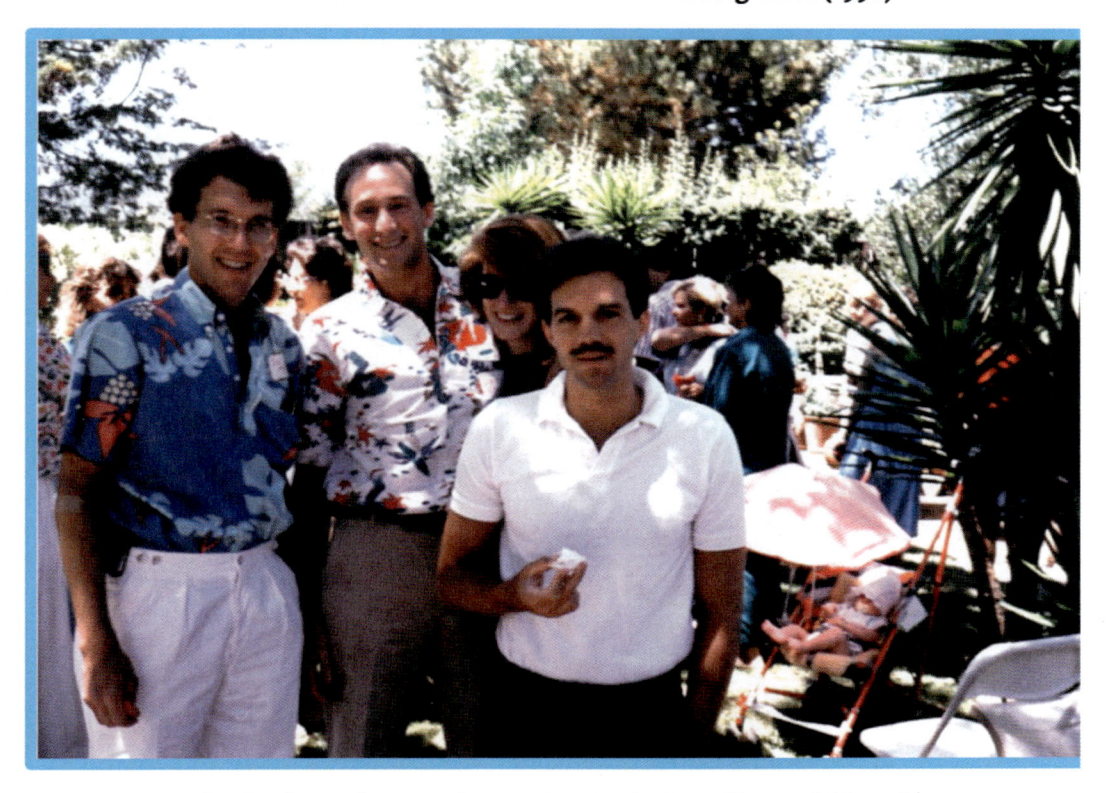

(L-R) John Archer, Leo Stemp, Pat Curtis, Dave Fitzgerald (1990)

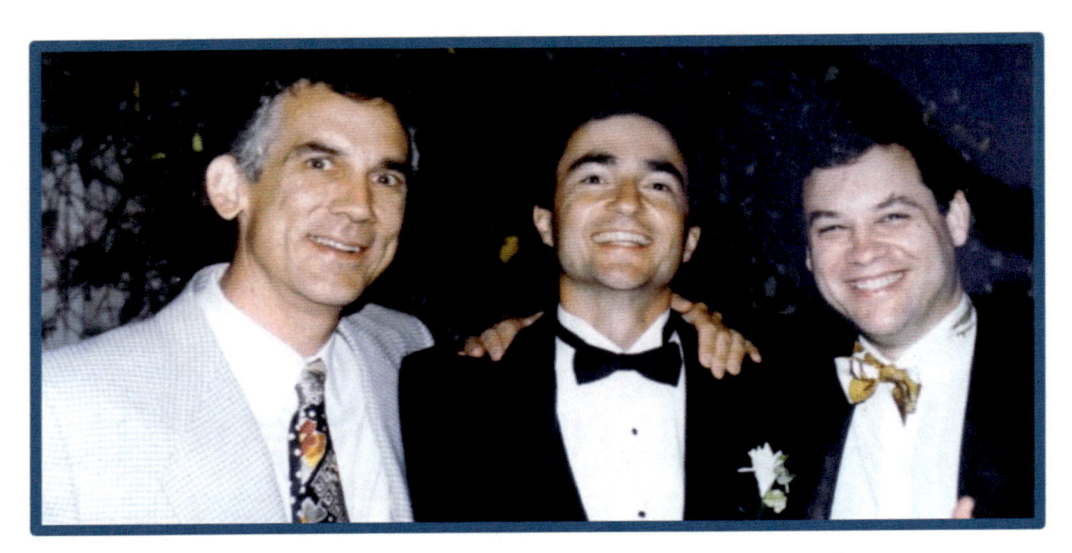

(L-R) Joe Andresen, Rick Novak, Milford Zasslow (1987)

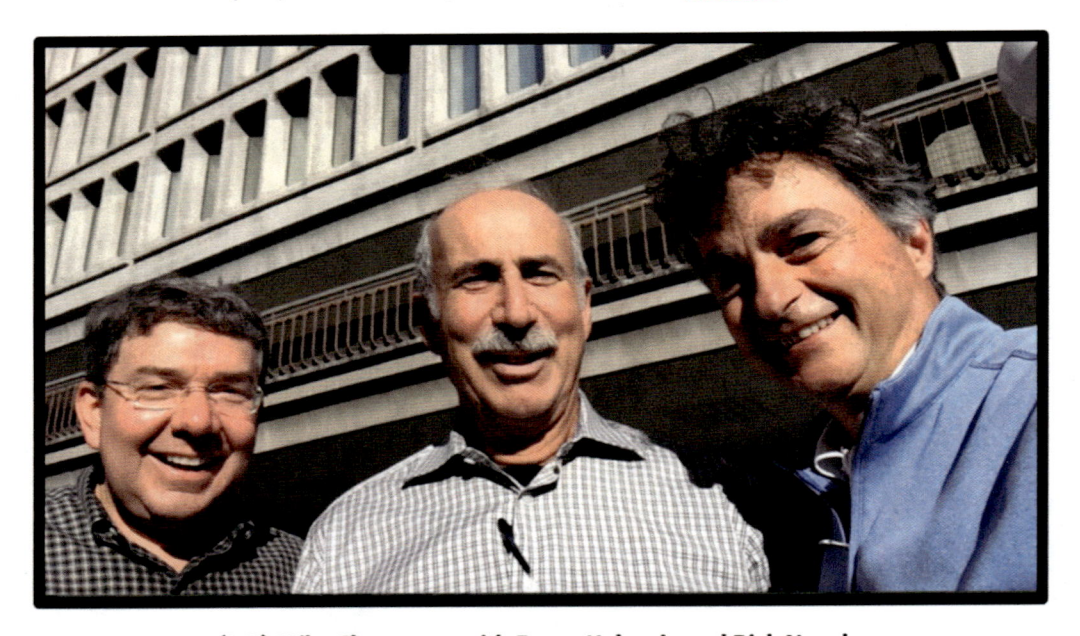

(L-R) Mike Champeau with Bruce Halperin and Rick Novak.

RESIDENTS (STARTING YEAR)

1983
David Stuart Anish
James Brian Bird
Michael Warren Champeau
James Tsung Chang
Brian Douglas Hershey
Paul Steven Hummel* (1984-1985)
Steven Charles Merlone* (1985-1986)
Ronald Gary Pearl
Michele Eileen Raney
Thomas Schares
Barry Nathaniel Swerdlow
Lorna Yoshi Yamaguchi
Paul Ying-Si Wong
Milford Alan Zasslow

1984
Brian Dirk Bohman*
Michael Dale Cully
Ann Arbetter Fischell
Steven Roy Ford
Thomas Lloyd Gaston
Neil Francis Marley
Richard John Novak
James Edward Pearson
Joshua Philip Prager (CA2)
Wendy Rabinov
Dana Wolf Rosenberg
Lisa Dianne Saunders
Leila Vieno Maria Siukola
John Henry Urbanowicz
Daniel Alan Waxer
Lawrence Babbit Weiss

1985
Leslie Comer Andes
Joseph Stanley Andresen
Edward Robert Baer
William George Brose* (1987-1988)
John Robert Cooper* (1986-1987)
Kelley Louis Crawford
Stephen Paul Fischer
Robert Mathew Hansen
Karel Merlin Kretzchmar
George Ichung Lee
Donald Miller Mason Jr
Ira Scott Segal
Gwendolyn Marie Stritter
Darrel Lee Tanelian
Amanda Dawn Tucker
Theodore Henry Tuschka

(X) Completed entire residency at Stanford
(X) Did portion of residency at Stanford
(X) Did not complete anesthesia residency
* Chief Resident (year)

1986
Bradley William Beebe
David Norman Buckley (CA3)
Sandra Reading Chaplan* (1988-1989)
Robert Joseph Cosgrove
Ray Holladay Engstrom
David Curtis Fitzgerald
Theresa Chun Flory
Rona Greenberg Giffard
Malcolm Warrington Howard (CA3)
Richard A. Jaffe
Robert Paul Kaye
Frederick Jonathan Long
Steven Laurence Marlowe
Kristi Lyn Peterson
Glenn Douglas Rennels
Steven L. Shafer
Lawrence Charles Siegel (CA3)
George E. Wakerlin Jr

1987
John Hoffman Archer* (1989-1990)
Carolyn Anita Bahl
Juliana Barr
Walter David Bernard
Patricia Elizabeth Curtis
Jean Gordon
Ernest Hayward Jr
Curtis Orland McMillan
Donald William Milne (CA3)
Friedrich Ekkehart Moritz
Carl Edward Noe (CA3)
Steven Travis Peake (CA3)
Marilyn Jeannie Roper
Dianne Mansfield Runyan
Lynn M. Scannell
Leo I. Stemp
Charles Henry Tadlock
Bradley Jonathan Thomas
Kristi Ann Watson

1988
Wayne Raleigh Anderson
Thomas White Cutter (CA1)
Ray Richard Gaeta
Allen George Gruber
Gerald A. Holguin
Steven Keith Howard
Shale Foster Imeson (CA3)
Ted Robert Kreitzman
Linda Rose Mignano
Emily Florence Ratner* (1990-1991)
Richard Snyder
Adrian George Tedeschi (CA3)
Christopher James Vasil
Vanessa Thien Vu
David Paul Whalen

1989
Daniel Raphael Azar
Kirtikumar Gopalji Desai (CA2, CA3)
James Crampton Finn III
David Minoru Fujii
John George Kelley
Peter Single Kosek
Blair Stephen Lee
Mei-Ven Chang Lo
Dennis Michael Lindeborg
Wai-Keung Loh
John Raymond Lubben (CA3)
Michael A. Mellenthin Jr (CA3)
Joel Anthony Peelen* (1991-1992)
Joseph Buford Pollard
Jon Wallace Propst
E. Price Stover

1990
Kariem Hakim Ali
Edward John Bertachini
Talmadge Dan Egan (CA3)
Paul James Elcavage
Michael Edwin Ennis
Steven Douglas Glacy (CA3)
Kimberly Anne Hanson
Thurman Eugene Hunt
George Lederhaas
William Cooper Longton
Edward Terry Riley* (1992-1993)
Berklee Robins
John Mark Schwab (CA3)
Clinton Lee Warne
Matthew Francis White
Elizabeth Joricia Youngs
Kenneth Paul Zuckerman

1991
Gregory Harnett Botz
Grace Chun
Jenifer Jo Damewood
Doris Mary Donoghue
Joseph S. Dunn (CA3)
Mark Allen Eggen
Lauren Anne Elliot
Catherine Lee Hamilton
Martha Cox Ho
Alex Macario* (1993-1994)
Thomas T. Nguyen
Fernando Fabian Okonski
Beemeth Tzaraoh Robles
Adam Jon Rubinstein
Joshua Ben Siegel
Helen Bao Tam
Bryan Peter Tunink

1992
Russell Hughes Allen
Kayvan Ariani
James M. Bell (CA2, CA3)
Helmuth Thorlakur Billy
Susan Kay Browne
Charles Anthony Boudreaux
Jeffrey Paul Clayton
Douglas Eugene Crockett
Michael Patrick Keating
Steven Paul Laitin
Richard Cary Mantin
John Edward Massey
Ricardo Barraza Ronquillo* (1994-1995)
Dean Stanton Walker

INDEX

[A]
Kariem Hakim Ali
167-169
Russell Hughes Allen
194
Wayne Raleigh Anderson
124
Leslie Comer Andes
58
Joseph Stanley Andresen
59-61
David Stuart Anish
9
John Hoffman Archer
110
Daniel Raphael Azar
147-149
Kayvan Ariani
194-196

[B]
Edward Robert Baer
61
Carolyn Anita Bahl
110-113
Juliana Barr
113-114
Bradley William Beebe
78
Diana Gillian Beeby
216
James M. Bell
204
Walter David Bernard
114
Edward John Bertachini
152
Helmuth Thorlakur Billy
204
James Brian Bird
9
Brian Dirk Bohman
20-21
Bruce Allen Bollen
205-206
Gregory Harnett Botz
173-174
Charles A. Boudreaux
197
William George Brose
62
Susan Kay Browne
196
David Norman Buckley
80-81

[C]
Michael W. Champeau
10-11
James Tsung Chang
11
Sandra Reading Chaplan
82-83
Grace Chun
174-176
Jeffrey Paul Clayton
197-199
John Robert Cooper
63-64
Robert Joseph Cosgrove
97
Kelley Louis Crawford
78
Douglas Eugene Crockett
199
Michael Dale Cully
21
Patricia Elizabeth Curtis
114
Thomas White Cutter
135

[D]
Jenifer Jo Damewood
176-178
Robin Davidson
218
Kirtikumar Gopalji Desai
145
Doris Mary Donoghue
190
Joseph S. Dunn
189-190

[E]
William F. Ebling
219
Talmadge Dan Egan
164-166
Mark Allen Eggen
178-180
Paul James Elcavage
152
Lauren Anne Elliot
180
Ray Holladay Engstrom
83-86
Michael Edwin Ennis
152-154

[F]
Henry Barrie Fairley
39-55
Lawrence Howard Feld
206
James Crampton Finn III
138
Ann Arbetter Fischell
21-23
Stephen Paul Fischer
65-66
David Curtis Fitzgerald
Theresa Chun Flory
87
Richard Joseph Flynn
218
Steven Roy Ford
23-25
David Minoru Fujii
138
Masahiko Fujinaga
219

[G]
Ray Richard Gaeta
124-125
Thomas Lloyd Gaston
25
Rona Greenberg Giffard
87-88
Steven Douglas Glacy
166
Jean Gordon
121

Allen George Gruber
135

[H]
Gordon Rowat Haddow
206-207
Catherine Lee Hamilton
180
Robert Mathew Hansen
67-68
Kimberly Anne Hanson
154-155
Ernest Hayward Jr
114-116
Brian Douglas Hershey
11
Martha Cox Ho
181-182
Gerald A. Holguin
125-126
Steven Keith Howard
127-130
Malcolm Howard
88
Thurman Eugene Hunt
155
Paul Steven Hummel
11

[I]
Shale Foster Imeson
135

[J]
Richard A. Jaffe
99-108

[K]
Robert Paul Kaye
89
Michael Patrick Keating
199
John George Kelley
139-141
Peter Single Kosek
142
Ted Robert Kreitzman
130
Karel Merlin Kretzchmar
69

[L]
Steven Paul Laitin
200
George Lederhaas
156
George Ichung Lee
69
Blair Stephen Lee
142
Harry Lemmens
191
Yuan-Chi Lin
207-209
Dennis Michael Lindeborg
142-143
Lawrence Litt
210-211
Mei-Ven Chang Lo
143
John Richard Loftus
211-212
Wai-Keung Loh
145
Frederick Jonathan Long
97
William Cooper Longton
157
John Raymond Lubben
145

[M]
Alex Macario
182-184
M. Bruce MacIver
220-221
Richard Cary Mantin
200-201
James Margary
216-217
Neil Francis Marley
38
Steven Laurence Marlowe
89
Donald Miller Mason Jr
69-70
John Edward Massey
201-202
Diana Beeby McGregor
216
Robert E. McKlveen
212-213

Curtis Orland McMillan
116
Michael A. Mellenthin Jr
145-146
Steven Charles Merlone
12
Linda Rose Mignano
130-131
Donald William Milne
118
Charles F. Minto
217
Friedrich Ekkehart Moritz
116
Robert Joseph Moynihan
213-214

[N]
Thomas T. Nguyen
190
Carl Edward Noe
119
Richard John Novak
26-27

[O]
Fernando Fabian Okonski
184-185

[P]
Steven Travis Peake
119
Ronald Gary Pearl
17-18
James Edward Pearson
37
Joel Anthony Peelen
143
Kristi Lyn Peterson
90-91
Joseph Buford Pollard
143
Joshua Philip Prager
27-29
Jon Wallace Propst
143-144
Audrey Gladys Pullens
222-223

[R]

Wendy Rabinov
29
Michele Eileen Raney
12-14
Emily Florence Ratner
131-133
Glenn Douglas Rennels
91-92
Edward Terry Riley
157-158
Berklee Robins
159
Beemeth Tzaraoh Robles
185-186
Ricardo Barraza Ronquillo
202-203
Marilyn Jeannie Roper
116
Dana Wolf Rosenberg
38
Adam Jon Rubinstein
186-187
Dianne Mansfield Runyan
121

[S]

Lisa Dianne Saunders
30-31
Lynn M. Scannell
121
Thomas Schares
14
John Mark Schwab
167
Ira Scott Segal
71
Barry C. Sellick
216
Audrey C. Shafer
214-215
Steven L. Shafer
94-96
Joshua Ben Siegel
187

Lawrence Charles Siegel
97
Leila Vieno Maria Siukola
32-34
Richard Snyder
133-134
Leo I. Stemp
120-121
E. Price Stover
144
Gwendolyn Marie Stritter
71-73
Barry Nathaniel Swerdlow
14-15

[T]

Charles Henry Tadlock
117
Helen Bao Tam
190
Darrel Lee Tanelian
74-75
Adrian George Tedeschi
135
Bradley Jonathan Thomas
117
Virginia F. Tse
221-222
Amanda Dawn Tucker
75-76
Bryan Peter Tunink
187-189
Theodore Henry Tuschka
76-78

[U]

John Henry Urbanowicz
34

[V]

Christopher James Vasil
134
Vanessa Thien Vu
134-135

[W]

George E. Wakerlin Jr
93
Dean Stanton Walker
203
John Walker
218
Clinton Lee Warne
159-160
Kristi Ann Watson
118
Daniel Alan Waxer
35-37
Lawrence Babbit Weiss
38
David Paul Whalen
135
Matthew Francis White
161
Paul Ying-Si Wong
15

[Y]

Lorna Yoshi Yamaguchi
15-16
Elizabeth Joricia Youngs
161-162

[Z]

Milford Alan Zasslow
16-17
John Zelcer
217-218
Kenneth Paul Zuckerman
163-164

ACKNOWLEDGEMENTS: The editors would like to thank Dr. Brian Bateman, Chair of the Department of Anesthesiology, Perioperative and Pain Medicine, for the support he has given to us for this and our other book projects. We also appreciate the work of Debbi Ramus and Carolyn Rebello who helped us contact many of the former residents, Fellows, and faculty members that are mentioned in this book. And most importantly, we wish to thank and recognize the individuals who submitted biographical information, and many contributed their personal memories and photographs. Without their help we could not have produced this book.

KARRIEM ALI	RONA GIFFARD	JOHN MASSEY
RUSSELL ALLEN	GORDON HADDOW	LINDA MIGNANO
WAYNE ANDERSON	ROBERT HANSEN	CHARLES MINTO
JOSEPH ANDRESEN	ERNEST HAYWARD	MICHELE RANEY
LESLIE ANDES	MARTHA HO	EMILY RATNER
KAYVAN ARIANI	GERALD HOLGUIN	GLENN RENNELS
DAN AZAR	STEVE HOWARD	ED RILEY
ED BAER	ROBERT KAYE	BERKLEE ROBINS
CAROLYN BAHL	JOHN KELLEY	BEEMETH ROBLES
JULIANA BARR	PETER KOSEK	RICK RONQUILLO
JAMES BELL	KAREL KRETZCHMAR	ADAM RUBINSTEIN
EDWARD BERTACINNI	GEORGE LEDERHAAS	LISA SAUNDERS
JIM BIRD	HARRY LEMMENS	THOMAS SCHARES
BRUCE BOLLEN	YUAN CHI-LIN	IRA SEGAL
GREG BOTZ	DENNIS LINDEBORG	AUDREY SHAFER
CHARLES BOUDREAUX	JOHN LOFTUS	STEVE SHAFER
BRYAN BOWMAN	WILL LONGTON	JOSHUA SIEGEL
BILL BROSE	BRUCE MACIVER	LEILA SIUKOLA
SUSAN BROWNE	RICK MANTIN	RICHARD SNYDER
NORMAN BUCKLEY	DONALD MASON	LEO STEMP
MICHAEL CHAMPEAU	DIANA MCGREGOR	GWEN STRITTER
JAMES CHANG	ROBERT MCKLVEEN	BARRY SWERDLOW
GRACE CHUN	CURTIS MCMILLAN	CHARLES TADLOCK
JEFFREY CLAYTON	MICHAEL MELLENTHIN	BRAD THOMAS
JOHN COOPER	STEVE MERLONE	VIRGINIA TSE
DOUG CROCKETT	LINDAA MIGNANO	BRYAN TUNINK
JENNIFER DAMEWOOD	DONALD MILNE	TED TUSCHKA
JOSEPH DUNN	CHARLES MINTO	JOHN URBANOWICZ
TALMADGE EGAN	FRITZ MORITZ	CHRIS VASIL
MARK EGGEN	ROBERT MOYNIHAN	VANESSA VU
RAY ENGSTROM	CARL NOE	GEORGE WAKERLIN
MICHAEL ENNIS	RICK NOVAK	CLINT WARNE
LAWRENCE FELD	FABIAN OKONSKI	DAN WAXER
ANNE FISCHELL	RON PEARL	MATTHEW WHITE
STEPHEN FISHER	KRISTI PETERSON	LORNA YAMAGUCHI
DAVID FITZGERALD	JOHN POLLARD	ELIZABETH YOUNGS
STEVE FORD	JOSHUA PRAGER	JOHN ZELCER
RAT GAETA	JON PROPST	KEN ZUCKERMAN
TOM GASTON	ALEX MACARIO	

Made in the USA
Columbia, SC
23 July 2024

575fbdf3-2807-480e-a916-a08a0d33e108R02